Cardiovascular Devices and Their Applications

Preface

I have always been impressed with the fact that there are few books describing medical devices and what they do: this book on cardiovascular devices addresses these two issues. There are many excellent reference works that describe cardiovascular instrumentation; however, most omit a discussion of the physiological and medical aspects of such devices. To remedy this defect, the presentations in this book seek to strike a balance between device description and the important physiology and pathophysiology associated with its use. Perhaps a better title for this book would be "Cardiovascular Devices—What They Do and How They Do It!"

This book is written for people who want to know about medical devices. Discussions of a large number of cardiovascular events and how they are measured, as well as descriptions of many therapeutic and assistive devices used in cardiology are presented. The discussions are designed for those who have a limited background in either the life or physical sciences. As such, this book should be of value to medical and paramedical persons at all levels, as well as those in the physical sciences who wish to enter the area of applied cardiovascular physiology. More specifically, the information presented here will be of practical value to medical and veterinary students, to nurses who are learning about the clinical applications of cardiovascular devices, and to physicians and others who are preparing for qualifying examinations. However, it should not be concluded that this volume is written only for the life scientist; on the contrary, it is written so that bioengineers, biomedical engineers, clinical engineers, and medical physicists can profit from the information it contains. Since the book covers the measurement of cardiovascular phenomena, it will also be of particular value to psychophysiologists and others who are interested in measuring cardiac functions.

Every opportunity has been taken to include quantitative data. Numerical calculations are presented to show how measured quantities are processed to provide useful clinical information. So often in the life science literature the intimate details of calculations are missing. The volume is designed to demonstrate that cardiovascular processes are amenable to quantification. There is no doubt that the era of descriptive biology is over, and it is time to provide quantitative examples of measurement and calculation.

Insofar as possible, each chapter is designed to be a complete presentation of a topic. Thus, it should be possible for the reader to use each as a reference for those topics of interest, without having to read others to acquire background information.

For me, the history of science has been a fascination, principally because it shows dramatically how our predecessors used sheer brain power and ingenuity to triumph over the lack of technology. At the end of each chapter I have made an attempt to share this fascination with the reader by including a historical postscript. Thus, each chapter contains descriptions of cardiovascular devices, the relevant physiology and pathophysiology, and a historical postscript.

The book starts out in Chapter 1 with a general survey of medical devices, both diagnostic and therapeutic, and includes a discussion of medical device legislation first enacted in the late 1930s.

Chapters 2–4 cover the direct and indirect measurement of blood pressure in humans. For the latter, recommendations are given for good practice. The clinically used methods for measuring cardiac output and blood flow are described in detail. Attention is given to the physics of blood flow and resistance, including the technique of reducing resistance by vessel dilation (angioplasty). Catheterization and cardiac shunts are covered in detail. An analysis is presented of the heart as a pump in terms of stroke work and power, and an evaluation of the heart as a pump is discussed in terms of the presently used cardiac function tests.

Cardiac valves, natural and prosthetic, are described in Chapter 5. The methods for measuring valve area are also developed. Chapter 6 covers the intraaortic balloon pump.

Simple electrocardiographic theory is presented in Chapter 7 along with numerous examples of recordings and recording techniques, including His-bundle electrocardiography.

Pacemakers are covered in Chapter 8 which deals with the various types, including exercise-responsive pacemakers. Closed-chest cardiac pacemaking is described briefly. A short section is devoted to energy sources—chemical and nuclear.

The defibrillator and the principles of defibrillation are presented in Chapter 9. The techniques and requirements for defibrillation with chest, direct-heart, and catheter electrodes are discussed. Coverage is also given to the newly introduced automatic implanted defibrillator.

Chapter 10 closes the book with discussions on electrical hazards of all kinds, ranging from 60-Hz leakage current to electrosurgical current. The hazards of explosion due to bowel gas and anesthetic gases are presented.

This chapter also describes isolated power systems, ground-fault interrupters, line-isolation monitors, and equipotential grounding. The cardiorespiratory responses due to accidental contact with power-line current are presented in some detail.

The material presented was drawn from a wide range of experiences with clinicians and scientists, starting with Wilder Penfield and Herbert Jasper, for whom I worked in Montreal from the mid-1940s to the early 1950s. They made neurosurgery and neurology come alive for me. The influence of Hebbel Hoff at Baylor Medical College in Houston was critical, because under his tutelage the world of cardiology unfolded and the history of medicine became a fascination that made progress appear very orderly. The 18-year experience with the summer course "Classical Physiology With Modern Instrumentation" at Baylor allowed me to meet, and in some small way contribute to the education of, more than 1000 clinicians, veterinarians, and basic and applied life and physical scientists. This experience exposed a world of fascinating problems, the solutions to which usually relied on medical devices.

Also at Baylor, the happy association with Lee Baker, Joe Bourland, Willis Tacker, John Rosborough, Arno Moore, Garland Cantrell, Tom Coulter, Cruz Martinez, Ernesto Arriaga, Carter Jordan, and Narvin Foster made it possible to develop teaching and research programs that led to the development of numerous instruments. Without the help of these dedicated people, much of my research would not have been possible.

The fortunate association with Carlos Vallbona and William Spencer, also at Baylor, showed me the severe cardiopulmonary and neurological sequelae of poliomyelitis. This association provided a rich experience in solving problems in clinical medicine.

I am grateful to the National Institutes of Health for inviting me to serve on one Study Section or another for over two decades. This activity placed me at the forefront of medical technology and science and presented the widest range of clinical cardiovascular problems. A shorter tour of duty with the FDA provided an equally rewarding experience in classifying medical devices.

To another governmental agency, NASA, I am grateful for the opportunity to serve as a consultant to the Mercury and Gemini spaceflights. Helping solve the problems of physiological monitoring during spaceflight was a rewarding experience and led to the early development of impedance respiration.

I thank John Hancock, Dean of Engineering at Purdue, and the Showalter Trustees for making it possible to come to Purdue. The Purdue experience with Willis Tracker, Joe Bourland, Charles Babbs, John Pearce, and Neal Fearnot reintroduced me to engineering with its new technologies for solving medical problems, as well as providing the opportunity to tackle many of the problems.

Finally, I wish to thank the many secretaries, typists, technicians, and students who helped me during many decades of collecting the material that constitutes this book. Special thanks are due to Chris Ramsey and Kim Gilbert for their assistance in processing the lecture notes that ultimately became this work on cardiovascular devices.

L. A. GEDDES

West Lafayette, Indiana
November 1983

Contents

Cardiovascular Devices and Their Applications

CHAPTER 1

Medical Devices

A medical device is a new term that is used to identify a wide variety of medical instruments. Since early history, human and animal physicians have used a wide variety of instruments to aid in the diagnosis of illness and to provide assistance in effecting a cure or providing life support after the disease process has abated. These facts were never been more elegantly stated than by Oliver Wendell Holmes, who wrote "Medicine appropriates everything from every source that can be the slightest use to anybody who is ailing in any way, or likely to be ailing from any cause. It learned from a monk how to use antimony, from a Jesuit how to cure the ague, from a friar how to cut for stone, from a soldier how to treat gout, from a sailor how to keep off scurvy, from a postmaster how to sound the Eustachian tube, from a dairy maid how to prevent smallpox, and from an old market woman how to catch the itch insect. It borrowed acupuncture and the moxa from the Japanese heathen, and was taught the use of lobelia by the American savage."

It is now appropriate to identify the uses to which these "appropriated" items were put. Antimony was reported to have been fed to hogs in the 15th century by Basil Valentine, a monk who noted that they fattened and showed astonishing vigor. Monks tried it on themselves with disastrous results, hence the name anti-moine (anti-monk). Its use nonetheless persisted, being endorsed by Louis XIV who was cured of a fever by it. Antimony, as tartar-emetic, was prescribed as an emetic at the onset of a fever.

The ague, or malarial fever, was cured by the Peruvian Indians by a tea made from the bark of the tree which was later named cinchona. A Jesuit father working among the Incas was cured of malaria by this tea administered by a medicine man. The Jesuit smuggled some of the bark back to Europe where it found its way into clinical use, later becoming known as quinine.

The friar who showed medicine how to cut for stone was Frere Jacques de Beaulieu, who wandered throughout France removing bladder stones by the ingenious surgical procedure he devised, which is now known as lateral lithotomy. The unique feature of his procedure was that it protected structures near the bladder from surgical damage. He had no medical training, little education, and performed his operations only in the presence of a physician or surgeon. As a reward for his services, he took only what was offered, and if it was excessive, he gave it to the poor.

The gout, an excruciatingly painful disease affecting the joints of extremities and in particular those of the great toes, was treated by Thomas Sydenham, a physician–soldier in Cromwell's army, who himself suffered from the disease. Recognizing that the disease "affected the rich more frequently than the poor and rarely attacked fools," he recommended rest, fresh air, and moderation in all things, particularly in diet and drinking habits.

Scurvy, caused by a deficiency of vitamin C, is a disease that used to decimate the crews of ships on long voyages. That a lack of fresh fruits, which we now know to be rich in the vitamin, was the origin of the disease in sailors was recognized by James Lind, a British Naval surgeon. Subsequently, the juice of lemons and limes was ordered served on British ships; hence the name "Limey" for British sailors.

The eustachian tube, connecting the oral cavity with the middle ear, equalizes the pressure across the eardrum. The postmaster who "sounded it"—placed a tube in it—was Edme-Gilles Guyot, of Versailles. He suffered from a chronic upper respiratory infection, which had entered the eustachian tube and obstructed it with mucus. Physicians gave him no hope of relief for the pain and progressive deafness produced by the inequaliy of pressure which then developed across the eardrum. Devising a small tube covered with leather and attached to a hand-operated pump, he succeeded in scouring his own eustachian tube and soon recovered his hearing.

The dairy maid who taught medicine how to prevent smallpox was Sarah Nelmes of Berkeley, England. Jenner noted that a milkmaid who developed a pustular eruption from milking a cow infected with cowpox was immune from smallpox. He made "vaccine" (*vacca* meaning cow) from the pustules of Sarah Nelmes and injected it into a small boy, James Phipps, who suffered only mild discomfort. A few months later he transferred to the boy virulent infection from a subject with smallpox. No disease followed, even after a second injection a few months later.

The old market woman who taught medicine about the itch insect was an unknown woman in Corsica who showed a Dr. Renucci that an insect was responsible for scabies, an intensely itchy disease of the skin characterized by short dark wavy lines accompanied by reddening and eruptions. The unknown Corsican woman had apparently opened several pustules and extracted the tiny red itch mite.

Acupuncture is an ancient oriental procedure for treating disease. The technique consists of inserting (hot or cold) needles of various metals into one or more of 365 specified points on the body. The aim of the treatment is to enter, at an appropriate site, one or another of the 12 vital invisible channels which carry the Yang (the active or male element) and the Yin (passive or female element). In health these elements or humors are supposed to be in equilibrium; their imbalance is the cause of disease. Acupuncture permits the escape of the element in excess and restores the balance. Now, of course, acupuncture is used for its pain-killing properties.

The moxa is also an ancient oriental treatment consisting of burning powdered leaves on various portions of the skin to produce blistering. Advocated for a variety of diseases, it acted as a counterirritant or a cautery and was supposed to extract or repel the vital humors, much like acupuncture.

Lobelia, the contribution of native Americans, is indian tobacco. From the dried leaves a drug was made that was used in the 19th century as an emetic, nauseant, expectorant, and antiasthmatic. It was occasionally used as a respiratory stimulant; but because of the dangers and the appearance of superior drugs, its use for this purpose has been abandoned. Interestingly enough, the use of lobelia has been proposed for control of the tobacco habit—that other gift of the American Indian.

History has well documented Holmes' statement regarding medicine's appropriative habit. Today, in addition to appropriating chemical agents, it borrows physical agents and, more importantly, stimulates their creation. Largely as a result of the "electronic revolution" following World War II (1939–1945), electronic devices were put to use for other than radio, radar, television, and communication purposes, resulting in a wide variety of electrical, electromechanical, and many pneumatic and mechanical devices that were designed to aid in the diagnosis of illness and in assisting in effecting therapy. With such a bewildering array of devices used in medicine, it is of value to create a classification scheme so that lay persons and those in or entering the field can have an understand-

TABLE 1.1. The Three Areas of Medicine

Diagnosis	Therapy	Rehabilitation
History Physical Examination Instrumental Data Physical Chemical	Chemical (Drugs) Surgery Physical Devices and energy	Application of assistive ortho- tic–prosthetic devices

ing of their function and thereby judge their value to a patient and to society.

Although the boundaries for classifying medical devices are not sharply defined, such devices tend to fall into one or more of three general categories: diagnostic, therapeutic, and assistive (or rehabilitative); Table 1.1 identifies the three medical procedures and characteristics of the devices in the three areas.

DIAGNOSTIC DEVICES

Diagnostic instruments are very common, because they are encountered when a physician first examines a patient. Perhaps the most familiar of these instruments is the stethoscope, which collects the feeble sounds made by some of the internal organs as they function and presents these sounds to the physician's ear. The timing and quality of the sounds of the beating heart and those produced by the movement of air in the respiratory and gastrointestinal tracts give important clues to the listener regarding the function of these systems. To measure blood pressure, an occluding cuff is wrapped around the upper arm and quickly inflated to a pressure high enough to occlude the artery under it. The pressure in the cuff is then lowered slowly. As blood spurts through the variably collapsing artery, a stethoscope is used to monitor the downstream arterial sounds, the appearance and disappearance of which tell the listener when to read the cuff pressure to determine the maximum (systolic) and minimum (diastolic) blood pressure without opening the vessel.

Body temperature is an indicator of the process of regulated burning of fuel (foods), which is called metabolism. A simple measuring instrument, the thermometer, provides important information on the severity and course of many diseases in which the balance between heat produced and lost is altered.

Helping the visual faculty are a variety of optical devices: some as simple as a mirror on a probe, others as complex as the compound microscope with its many hundredfold magnifying properties. The ophthalmoscope, bronchoscope, gastroscope, and proctoscope are optical instruments that allow peering into the eye or ear, examination of the walls of the respiratory tract, stomach, bladder, and lower digestive tract, permitting visualization of these organs as they function in their relatively inaccessible locations.

Other structures and organs are much more inaccessible and must be transilluminated for visualization. The low-energy X-ray beam is used to advantage here, but because the eye is insensitive to this type of electromagnetic energy, the photographic surface or fluorescent screen is employed to convert the absorption image to a visible one. Low-energy ultrasound waves are also used to produce transmission or reflectance density shadowgrams of internal structures. Similarly, thermograms, or photographs of the radiant heat emitted by the body, indicate in a dramatic manner the temperature distribution in various regions of the body surface.

Many normal and abnormal organs selectively take up radioactive isotopes injected into the vascular system, building up within them in a short time a concentration of the material that can be located with instruments which detect radioactivity. Total count and count-rate meters, along with photographic emulsions and arrays of radiation sensors, reveal the presence of this type of radiation.

The functioning of many organs is accompanied by the appearance of electrical potentials. The heart, brain, nerves, skeletal and smooth muscles, and even the eyes and ears produce signals that have characteristic forms in health which are altered by disease. These low-amplitude signals, when enlarged and displayed on paper tape or on oscilloscope screens, yield important diagnostic information.

Another physical instrument is the spirometer, used to determine the oxygen consumed and the volume of air moved during respiration. The thyroid gland regulates oxygen consumption; thus the oxygen uptake serves as a quantitative measurement of thyroid activity. Diseases also alter the oxygen uptake, which is quantitated by the spirometer.

From these examples it can be seen that the diagnostic instrument functions in a variety of interesting ways. It frequently provides selectivity, calibration, and amplification. It often places the observer's senses in inaccessible environments; while at other times it provides the clinician with new sense organs. Diagnostic instruments can truly be called extenders of the human senses.

Diagnostic instruments may be used for purposes other than diagnosis. After the institution of a therapeutic program, diagnostic instruments are frequently used to monitor the efficacy of the applied therapy, providing useful information relative to the response to therapeutic agents. In this role, they serve as an early warning system, affording the opportunity to prevent crisis. The many patient-monitoring systems now in use are assemblages of diagnostic instruments designed to follow the variations of a few select physiological events believed to be most meaningful in reflecting the recovery from an illness.

THERAPEUTIC DEVICES

Once the diagnosis is made, appropriate therapeutic procedures are instituted. Drugs constitute the most extensively used therapy; but even with this form of therapy, instruments are of importance because many chemotherapeutic agents are introduced into the body with the aid of physical instruments, the most familiar is the hypodermic needle and syringe. Its first use was by the noted architect Sir Christopher Wren, who adapted it from the ancient enema syringe. Another injecting device is the high-velocity jet, which drives dissolved substances through the skin. Likewise, drugs are delivered as a mist produced by ultrasonic generators.

In addition to chemotherapeutic agents, the therapist has recourse to physical systems that produce various types of energy. In general, such devices either stimulate or inhibit active cells or alter their function.

Therapeutic devices are used to control or cure an illness. However, some of these devices are required to sustain function after the disease process has been arrested. Thus, there is an indistinct boundary between therapeutic devices, which are used or installed by the physician, and rehabilitative devices, which are used by the patient to compensate for lost function after the disease process has been arrested.

A host of familiar and unfamiliar therapeutic instruments are in use. Among these are a variety of devices that produce radiant energy, the most familiar being the high-voltage short-wavelength X-ray beam which alters the growth pattern of cancerous cells. Longer in wavelength is ultraviolet radiation with its germicidal and sun-tanning properties. In the visible region, the high-intensity coherent beam of the laser is now used as a precise cautery to cement (spot-weld) detached retinas and to perform surgical cutting. Radiation in the longer-wave infrared spectrum is used for heating tissues within the body, thereby enhancing circulation in the irradiated area. Radio waves, produced by the diathermy, provide resistive and dielectric heating to achieve the same result. Another widely used therapeutic device is the electrosurgical instrument that applies accurately controlled radio-frequency energy to a small-area active electrode in contrast with living tissue. With low current, the tissue under the active electrode is dehydrated. With higher current, protein coagulation occurs; this property aids in the control of bleeding. With even higher current, the tissues are cut and divide as the active electrode is advanced. Introduction of the electrosurgical instrument in the early 1900s permitted surgeons to cut and coagulate tissue which could not be excised by the scalpel alone due to excessive bleeding.

Ultrasonic generators operate in the megahertz to fraction of a megahertz range. When applied with low intensity, these vibrations produce heat and alter metabolism and circulation at the cellular level. With higher-intensity focused sound waves, a cutting action is produced, and this effect has been exploited in surgery. Sound energy in the audible range is used to produce analgesia in some dental procedures. Stereophonic sound, mixed with white noise, applied to two closely fitting earphones appears to lessen the appreciation of dental pain.

A variety of devices that produce an electrical output have been used therapeutically. The electrical stimulator, which generates pulses of current, is used to exercise paralyzed muscles while nerve regeneration is taking place. A current pulse of many amperes is passed through the chest to arrest ventricular fibrillation, an arrhythmia that results in a cessation of the pumping action of the heart and loss of blood pressure. With more than 3 minutes of circulatory arrest, irreversible damage results in the brain; thus defibrillation is an emergency therapy. Currents of several amperes are passed through the head in electric-shock therapy for certain psychiatric disorders. Interestingly enough, a lower intensity sine- or square-wave current passed through the head produces a sleeplike state. This phenomenon was used clinically for a short time in foreign countries, but the basic research has not been performed, so its status is still unsettled.

In some disease states, and often as a result of aging, the ventricles of the heart lose their drive and beat too slowly. Under these conditions, single shocks delivered rhythmically to the ventricles produce contractions. Stimulators for this purpose are called cardiac pacemakers. In some cases cardiac pacemaking is required temporarily; in others, pacemakers are permanently implanted. Most modern pacemakers monitor the heart and deliver a stimulus only in the absence of a heart beat. Another therapeutic instrument, which often sees prolonged service beyond the hospitalization period, is the iron lung in which a patient is placed to provide lung ventilation during the acute phase of a disease that paralyzes the muscles of respiration or affects the respiratory center within the brain.

The heart–lung machine, which takes over the pumping action of the heart and the gas-exchange function of the lungs, is a therapeutic instrument used in surgical repair of the heart or its larger vessels. With the heart–lung machine, the brain, heart muscle, and other vital organs are not deprived of oxygenated blood while vessels are closed for repair or replacement. On completion of the surgery, the patient is slowly withdrawn (weaned) from the machine. At present, such machines can take over the function of the heart and lungs for up to about 4 hours. There is no doubt that improvements in this equipment will extend the permissible bypass period.

Ion and fluid balance are maintained by the kidneys, but when they are diseased, they can no longer perform this function. Artificial kidneys or dialyzers have been developed which remove or add substances to the bloodstream while the diseased kidneys are recovering. At present, there are patients living with virtually no kidney function. To remove the wastes from the bloodstream, such patients must check into a special treatment center every 3 days or so and be connected to the dialyzer, or obtain a unit for home dialysis. In the dialyzer, blood contacts one surface of a thin membrane and the dialysis fluid contacts the other surface. The chemical gradients effect the transfer of materials in one direction or the other. Connection to the dialyzer has been facilitated by surgically implanting tubes into an artery and vein which are easily coupled to the "artificial kidney." Home dialysis is becoming an increasingly popular technique.

Implanted Therapeutic Devices

There are an increasing number of implanted therapeutic devices being created. The most familiar example is the cardiac pacemaker. However, other examples are the dorsal-column stimulator, the auditory prosthesis, and the bone-growth stimulator. The dorsal-column stimulator is a tiny radio receiver that is connected to electrodes on the dorsal (posterior) columns of the spinal cord. Stimulation of these nerve fibers, effected by a small external transmitter, reduces or abolishes pain in a region beyond the electrodes. The auditory prosthesis is another type of implanted radio receiver having electrodes connected to an auditory nerve in a deaf person (with a functional auditory nerve). Environmental sound is detected by a microphone which delivers its signal to a stimulus coder, which in turn activates a skin-surface transmitter that telemeters the signal to the implant. Although progress is slow in establishing communication with the deaf in this way, the initial results are very encouraging, and many auditory prostheses are used today. The implanted bone-growth stimulator is a small constant direct-current source. Electrodes applied to a fracture site promote fracture union remarkably well. The same technique can be used to stimulate bone growth in the young subject.

Perhaps the largest area of activity relates to the creation of implanted drug-dispensing devices. Already there is an implant for the slow delivery of heparin, an anticoagulant, which has been reported by Blackshear et al. (1975). On the horizon are implanted drug-delivery systems for insulin, antiarrhythmic drugs, and drugs to reduce blood pressure. Presently available implants permit refilling the drug reservoir with a hypodermic needle and syringe. Research is underway to set the rate of delivery of such drugs by external telemetry.

Automatic (Servo) Control Devices

Increasing numbers of diagnostic and therapeutic devices are being joined in a closed-loop feedback system to control automatically a body function. Surprisingly, this concept is by no means new; its first demonstration was reported by Bickford (1950, 1951), who used the electroencephalograph (EEG) to control the depth of anesthesia. Beyond a certain depth of anesthesia, the dominant frequency of the EEG decreases. Using appropriate filtering circuitry to process the EEG signal, Bickford created a system that controlled the infusion of an intravenous anesthetic.

EEG control of anesthesia is fraught with difficulties. For example, not all anesthetics affect the EEG frequency spectrum in the same way. In addition, there are other factors, such as reduced brain perfusion, that affect the EEG. For these reasons, the EEG has not been pursued as a controller of the depth of anesthesia.

Electromyographic (EMG) potentials have been used to control assistive devices in a closed-loop mode. Montgomery (1957) used the EMG from residual respiratory muscles in a postpolio patient to control the cycling of a chest (cuirass) respirator. At the start of inspiration, the EMG triggered the respirator to produce inspiration. When the EMG potentials ceased, the respirator was triggered to cause expiration. A failure of the EMG to occur at a preset time caused the respirator to cycle automatically. The modern analog for this action is in the demand pacemaker.

The EMG was also used by Geddes et al. (1959) to provide motion in paralyzed limbs of polio patients. The EMG from small groups of residual muscles was used to open a solenoid valve to allow inflation of the McKibben artificial muscle, which is a bladder in a woven sleeve. Inflation of the bladder causes the sleeve to increase in diameter and decrease in length. The decrease in length was used to move an arm brace on the patient. Contraction of one group of muscles triggered "contraction" of the artificial muscle; contraction of a different group of muscles triggered "relaxation" of the artificial muscle. In this way the artificial muscle could be left in any state of contraction or relaxation without the need for EMG signals or inflating gas.

Blood sugar was controlled automatically in humans by Kadish (1964). The system consisted of an autoanalyzer to measure the blood sugar level and two motor-driven syringes, one for insulin (which reduces blood sugar) and the other for glucagon (which increases blood sugar). The control system triggered the release of insulin or glucagon when the blood sugar exceeded 150 or fell below 50 mg%. The system was used on normal and diabetic human subjects.

Automatic control of blood glucose at the bedside by the controlled injection of insulin is becoming quite common. There are commercially available devices for this purpose. An excellent review of the technology was presented by Albisser (1979), one of the first creators of such a device for bedside use.

There is an important subtlety relating to the control of blood sugar by controlled insulin injection. Whereas there is the need for a basal level of insulin, there is a sudden increased need at the start of a meal when the blood sugar starts to rise rapidly. Because existing automatic insulin-delivery systems have difficulty in accommodating this need (owing to delays in the system), Kraegen et al. (1981) created a dual-algorithm controller that permits manual initiation of the programmed release of insulin designed to prevent the blood sugar from rising excessively. In this way, the tonic and phasic needs for insulin are accommodated.

Automatic control of blood pressure at the bedside was reported by Schade (1973), who used an adaptive-control algorithm, implemented by a digital computer located at some distance from the hospital. Since then, many have researched the subject and perhaps Sheppard et al. (1980) have had the most experience with such a system. They used a proportional-integral-differential (PID) algorithm to control the blood pressure in postcardiac surgery patients by the intravenous infusion of nitroprusside. At present the system has been used on more than 10,000 patients.

Automatic Implanted Therapeutic Devices

Many of the automatic (closed-loop feedback) systems just described are eligible for implementation as implanted devices. The only drawback in taking this final step is the lack of suitable implantable transducers to sense the events being measured and controlled. At present there is considerable research in this important area.

Despite the lack of implantable transducers, there are a few automatic implantable therapeutic devices. Perhaps the most familiar is the demand pacemaker, which sits idle if the ventricles are beating and, if not, delivers rhythmic stimuli as needed. The transducer to detect a spontaneous (or normal) beat is the same pair of electrodes that is used for pacing. The current annual sales of pacemakers is on the order of 100,000. Details of the operation of pacemakers are presented in Chapter 8.

Another automatic implanted therapeutic device is the automatic defibrillator. This device monitors ventricular activity continuously and, when fibrillation occurs, delivers a strong (defibrillating) shock to the ventricles. There are now more than two dozen patients with such implants (Mirowski et al., 1980).

Research is underway to create an automatic implantable blood-pressure controller, because hypertension is so prevalent in western countries. It is estimated that 20% of the U.S. population is hypertensive, and only about one-quarter of these are on adequate therapy. Obviously, the creation of an implantable pressure transducer is occupying the attention of many.

Another area in which an automatic implantable device is needed is for the treatment of diabetes. Vigorous research is underway to create an implantable glucose sensor.

It is difficult to predict where the breakthroughs will occur in the creation of automatic implantable therapeutic devices. The ingenious innovator may well find unusual ways of sensing the event to be controlled or an event closely related to it.

ASSISTIVE OR REHABILITATIVE DEVICES

After an illness has been cured or after a disease process has been arrested, there often remains a deficit in function; assistive devices are needed to restore or compensate for lost function. Deficits also occur naturally with advancing age. As the result of medical progress, the percentage of senior citizens will increase, and assistive devices for this group will assume a more important role in their medical care. Prior to discussing assistive devices for patients who have survived a life-threatening illness, it is worthwhile examining some of the assistive devices needed for the deficits of age.

Particularly prominent in aging is a hearing defect. Reliable estimates indicate that 12 million adults and 3 million children in the United States have a hearing problem, although few of these are deaf. Only about 500,000 people in the United States use hearing aids, but it is estimated that 6 million could benefit from their use. Either for economic reasons or vanity, these people are forced to live in a world of relative silence and are deprived of acoustic information from their environment. It is a simple task to make a miniature amplifier to intensify sounds, but matching the device to the patient presents many special problems far beyond the fields of electronics and acoustics. The task of providing an appropriate frequency response curve and an automatic gain control are dwarfed by problems in the psychological sphere.

One of the biggest handicaps of the blind person is the inability to move from place to place in safety. In one survey, it was found that about 70% of the blind use canes and 30% depend on sighted persons as guides. Only about 1% of the blind use seeing-eye dogs for guidance and about as many more could employ them. There is a considerable need for devices to communicate information about the environment to the blind person. Several guidance devices are under development: one is a portable sonar, a second is an optical distance-measuring instrument, and a third is a capacity-type proximity indicator. All are in the developmental stage, and some show considerable promise.

Research is being conducted to determine if visual images can be perceived by direct patterned stimulation of the calcarine cortex of the brain. To date, only phosphenes (bright dots) and a very crude image of a cross have been perceived by a human subject. If it turns out that temporal and spatial stimulus patterns can be developed which conjure up visual image, development will occur of this type of visual prosthesis for those without functioning retinas or optic nerves.

All are familiar with crutches and walkers which are assistive devices that are used when control of the muscles of locomotion is temporarily or permanently impaired. In many, a severe lack of muscle power, or adequate nervous control of the muscles, makes locomotion or movement difficult or impossible. In the United States, paralytic diseases and trauma account for 500,000 persons with severe paralysis in both arms and legs. Damage to the blood supply of the brain, mainly resulting from arterial disease, has produced 2 million people who are paralyzed on one side of their body. Another 500,000 persons with cerebral palsy have lost effective control of their muscles. Approximately 4 million people are now living with crippling rheumatoid arthritis. In this country there are now 500,000 people living with multiple sclerosis, a disease that affects the coordinating centers for sensation and muscular motion. The deficits found in these subjects are severe and merit attention because the disease strikes the young adult population in the 18–45-year group. The life expectancy from onset of symptoms is about 25 years, so that appropriate assistive devices might be expected to increase very significantly this group's well being and productivity.

An unknown number use artificial arms or legs, and there are probably more who could benefit from their use. Assistance to this group of patients falls within the relatively new medical specialty called physical medicine and rehabilitation. Two classes of devices are applied to help these patients regain some function. Those aids that provide alignment and support function are called orthoses, while substitute parts are called prostheses. One of the common denominators in this group of patients is that there is usually some movement which can be harnessed to move paralyzed parts or artificial replacements. There are several types of artificial muscles that are beginning to be applied to orthotic and prosthetic devices. Trace movements from other parts of the body are detected and used to control the "contraction" and "relaxation" of these artificial muscles. The goals in the application of such devices are to provide for self-care and to create function which will assist in earning a livelihood.

Locomotion is presently provided for subjects with a loss of leg muscles by manual or motor-driven wheel chairs. Automobiles fitted with hand controls also permit paraplegic persons to get around. Many diseases produce a loss of respiratory muscle power. In such cases, the iron lung or chest respirator (cuirass) provides intermittent negative pressure around the body from the neck down, or over the chest; both devices provide inspiration. Removal of the negative pressure allows the elastic recoil of the rib cage to take place and expiration results.

Special attention is being focused on the increasing number of patients with spinal-cord damage. With this type of injury, there is a loss of voluntary control of the muscles below the region of injury; there is also a loss of sensation in the same parts. Although the muscles are paralyzed, their innervation is intact. If nothing is done, the muscles will atrophy due to disuse. However, the muscles can be made to contract by placing electrodes on the skin at the appropriate sites and applying stimuli to the desired motor nerves. Since sensation is lost, the stimuli cannot be perceived, but the muscles can be made to contract. Rhythmic stimulation can exercise muscles and increase their mass and strength quite dramatically (Petrofsky, 1983).

The idea of stimulating motor nerves in cord-paralyzed patients using skin-surface electrodes is gaining popularity. Although nerve trunks carry fibers that innervate both flexor and extensor muscles, by strategic placement of skin-surface electrodes it is becoming possible to obtain patterned movement by appropriate programmed delivery of the stimuli to multiple electrodes. Petrofsky (1983) has been able to have a paralyzed person pedal a bicycle using this technique. The first primitive motions resembling walking have also been taken.

It is likely that a finer control of patterned movement will be obtained in paraplegic and quadriplegic patients with implanted receivers connected to electrodes on selected nerves. Each implant would be passive, and the stimuli can easily be transmitted by a radio-frequency carrier. This technique was developed in the very early days of cardiac pacemaking, and it will likely be used to obtain patterned movement in paralyzed upper extremities because of the obvious immediate benefit to such patients.

Because use of many of the therapeutic devices continues beyond the period of medical crisis, the same devices become assistive or rehabilitative devices. Perhaps the most prominent of these are the "artificial kidney" or dialyzer and iron lung. Numerous other examples could be cited. However, the most important point about the application of assistive or rehabilitative devices relates to their ability to permit the patient to return to society and improve the quality of his or her life. Ideally, rehabilitative devices should, as one of their goals, provide the patient with the opportunity to become self-sufficient and self-supporting. Attainment of this latter goal may or may not include restoration of the lost function or even locomotion.

Those who wish to participate in medical progress can select one or more of these three areas and make contributions. Biomedical engineers are trained physical scientists who work in all three areas. Physicists, chemists, and mathematicians (including computer experts) also find niches for themselves in all three areas of medical endeavor. One of the newest to serve medicine is the clinical engineer, who is concerned with the safety and efficacy of all medical devices used within hospitals. Not only are training programs in existence for clinical engineers, but at least two professional groups have certification programs for these newcomers to the medical scene.

MEDICAL DEVICE LEGISLATION

By 1938 in the United States, it became recognized by the lawmakers that the public needed protection against unscrupulous vendors of a variety of medical products. The main concern at that time related to truthful labeling, that is, claims made for the product and the need to remove fraudulent items from the market. In 1938, the Food and Drug Administration (FDA) was given the authority for seizure, injunction, or criminal prosecution with respect to "adulterated" or "misbranded" devices. Although numerous cases were tried and many products were removed from the market, the postwar medical instrumentation boom created new jurisdictional problems. After the mid-1940s an enormous variety of medical devices became available to physicians. A large number of these devices made no claims regarding safety and efficacy. It is very important to note that many devices played life-saving roles in the hands of physicians. However, many had technological flaws. For example, the *Federal Register* of March 9, 1976, noted that "a committee chaired by Dr. Theordore Cooper, then Director of the National Heart Institute, issued a report indicating that in the 10 years prior to 1969 medical devices caused 10,000 serious injuries and over 750 deaths." An intrauterine device marketed in the early 1970s was linked to 16 deaths and 25 miscarriages. Significant defects in cardiac pacemakers had resulted in 34 voluntary recalls, involving 23,000 units.

Taking note of these facts, the lawmakers passed the medical device legislation amendments bill of 1976 (HR-11124, *Federal Register*, March 9, 1976), which was signed into law. The bill amended the federal Food, Drug, and Cosmetic Act to give it jurisdiction over the safety and effectiveness of medical devices intended for human use in the United States.

First, the bill required the Food and Drug Administration to classify all devices into regulatory categories based on the types of controls necessary to ensure the safety and efficacy of devices. The categories are class I—general controls; class II—performance standards; and class III—premarket approval.

Classification of a device into class I—general controls—means that it shall be subject to the existing and new general controls relating to adulteration, misbranding, banning, reporting, registration, restrictions on sale and distribution, and requirements for good manufacturing practices, except that FDA can exempt devices from some general controls. In general, class I devices are nonhazardous by their nature and good manufacturing practice controls their quality.

If placed in class II—performance standards—a device shall be required to meet an applicable standard on such date as is prescribed by the FDA but not before 1 year after the date on which the standard is established. The major general controls will continue to apply to the device unless superseded by the standard. In effect, it means that enough data relative to safety and efficacy are available to accurately describe and control devices in this category. An important subtlety of class II is that safety and efficacy can be defined on the basis of published scientific data.

If placed in class III—premarket approval—and it is a new device, the device may not be marketed until it meets premarket approval requirements. If it is a device that is on the market before the date of enactment, a regulation must first be promulgated to require premarket approval and then the device manufacturer has until the later of 30 months after its classification or 90 days after the promulgation of the regulation to file an application.

The bill required establishment of expert panels to assist the FDA in classifying devices and required that panels submit recommendations for classification of marketed devices within 1 year of enactment. Most of the classification panels have completed their task of placing devices into class II or III.

There are special provisions for implantable devices and devices for supporting or sustaining life. The bill required panels to recommend that devices intended to be implanted in the human body which are on the market prior to the date of enactment of the bill—or which are substantially equivalent to such devices—be classified into class III—subject to premarket approval—unless they determine that such classification is not necessary to provide reasonable assurance of safety and effectiveness. It also required that all devices including implantable devices not on the market prior to the date of enactment—and not substantially equivalent to devices on the market before such date—undergo premarket approval before they may enter the market.

The bill prescribed procedures whereby qualified groups may develop proposed standards or submit existing standards to be utilized by the FDA in promulgating performance standards applicable to class II devices.

The FDA is authorized to exempt a device from the requirements of the bill if the device is intended solely for investigational use and if the proponent of the device submits a plan demonstrating that the testing of the device will be supervised by an institutional review committee, ensures appropriate patient consent, and maintains certain records and reports. The protocol must be scientifically sound, and the benefits and knowledge to be gained must outweigh the risks to the patient.

The bill authorized proponents of devices classified into class III to submit product development protocols (PDP) in lieu of applications for premarket approval. This exception authorizes a procedure whereby the development of data necessary to secure premarket approval are, in effect, merged. The PDP exception requires submission of a protocol for testing, and approval of the protocol by the FDA. Upon a finding by the FDA that the protocol has been completed, the device is considered as having an approved application for premarket approval.

The bill authorized the FDA to ban a device which presents a substantial deception or substantial risk of illness or injury; to require notification and repair, replacement, or refund in appropriate circumstances in connection with medical devices; and to require maintenance of records and reports by manufacturers and distributors of medical devices. It authorized FDA inspection of such records and reports and authorized the FDA to prescribe good manufacturing practices for device manufacturers.

The bill authorized "custom devices"—devices especially ordered for patients or intended for use solely by an individual physician or other specially qualified person—to deviate from performance standards and requirements for premarket approval.

REFERENCES

Albisser, A. M. (1979). Devices for the control of diabetes mellitus, *IEEE Proc.*, **67**, 1308–1320.

Bickford, R. C. (1950). Automatic electroencephalographic control of general anesthesia, *EEG Clin. Neurophysiol.*, **2**, 93–94; (1951), **3**, 83–86.

Blackshear, P. J., Narco, R. L., and Buchwald, H. (1975). One year continuous heparinization in the dog using a totally implantable infusion pump, *Surg. Gyn. Obst.*, **141**, 176–186.

Geddes, L. A., Moore, A. G., Spencer, W. A., and Hoff, H. E. (1959). Electropneumatic control of the McKibben muscle, *Ortho. Pros. Appl. J.*, **13**, 33–36.

Kadish, A. H. (1964). Automatic control of blood sugar. *Am. J. Med. Electron.*, 81–86 (April/June).

Kraegen, E. W., Chisholm, D. J., and McNamara, M. E. (1981). Timing of insulin delivery with meals, *Hormone Metab. Res.*, **13**, 365–367.

Mirowski, M., Reid, P. R., Mower, M. M., Watkins, L., Gotz, V., Schauble, J. F., Langer, A., Heilman, M. S., Koelnik, R. A., Fischell, R. F., and Weisfeldt, M. (1980). Termination of malignant ventricular arrhythmias with an implanted automatic defibrillator in human beings, *N. Engl. J. Med.* **303**, 322–324.

Montgomery, L. H. (1957). Electronic control of artificial respiration, *IRE Conv. Rec.*, Part 4, 90–93; *Electronics*, **30**, 180.

Petrofsky, J. S. (1983). Current concepts in functional electric stimulation. in spinal cord injuries. In *Medical Engineering*, D. Ghista (Ed.), Charles Thomas, Springfield, Ill.

Petrofsky, J. S. (1983). Microprocessor-controlled stimulation of paralyzed muscle. In *Computer Aids for the Handicapped*, Charles Thomas, Springfield, Ill.

Schade, C. M. (1973). Automatic therapeutic control system for regulating blood pressure, *Proc. San Diego Biomed. Eng. Symp.*, **12**, 47–52.

Sheppard, L. C., Kouchoukos, N. T., Kirklin, J. W., Shotts, J. F., Wallace, F. D., and Allen, J. E. (1980). Computer controlled infusion of vasoactive agents—six year's experience, *Computers in Cardiology*, Williamsburg, VA; *Ann. Biomed. Eng.* **8**, 431–444.

CHAPTER 2

Blood Pressure and its Direct Measurement

TRANSDUCER TYPES

There are two types of electrical transducer for the direct measurement of blood pressure: one is the catheter-type transducer and the other is the catheter-tip transducer. Frequently, the word manometer is used to designate a blood-pressure-measuring device. The word "manometer" is derived from the Greek *manos* which means "thin or rare," because manometers were first used for measuring the pressure of air or gases. The older mercury or water-filled manometers are still in use when static or slowly varying pressures are to be measured. The various types of transducers will be described in this chapter, following a section on pressures in the circulatory system.

PRESSURES IN THE CIRCULATORY SYSTEM

Prior to discussing transducers for blood pressure, it is of value to illustrate the pressures they measure in the vascular system. The maximum and minimum arterial pressures are called systolic and diastolic, respectively. Figure 2.1*a* illustrates these pressures. Because the heart is a valved stroke pump, its chamber pressures are quite different than those in the outflow tracts. Although aortic pressure is typically 120/80 mm Hg, left ventricular systolic pressure is slightly above 120 mm Hg and diastolic

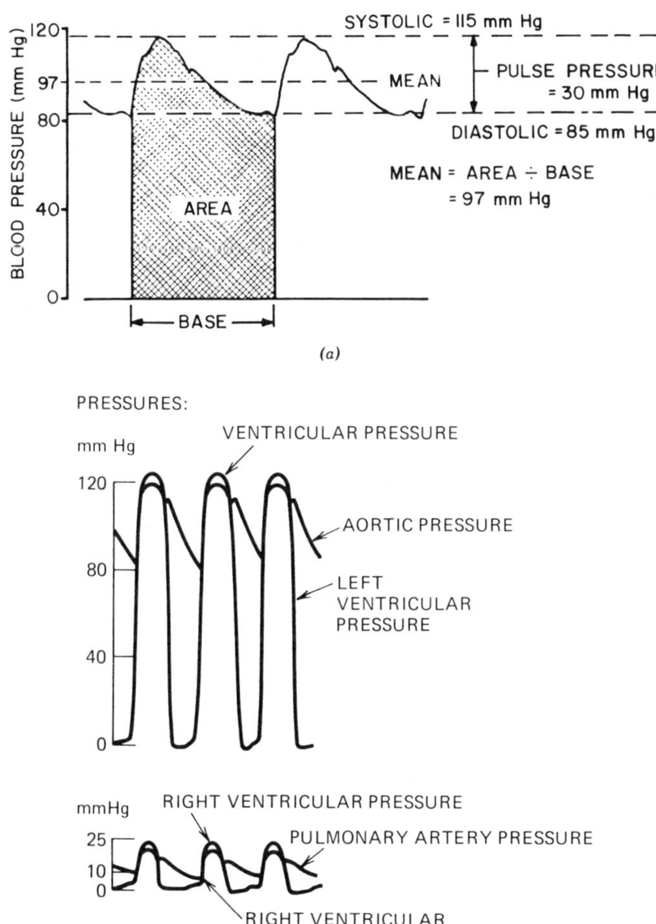

FIGURE 2.1. (*a*) Arterial pressure and (*b*) ventricular, aortic, and pulmonic pressures.

pressure is very nearly zero as shown in Figure 2.1*b*. The next highest pressures are associated with the right side of the heart. Pulmonary artery pressure is typically 25/10 mm Hg, and the right ventricular systolic pressure is slightly above 25 and diastolic pressure is nearly 0 mm Hg, as shown in Figure 2.1*b*.

An important concept to be understood is mean blood pressure, which is not the arithmetic average of systolic and diastolic pressures. True mean arterial pressure is the static pressure that is equivalent to a changing pressure. True mean pressure is found by dividing the area under a

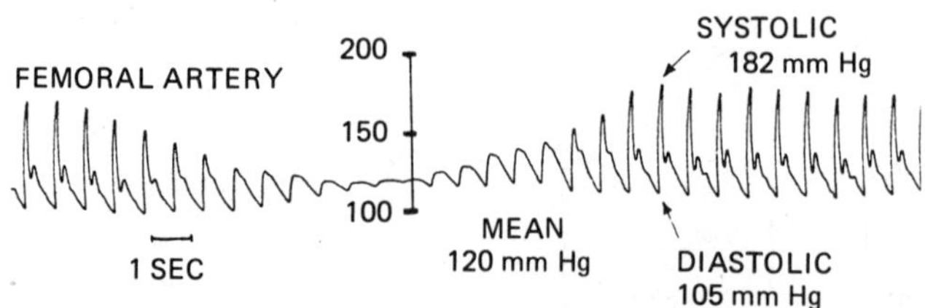

FIGURE 2.2. Mean arterial pressure recorded by gradually decreasing the diameter of the catheter leading to the transducer.

single pulse wave by the width of the pulse, as shown in Figure 2.1*a*. In practical situations, true mean arterial pressure falls between diastolic pressure plus about 20–40% of the pulse pressure, which is the difference between systolic and diastolic pressure. Mathematically, $\bar{P} = D + k(S - D)$, where $\bar{P}$ is mean pressure, D is diastolic pressure, S is systolic pressure, and k is a factor that ranges between about 0.2 and 0.4, depending on the form of the pulse wave. In the brachial artery, k is about one-third. A record showing the relationship of mean pressure to systolic and diastolic pressure is shown in Figure 2.2. This record was made by progressively reducing the speed of response of the transducer (by pinching the catheter), making it capable of registering mean pressure only. Note that mean pressure is well below the midpoint of the pulse pressure.

Mean pressure decreases from the aortic valve to the capillaries. Figure 2.3*a* diagrams a typical sequence. In the femoral and dorsalis pedis arteries, pulse pressure is usually larger than in the ascending aorta as shown in Figure 2.3*b*, which lists k values for each waveform.

The lowest pressures are found in the venous system. Venous pressure is so low that its magnitude is influenced markedly by body position (gravity effect) and respiration. Because a pressure of 10 mm Hg is developed by a column of blood 13.6 cm high, it is important to choose a reference pressure for measurement. The reference for blood pressure is the level of the right atrium. Venous pressure is measured with the subject in a horizontal position.

Central venous pressure is usually measured in the right atrium or the jugular bulb in the neck. This pressure rarely exceeds 10 mm Hg; it is usually a few centimeters of H_2O. With inspiration, the jugular venous pressure falls due to the negative intrathoracic pressure. With expiration, jugular venous pressure rises because of positive intrathoracic pressure. This sequence of events can be seen easily in singers. During inspiration the neck veins collapse, and during expiration, when vocalizing occurs, the veins bulge. In addition to the respiratory variations in jugular pressure, there are pulsatile changes which are recordable. Since there are no

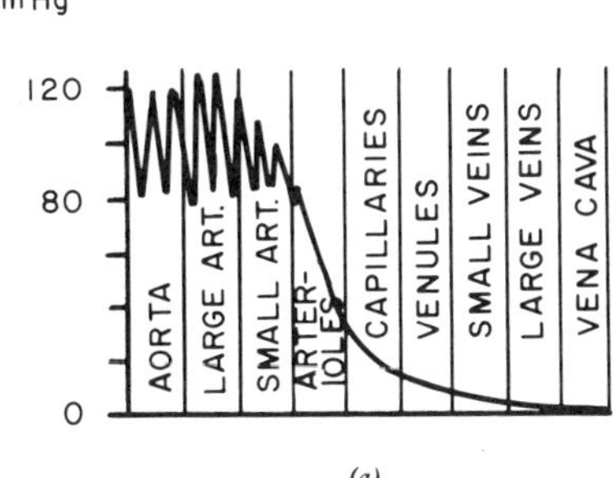

(a)

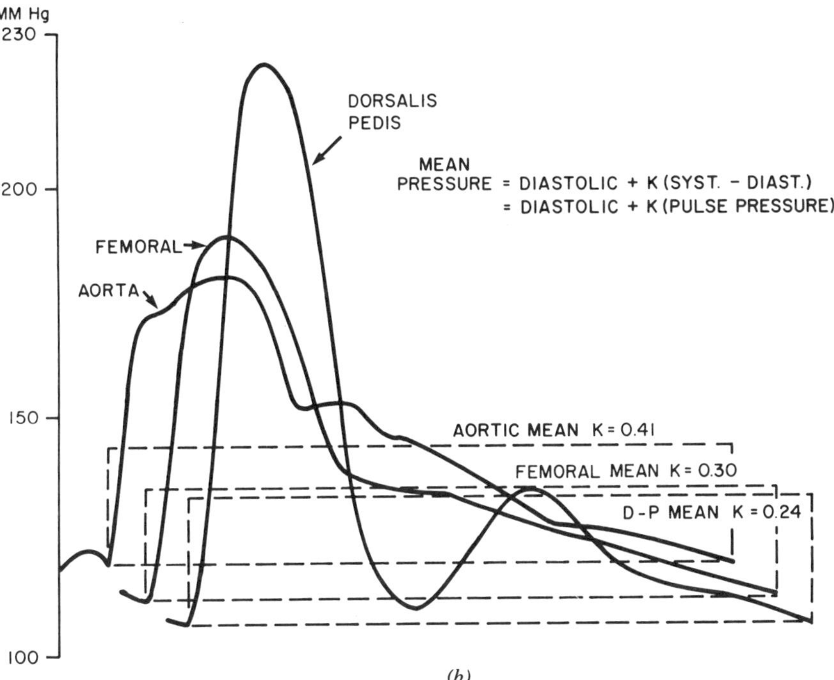

(b)

FIGURE 2.3. (*a*) Systemic pressure and (*b*) pulse waves recorded from the aorta (A), femoral (F), and dorsalis pedis (DP) arteries.

valves between the right atrium and the jugular vein, right atrial systole causes a pressure pulse to appear in the neck veins (the "a" or atrial wave). There is also an arterial pulse transmitted indirectly to the jugular vein (the "c" or carotid wave). At the end of the ventricular systole, rapid passive filling of the right ventricle occurs and right atrial pressure suddenly falls, producing the "v" or venous wave in the jugular pressure record. Figure 2.4 illustrates a typical jugular pressure record. Venous

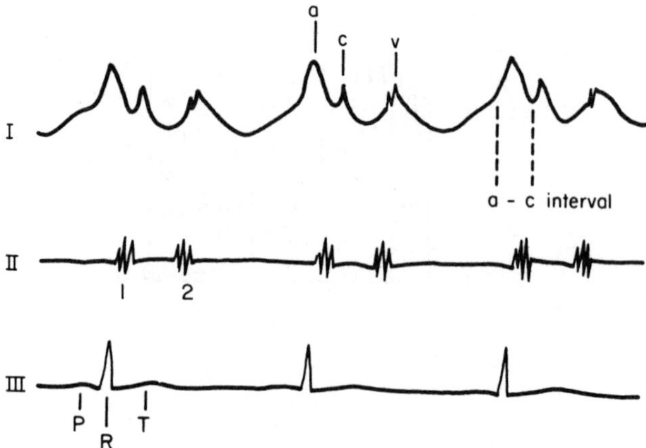

FIGURE 2.4. The jugular venous pulse (I), the heart sounds (II), and the ECG (III).

pressure is a very sensitive indicator of the ability of the heart to pump the blood that is returned to it. An increase in venous pressure is indicative of failure of the right heart to pump adequately. Elevation in venous pressure is seen in a variety of cardiovascular diseases.

THE MERCURY MANOMETER

The first measurement of blood pressure in the laboratory used the mercury U-tube manometer, which is illustrated in Figure 2.5*a*. It was from this device that the units for measuring blood pressure were derived. Note that the pressure is always the difference in height (*H*) of the mercury in the two arms of the manometer (Figure 2.5*b*). Stated another way, the pressure in mm Hg is always equal to height of the column of mercury supported by the blood pressure. The mercury manometer cannot reproduce faithfully systolic and diastolic pressures; however, it can be used to display mean pressure.

As stated in the preceding paragraph, the pressure in a fluid-filled U-tube manometer is always equal to the difference in height in the two arms of the U. However, it is important to note that a millimeter scale is often mounted beside one arm. In such a situation pressure is read by the displacement of the level of mercury in one arm. The true pressure is equal to twice the displacement in millimeters, provided the two arms of the U-tube have the same cross-sectional area. If the two arms of the U-tube have different cross-sectional areas, as shown in Figure 2.5*c*, the true pressure is still the difference in height between the mercury in the

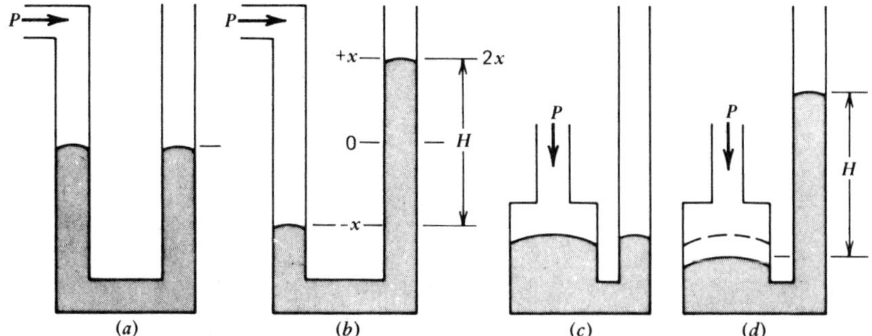

FIGURE 2.5. Various U-tube manometers. The pressure is always the difference in height in the two arms of the U. Note that with equal cross-sectional areas the pressure is twice the rise (or fall) in one tube. With unequal areas, the rise in one tube is much greater than in the other. The pressure is always equal to the height (H) of the column of mercury that is supported.

two arms. In practice, however, a scale is usually mounted beside the tube of narrower cross-sectional area. Thus the distance between the millimeter marks will be less than 1 mm and will depend on the ratio of the tube cross-sectional areas, because the zero reference in the large-diameter reservoir moves down by an amount related to the area ratio.

In mercury manometers with arms having different cross-sectional areas, it is essential that the reservoir be filled so that the level of mercury in the smaller tube is at the zero mark on the scale. If the reservoir is not filled adequately, that is, the mercury is below zero, a serious error results. This type of error, which is commonly encountered with portable manometers, is called a "zero error."

When a long vertical tube is connected to an artery or vein, blood will rise in the tube to a height that is dependent on the pressure. To calculate the pressure in mm Hg, it is only necessary to know the height of the column above the heart, the density of blood, and the density of mercury. The following example will illustrate the calculation.

When Stephen Hales first measured blood pressure in the horse, he connected a femoral artery to a vertical glass tube. Blood rose 8 ft 4 in. above the level of the heart. To express this height in mm Hg, it is first necessary to convert the height to millimeters (8 ft. × 12 in./ft + 4 in. = 100 in. × 25.4 mm/in. = 2540 mm of blood). The specific gravity of mercury is 13.6 and that of blood is 1.03. Therefore, the mean arterial pressure was

$$\frac{2540}{13.6} \times 1.03 = 192.4 \text{ mm Hg}$$

In general, the mean pressure ($\bar{P}$ in mm Hg) represented by a column H cm in height of a fluid with a specific gravity S is

$$\bar{P} = \frac{10\ HS}{13.6}$$

It is interesting to recognize that the diameter of the column of fluid is unimportant. A good rule of thumb is that a 1-in. height of water represents 1.87 mm Hg. This figure is important when measuring blood pressure with fluid-filled catheters which are connected to transducers that are not at the same level as the right atrium. If the transducer is below this reference point, the measured pressure is falsely high; if above, the pressure is falsely low. By measuring the difference in height between the transducer and the right atrium, the appropriate correction can be applied, that is, 1.87 mm Hg/in. difference in height.

BLOOD-PRESSURE TRANSDUCERS

All modern blood-pressure transducers operate on the principle of the electrical detection of the deflection of an elastic member exposed to blood pressure. A wide variety of methods are used to convert this deflection to an electrical signal. Before the electronic era, deflection of the elastic member was reproduced by using a mirror that reflected a light beam onto a moving photosensitive paper. In the early 1900s, such devices succeeded manometers in which a writing lever was coupled directly to the elastic member; Mercury manometers are still the standard instrument for calibrating blood-pressure transducers.

Catheter-Type Transducers

The principle underlying the operation of the catheter-type pressure transducer is characterized in Figure 2.6*a*. The traditional elastic member (diaphragm) exposed to blood pressure is represented by a piston, which is loaded by a sping K. The application of a pressure $P(t)$ causes a small amount of fluid (ΔV) to enter the transducer dome as the piston is displaced (ΔX). Often, a long fluid-filled catheter (Figure 2.6*b*) is used to couple the transducer to the pressure to be measured. It is the deflection of the elastic member (usually a diaphragm) that is detected electrically to produce a signal which identifies the applied pressure $P(t)$.

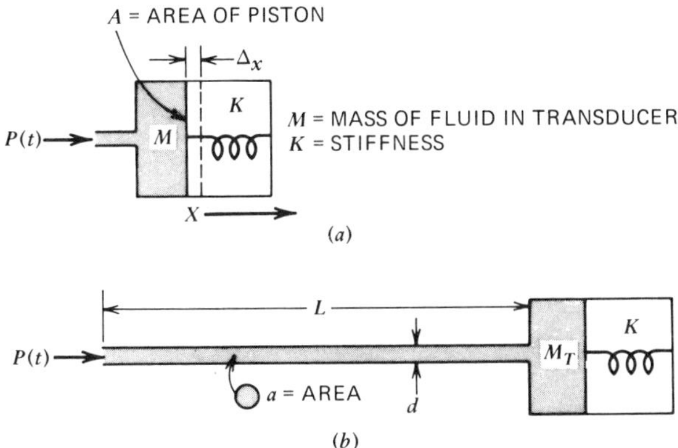

FIGURE 2.6. Principle employed in the catheter-type pressure transducer. The elastic diaphragm has been represented by a piston operating against a spring K. Application of a pressure $P(t)$ causes a small amount of fluid (ΔV) to enter the transducer. Detection of the deflection of the diaphragm (i.e., displacement of the idealized piston ΔX) is accomplished electrically to produce a recordable signal.

Strain-Gauge Transducers

The most popular pressure transducers employ strain gauges, that is, conductors that increase their resistance when stretched. Strain is defined as the fractional increase in length. Three of the popular types of strain-gauge pressure transducers are shown in Figures 2.7*a*–2.7*c*. In these devices the strain-gauge elements are arranged in a bridge circuit in which strain in the same direction is applied to opposite arms of the bridge. Because temperature changes affect resistance, all four strain gauges are affected equally, and the bridge remains balanced despite variations in temperature.

Figure 2.7*a* illustrates the Statham pressure transducer. Pressure applied to the corrugated diaphragm increases the tension in wires 2 and 3 and decreases it in wires 1 and 4. These tension changes produce a change in resistance and unbalance the Wheatstone bridge constituted by 1, 2, 3, and 4, thereby providing a signal proportional to pressure. A typical sensitivity is about 5 μV per volt of excitation per mm Hg of pressure.

Figure 2.7*b* illustrates the Bell and Howell strain-gauge pressure transducer. The strain-gauge wires are wrapped around posts mounted on a spring member in the form of a cross. Pressure applied to the diaphragm is coupled to the center of the spring member which bends, causing tension to increase in the strain-gauge wires above the elastic member and to decrease in those below it. The strain-gauge elements are arranged in a

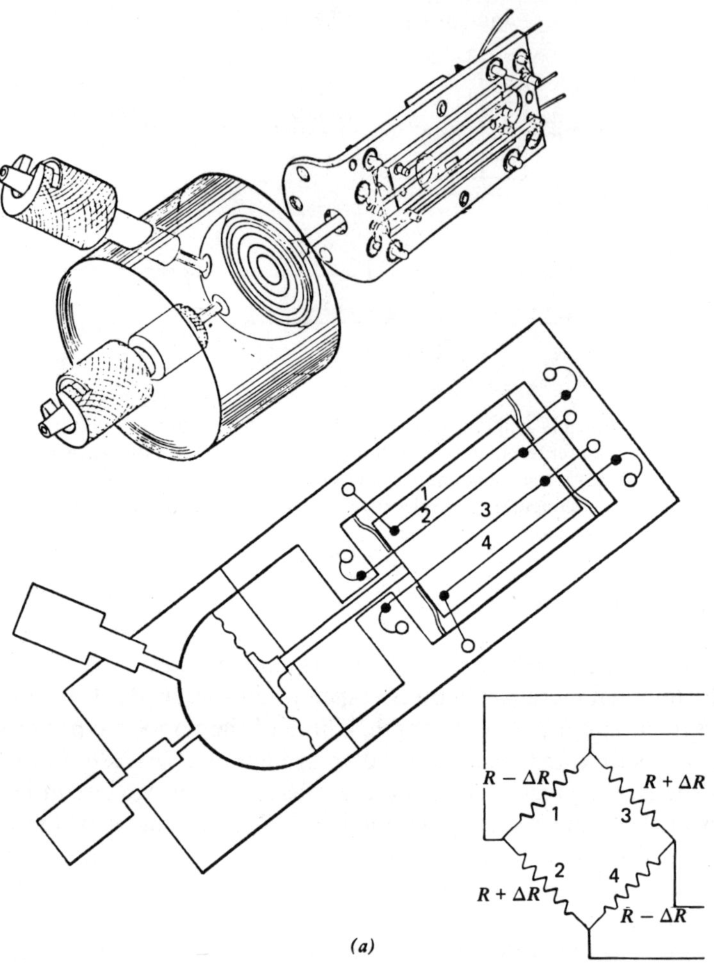

FIGURE 2.7*a*. Strain-gauge pressure transducer. [Courtesy Gould (Statham) Instruments, Oxnard, CA.]

bridge circuit, and the output is about 5 μV per volt of excitation per mm Hg of pressure.

Figure 2.7*c* illustrates a newly introduced disposable, solid-state, pressure transducer, consisting of a silicon diaphragm to which are bonded four strain-gauge conductors. The silicon diaphragm is coated with an insulating material and additional electrical isolation is provided in the electronic circuit that drives it. The unit is hermetically sealed, and the back side of the silicon diaphragm communicates with atmospheric pres-

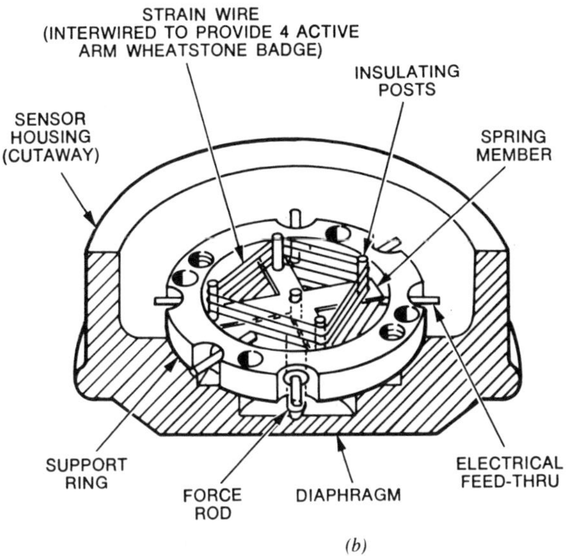

(b)

FIGURE 2.7*b*. Strain-gauge pressure transducer. (Courtesy Bell & Howell Co., Pasadena, CA.)

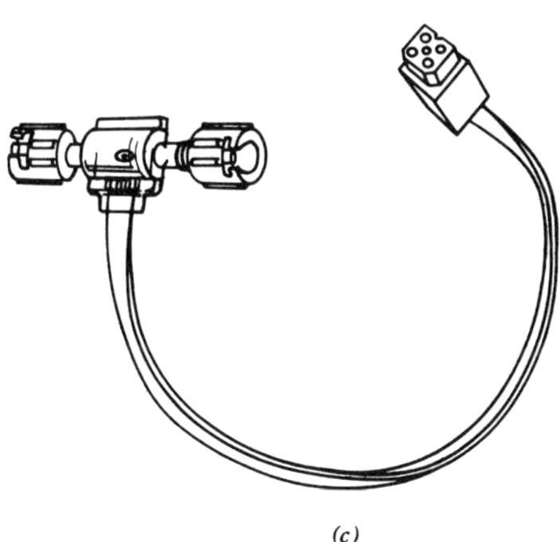

(c)

FIGURE 2.7*c*. The disposable, solid-state pressure transducer in which the four strain-gauge elements are deposited on the diaphragm. The central hole in the connector communicates with the back of the diaphragm. (Courtesy Cobe Laboratories, Denver, CO.)

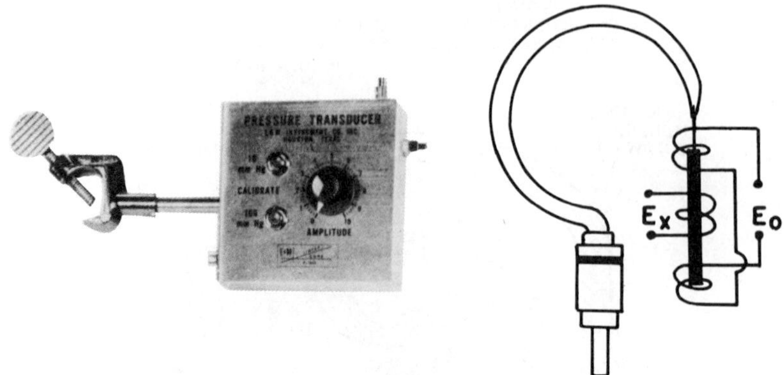

FIGURE 2.8. The linear variable differential transformer (LVDT) used to detect the deflection of a Bourdon tube exposed to pressure. (Courtesy Narco Bio Systems, Houston, TX.)

sure via a tube in the cable carrying the wires from the bridge to the connector. The output is 8 μV per volt of excitation per mm Hg pressure.

Linear Variable Differential Transformer Transducer

The linear variable differential transformer (LVDT) is also used in pressure transducers. The LVDT consists of a three-winding transformer with a movable core which is connected to the elastic member that is deflected by pressure. Figure 2.8 illustrates one type of LVDT pressure transducer in which the elastic member is a short Bourdon tube. The central winding of the LVDT is energized by an alternating current (E_x) and the two outer windings are connected in series opposition, making the output (E_o) zero when the elastic member is undeflected. The application of pressure to the transducer moves the core from its central position and the voltages induced in the two outer windings become unequal; hence, there arises an alternating voltage (E_o) that is proportional to pressure. This voltage is processed to provide a direct voltage or current, the magnitude of which is proportional to the applied pressure.

Capacitive Transducer

The capacitance-change principle was used in the early days of transducer development. With this method, the elastic member is one of the plates of the capacitor; the other plate is fixed and nearby. The application of pressure decreases the spacing between the plates and thereby increases the capacitance, which changes the frequency of a tuned circuit or the balance of a bridge. Suitable processing circuitry is used to provide a recordable signal. Because of practical difficulties (e.g., the small signal produced and the sensitivity to temperature changes), the capacitance principle became less used in transducers for blood-pressure measurement. However, these defects have been eliminated in present-day capacitance manometers.

Absolute-Pressure Transducer

It is important to recognize that pressure measurement must always have a reference. With blood-pressure transducers outside of the body, the reference is ambient atmospheric pressure. When a pressure transducer is totally implanted, it must be sealed and the reference pressure must be defined. If the chamber behind the elastic member is sealed, the reference is the ambient pressure when the seal was made; however, the volume of air in this space will change if the temperature changes, as well as with a change in barometric pressure. To avoid this problem with implanted pressure transducers, the space behind the elastic member is evacuated, and the pressure reading is now referred to 0 mm Hg, that is, absolute zero pressure, rather than atmosphere pressure, which is typically 760 mm Hg.

Operating Characteristics of Catheter-Type Transducers

Although a pressure transducer is simple in concept, the factors that govern its response are not obvious. It is the relationship between three quantities—mass, stiffness, and viscous drag—that determine the dynamic response of a pressure transducer to an applied pressure. The mass is composed of all of the moving components, that is, fluid in the transducer dome and its interconnecting catheter, as well as that of the elastic member and any masses connected to it. The stiffness pertains to the force needed to deflect the elastic member (diaphragm). This factor, which is really a compliance, is specified in terms of the volume displacement, which is the number of cubic millimeters of fluid that enters for the application of 100 mm Hg of pressure. Viscous drag, which provides damping, is a force having a magnitude that depends on velocity of movement. In blood-pressure transducers, the viscous damping arises from fluid flow into the transducer with the application of pressure. Note that viscous drag will be proportional to the rate of change of applied pressure.

From the foregoing it should be obvious that the fluid-filled pressure transducer is analogous to a mass–spring system with viscous damping.

The following differential equation describes the operation of a blood-pressure transducer:

$$M\frac{d^2x}{dt^2} \quad + \quad R\frac{dx}{dt} \quad + \quad Kx \quad = \quad P(t)$$

$$\begin{pmatrix}\textit{mass} \times \\ \textit{acceleration}\end{pmatrix} + \begin{pmatrix}\textit{viscous} \\ \textit{drag}\end{pmatrix} + \begin{pmatrix}\textit{stiff-} \\ \textit{ness}\end{pmatrix} = \begin{pmatrix}\textit{applied} \\ \textit{pressure}\end{pmatrix}$$

where M = effective moving mass
x = distance moved
R = viscous drag factor
K = stiffness (expressed as volume displacement).

If the transducer is used without a long fluid-filled catheter, solution of the differential equation is easy. However, in a practical case, the fluid in the transducer has a mass with its own velocity; the same is true for the fluid in the catheter. Therefore, both components need to be considered. It usually turns out in a practical case that the dominant component is the fluid in the catheter.

Resonant Frequency

With any mass–spring system, if the viscous forces are made small, the system will oscillate for a long time following presentation of an applied force. Such a response is exhibited by pressure transducers. The resonant frequency (f_r) of a pressure transducer is obtained by solving the differential equation for zero viscous drag (i.e., no damping, $R=0$). Referring to Figure 2.6*a* in which a spring-loaded piston is used to represent the diaphragm and the stiffness is K, the application of a pressure (ΔP) results in the creation of a force equal to ΔPA, where A is the area of the piston. The piston will move by an amount ΔX, therefore,

$$\Delta PA = K\Delta X$$

from which the stiffness K is as follows:

$$K = \frac{\Delta PA}{\Delta X}$$

Multiplying by A/A gives

$$K = \frac{\Delta PA^2}{A\Delta X}$$

Now $A\Delta X$, is the volume entering the transducer; therefore,

$$K = \frac{A^2 \Delta P}{\Delta V}$$

The volume displacement (V_d) is $\Delta V/\Delta P$, therefore

$$K = \frac{A^2}{V_d}$$

In such a transducer system, the resonant frequency (f_r) is as follows:

$$f_r = \frac{1}{2\pi}\sqrt{\frac{A^2}{MV_d}}$$

where A = the area of the piston
M = the mass of the moving parts
V_d = the volume displacement.

Sometimes the term "volume elasticity" (E in dyne/cm^5) is used to describe the stiffness of the elastic member. The volume modulus of elasticity is the reciprocal of volume displacement; V_d in mm^3/100 mm Hg is equal to $1.333 \times 10^8/E$. Typical transducers for blood pressure have a volume displacement on the order of 0.01–0.03 mm^3/100 mm Hg. Using the volume elasticity, the resonant frequency is

$$f_r = \frac{1}{2\pi}\sqrt{\frac{A^2E}{M}}$$

It is useful to recognize that the resonant frequency is inversely dependent on the mass (M) and volume displacement (V_d); a small mass and small volume displacement favor the creation of a high natural resonant frequency.

The importance of an adequately high natural resonant frequency (f_r) can be appreciated by considering the application of a sudden and sustained rise in pressure (Figure 2.9*a*, i.e., a step function) to systems with low and high natural resonant frequencies. In Figure 2.9*b* the resonant frequency is low and in 2.9*c* it is high. Note that the time to reach the magnitude of the applied pressure (1.0) is shorter for the system having the higher resonant frequency (Figure 2.9*c*). The fact that there is a 100% overshoot merely reveals that there is no viscous drag (i.e., no damping). Recall that a small volume displacement and a small moving mass will favor a high resonant frequency and the ability to respond rapidly.

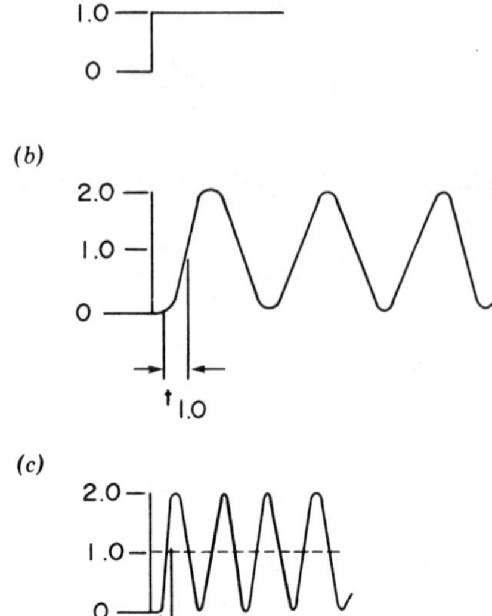

FIGURE 2.9. Response to a (*a*) step function of applied pressure to a transducer with a (*b*) low and (*c*) high natural resonant frequency and with no damping.

Blood-pressure transducers are not used alone; usually a fluid-filled catheter communicates the pressure to the transducer, as shown in Figure 2.6*b*. The moving mass is now composed of the mass of the fluid in the transducer (M_T) and that in the catheter (M_c). However, both fluids have different velocities, that in the catheter being higher than that in the transducer. By conserving kinetic energy and assuming laminar flow in the catheter, it is possible to show that the effective mass of the fluid in the catheter is $\frac{4}{3}M_c$.

Again by conserving kinetic energy it is possible to show that the effective moving fluid mass (M_{eq}) for the catheter–transducer system is as follows:

$$M_{eq} = \frac{4}{3} M_c \left(\frac{A}{a}\right)^2 + M_T$$

where M_c and M_T are the masses of fluid in the catheter and transducer, respectively; and A and a are the areas of the transducer diaphragm and catheter, respectively.

In a practical situation, a typical transducer diaphragm may be 1.0 cm in diameter and hold 1 mL (i.e., $M_T = 1$ g), of fluid in the dome. A #7F catheter has a diameter of 0.117 cm and is 100 cm long. Therefore, the area ratio squared $(A/a)^2$ is 5336. The mass of fluid in the #7F catheter (M_c) is 1.07 g; therefore, the effective moving mass is as follows:

$$M_{eq} = \frac{4}{3} M_c \left(\frac{A}{a}\right)^2 + M_T$$

$$M_{eq} = \frac{4}{3} \times 1.07 \times 5336 + 1.0 = 7613 + 1.0$$

It is clear that the effective mass of the fluid in the catheter exceeds that in the transducer; the latter can therefore be neglected when a long fluid-filled catheter is used.

The natural resonant frequency of the catheter–transducer system then becomes

$$f_r = \frac{1}{2\pi} \sqrt{\frac{A^2}{M_{eq} V_d}}$$

and substituting for M_{eq} (which neglects M_T), the following is obtained for the natural resonant frequency:

$$f_r = \frac{d}{8} \sqrt{\frac{3}{\pi L \rho V_d}}$$

where d = the catheter diameter
L = the catheter length
ρ = the density of the fluid filling the catheter
V_d = the transducer volume displacement.

The foregoing expression makes it clear that a large diameter, short catheter and a small volume displacement favor the creation of a high natural resonant frequency.

Damping

Viscous damping is always present and is due to the movement of fluid into and out of the transducer–catheter system. As stated previously, viscous damping represents a retarding force that is proportional to the velocity of movement of the fluid in the transducer–catheter system; it can be increased by using a long, small-bore catheter to communicate the pressure to the transducer. The effect of increasing the damping is shown in Figure 2.10*a* for the application of a step function of pressure. Note that with no damping (Figure 2.9) there is a 100% overshoot and the system oscillates. Figure 2.10*a* shows that as the damping is increased the percentage overshoot decreases and the time to reach 100% of the applied pressure (rise time) increases. Obviously, a desirable goal is to achieve as short a rise time as possible without overshoot. Unfortunately these two desiderata are incompatible since, as shown in Figure 2.10*a*, only when the damping is critical (1.0) is there no overshoot; but under this condition the rise time is long, especially when compared to that when a 5% overshoot is permitted which occurs with a damping of 0.7. Figure 2.10*b* illustrates how the overshoot and rise time depend on damping.

For a fluid-filled catheter–transducer system, the damping factor (D) is given by the following (Geddes, 1970):

$$D = \frac{16n}{d^3}\sqrt{\frac{3LV_d}{\pi\rho}}$$

where n = the viscosity of the fluid
ρ = the density of the fluid
d = the diameter of the catheter
L = the length of the catheter
V_d = the transducer volume displacement.

From the foregoing expression, which was derived on the basis of the effective mass of the fluid in the catheter being dominant, it should be clear that in order to achieve the desired damping (e.g., 0.7 or slightly more) there is a critical relationship between catheter dimensions and transducer volume displacement. In practice, transducers with volume displacements on the order of 0.01–0.03 mm^3/100 mm Hg are used with catheters that are not necessarily matched to provide a damping of 0.7 or more. This point will be discussed following a presentation of the sinusoidal frequency response of catheter–transducer systems.

Frequency Content of Pressure Waves

The full meaning of the sine-wave frequency response of a blood-pressure-measuring system can best be established by a presentation of the concepts underlying the Fourier series, which states mathematically that any periodic complex (nonsinusoidal) wave can be synthesized from a series consisting of a constant plus a series of harmonically related sine

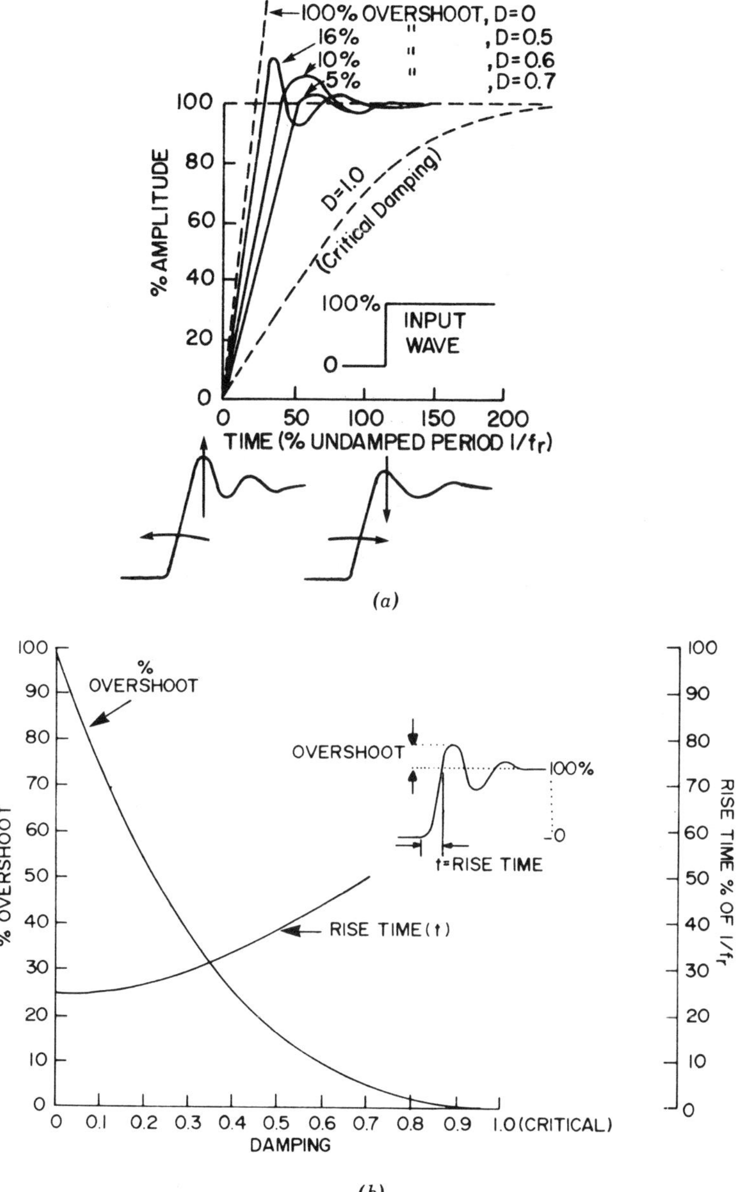

FIGURE 2.10. The effect of damping on (*a*) overshoot and (*b*) rise time for the application of a step function of pressure to a transducer.

and cosine waves. It is the type of waveform that dictates the amplitudes of the components (constant and amplitudes of the sine and cosine waves), some of which may be zero.

Rather than presenting the Fourier series formally, the important concepts can be illustrated by synthesis of a blood-pressure pulse waveform, as shown in Figure 2.11*a*. The original pressure wave (a) was synthesized from a series of sine waves having the amplitudes shown on the figure. Note that by adding the amplitudes of six harmonics, the reproduction (b) is reasonably good. Note also that the higher harmonics, that is, sine waves with higher multiples of the cardiac frequency, contribute progressively less to the synthesis of the pulse. The degree of reproduction can be improved by adding more harmonic components.

Recall that sine (and cosine) waves have no average value; but blood pressure has. Therefore, the baseline (0–0) for the sine waves is mean blood pressure, that is, the constant term in the Fourier series.

Many different blood-pressure waveforms have been analyzed for their sine-wave-frequency components. Figure 2.11*b* presents the relationship between harmonic amplitude and harmonic number. In all cases, it is clear that the higher-frequency components contribute proportionally less to synthesis of the pressure waveform. A good rule-of-thumb is that inclusion of up to about the tenth harmonic provides a good reproduction of the blood-pressure wave.

Transducer–Catheter Response

The frequency response of a fluid-filled catheter–transducer system can be measured by applying sinusoidal hydraulic pressure waves of constant amplitude and differing frequencies and measuring the electrical output of the transducer. The type of graph (i.e., amplitude versus sinusoidal frequency) that is obtained depends on the resonant frequency and damping of the system. Figure 2.12 illustrates typical results for catheter–transducer systems having 0, 0.5, 0.6, 0.7, and 1.0 (critical) damping. It is quite clear that with zero damping, as the frequency of the applied pressure wave approaches that of the resonant frequency of the system, the amplitude becomes larger and larger. With zero damping (which is impossible) the response would be so large that the system would be destroyed. However, it is possible to create a system with very little viscous damping, and the amplitude at resonance could be very large indeed.

With increased damping, the sinusoidal frequency response becomes more uniform. With a damping factor of 0.7, it is almost flat. With critical damping (1.0), the frequency response falls off very rapidly with increas-

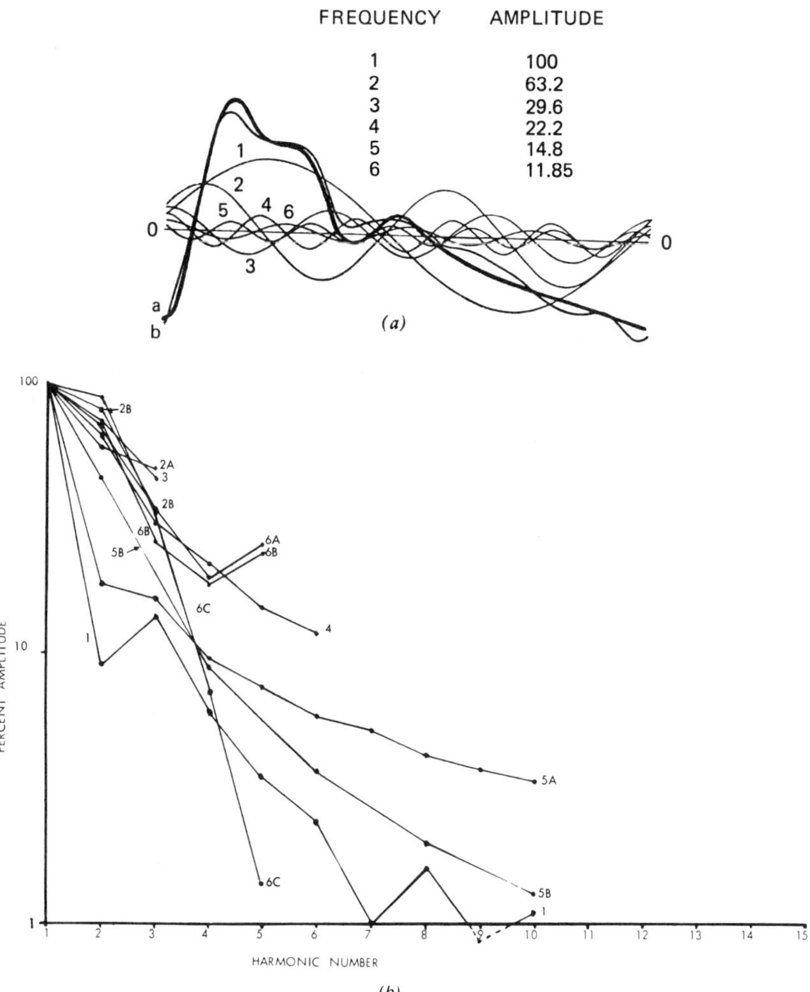

FIGURE 2.11. (*a*) Synthesis of a blood-pressure wave using harmonically related sine waves. (*b*) Illustrates the harmonic amplitudes for various blood pressure waves. [1, left ventricle; 2A, central pulse; 2B, peripheral pulse; 3, subclavian pulse; 4, arterial pulse; 5A, pulmonary artery; 5B, right ventricle; 6A, ascending aorta; 6B, abdominal aorta; 6C, femoral artery. [From Geddes, L. A. (1970). *The Direct and Indirect Measurement of Blood Pressure,* Year Book Medical Publishers, Chicago.]

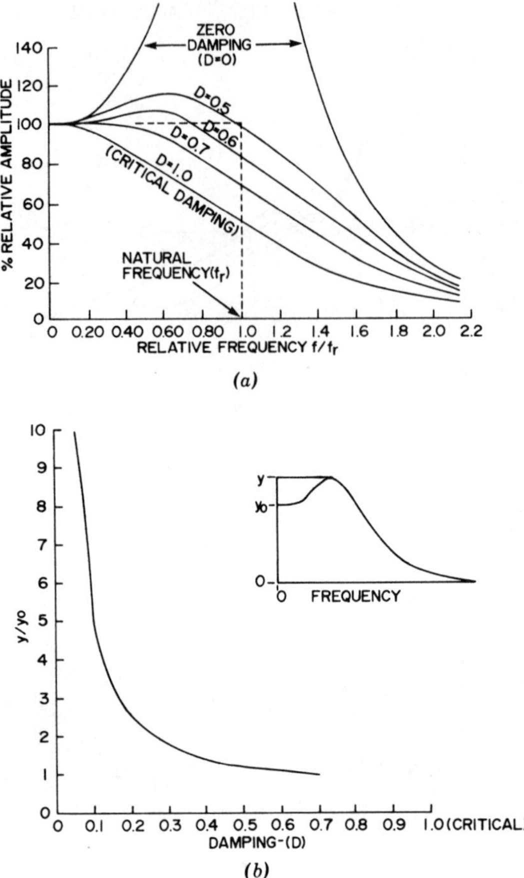

FIGURE 2.12. Sine-wave frequency response of a transducer system having different degrees of damping.

ing frequency as is shown in Figure 2.12*a*. Figure 2.12*b* describes the rise in the sine-wave frequency response with different degrees of damping (*D*).

Recall that in the previous section it was stated that provision for full reproduction up to the tenth harmonic provides reasonable waveform fidelity. Therefore, it is seen that the natural resonant frequency of the catheter–transducer system must be about twice this value, so that with a damping factor of about 0.7, the sine-wave frequency response will be virtually uniform up to the tenth harmonic of the cardiac frequency.

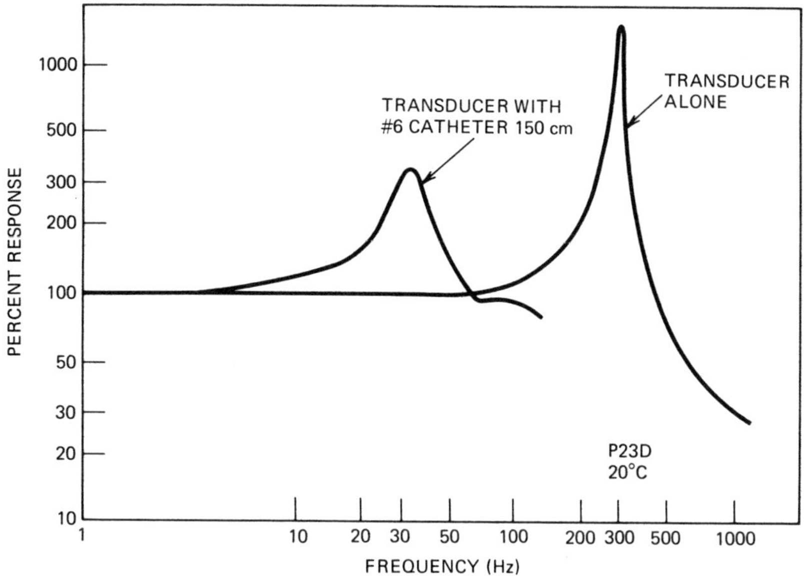

FIGURE 2.13. Sinusoidal frequency response of typical blood-pressure transducers. [Redrawn from Noble, F. W. (1957). *IRE Trans. Bio-Med. Elect.*, **PGME 8,** 38–45.]

Frequency Response of Typical Transducers

It is of value to examine the frequency-response characteristic of a typical pressure transducer without a catheter attached. Figure 2.13 reveals that a fluid-filled transducer by itself is highly underdamped and has a resonant frequency around 300 Hz.

When a fluid-filled catheter is connected to a transducer, the viscous drag due to movement of the fluid in the catheter and transducer provides considerable damping; Figure 2.13 illustrates this point. The resonant peak for the transducer alone was about 300 Hz and the damping was about 0.03. When the catheter was added, the peak in the sinusoidal frequency response moved to 35 Hz (owing to the increase in the effective mass) and the damping was increased to about 0.15 (owing to the increased fluid friction).

The performance characteristics illustrated in Figure 2.13 merit some comment in terms of what they will do to the reproduction of a blood-pressure wave. Suppose that the heart rate is 120 beats per minute (2 beats per second); the tenth harmonic is therefore 20 Hz. The amplitude of the tenth harmonic of a typical blood-pressure wave is on the order of

1–5% of the fundamental (Figure 2.11*b*). Therefore, addition of the tenth harmonic (20 Hz) by 50% more amplitude then it should have will not significantly distort the pressure waveform. In general, therefore, if there is a resonant peak in the overall sine-wave frequency response of the catheter–transducer system, the significance depends on the amplitude of the harmonic having that frequency. Obviously, if the resonant peak is well beyond the tenth harmonic of the cardiac frequency, little distortion is expected.

At present, there is great difficulty in obtaining high-fidelity pressure recordings with tiny catheters placed in the vessels of very small subjects. Systolic and diastolic pressures may not be accurately displayed in these cases, even with the best commercially available transducers. In this application, a transducer with the smallest volume displacement is required. In general, if a clear dicrotic notch is seen, the systolic and diastolic pressures can be assumed to be reasonably well reproduced.

Air Bubbles

The performance of a high-quality pressure-recording system can be deteriorated dramatically if a tiny air bubble is present in the catheter–transducer system. Air is compressible, and the presence of such a bubble increases the volume displacement of the system, which, in turn, increases the damping and prolongs the rise time. Bourland (1978) demonstrated this fact elegantly by using an intravascular catheter-tip pressure transducer which measures pressure at the catheter tip as the reference, and a standard catheter–transducer system to measure the same pressure at the same site.

Figure 2.14 presents a two-channel record of canine arterial pressure recorded with a #6F catheter and transducer and a catheter-tip transducer. Note that the waveforms are virtually identical and that the times for the systolic peaks are the same, as identified by the vertical line. Then, a small air bubble was injected into the transducer dome; the result is shown in Figure 2.15. Note that the amplitude of the dicrotic wave is less in the catheter–transducer recording and that there is a 42 msec delay between the systolic peak for the catheter-based system.

The foregoing illustrates that increasing damping not only reduces the amplitude of the rapidly changing parts of a wave, but also adds a time delay. This latter fact is of paramount importance if time measurements and their relation to other cardiac events are to be made on the blood-pressure wave.

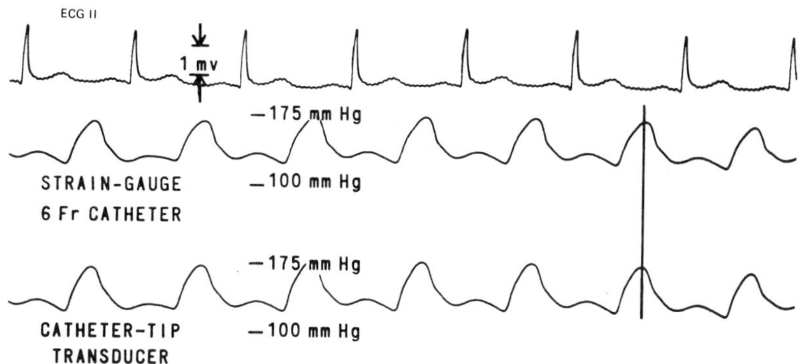

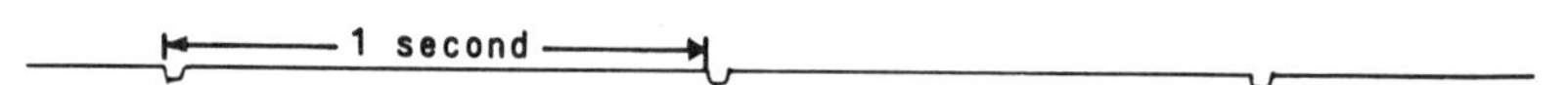

FIGURE 2.14. Lead II ECG and canine carotid blood pressure recorded with a fluid-filled catheter connected to a strain-gauge transducer and with a catheter-tip transducer. Note the similarity of the records and the time correspondence identified by the vertical line. (Courtesy J. D. Bourland, Purdue University, 1978.)

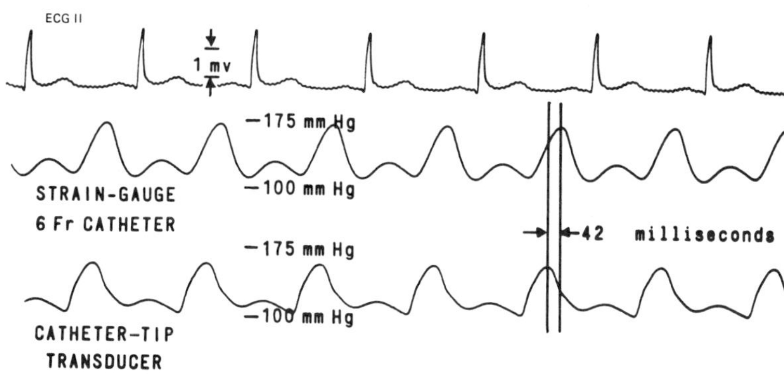

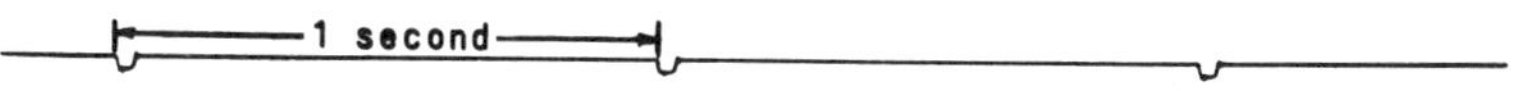

FIGURE 2.15. Lead II ECG and canine carotid blood pressure recorded with a fluid-filled catheter connected to a strain-gauge transducer containing an air bubble, and a catheter-tip transducer. Note the decreased amplitude of the dicrotic wave and the 42 msec time delay in the catheter record. (Courtesy J. D. Bourland, Purdue University, 1978.)

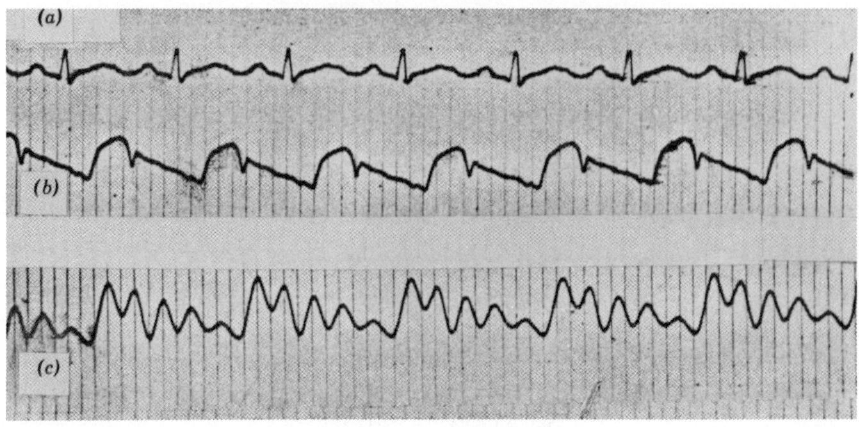

FIGURE 2.16. Catheter whip. (*a*) Illustrates the ECG; (*b*) illustrates a high, quality recording, and (*c*) illustrates catheter whip. [Redrawn from Piemme, T. E. (1963). *Prog. Cardiovasc. Dis.*, **5**, 574–594.)

Catheter Whip

Catheter whip is the term used to describe the appearance of low-frequency oscillations in a record produced by flailing of the catheter in a large-diameter blood vessel. Piemme (1963) presented a record demonstrating catheter whip obtained with a #5F catheter connected to a strain-gauge transducer. Figure 2.16*a* illustrates the ECG, Figure 2.16*b* illustrates a high-fidelity record of arterial pressure obtained with a catheter-tip transducer, and Figure 2.16*c* illustrates the presence of catheter whip.

Catheters and Needles

Vascular pressures are communicated to pressure transducers via catheters and needles. Table 2.1 lists standard catheter dimensions and Table 2.2 presents the dimensions of standard needles. For catheters, the outer diameter, in millimeters, is approximately one-third of the F (French) size. However, there is no such handy rule for identification of needle diameter from the gauge size.

Disposable Transducer Domes

Recently, presterilized, disposable transducer domes have become available for a variety of transducers. The dome contains a thin, compliant

TABLE 2.1. Catheter Dimensions[a]

	Thick-Walled Catheter		Thin-Walled Catheter	
Catheter Size "F"	Outer Diameter (mm)	Lumen Diameter (mm)	Outer Diameter (mm)	Lumen Diameter (mm)
3F	1.00	0.36	—	—
4F	1.33	0.46	1.33	0.58
5F	1.67	0.66	1.67	0.86
6F	2.00	0.91	2.00	1.17
7F	2.33	1.17	2.33	1.47
8F	2.67	1.42	2.67	1.73
9F	3.00	1.63	3.00	1.98
10F	3.33	1.83	3.33	2.24
11F	3.67	2.11	3.67	2.49
12F	4.00	2.39	4.00	2.74
14F	4.67	2.90	4.67	3.25

[a] From catalog of the U.S. Catheter & Instrument Company, Glens Falls, N.Y.

TABLE 2.2. Hypodermic Needle Sizes[a]

Size (Stubs gauge)	Outer Diameter (mm)	Lumen[a] Diameter (mm)
11	3.17	2.45
12	2.75	2.15
13	2.4	1.8
14	2.1	1.6
15	1.83	1.37
16	1.65	1.2
17	1.47	1.06
18	1.25	0.94
19	1.06	0.76
20	0.9	0.63
21	0.8	0.56
22	0.7	0.455
23	0.63	0.38
24	0.55	0.355
25	0.5	0.305
26	0.455	0.305
27	0.4	0.25

[a] From *Medical Physics,* (1950), **2,** 409.

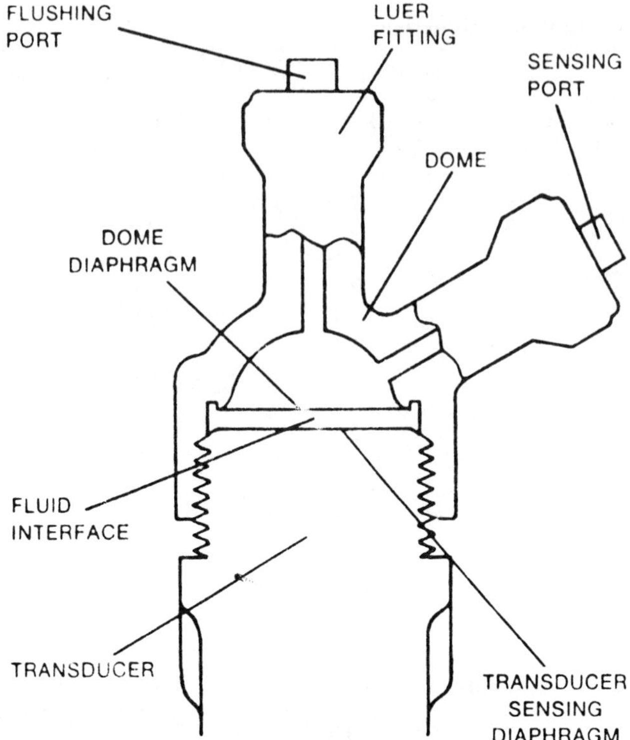

FIGURE 2.17. Disposable pressure transducer dome.

membrane that separates the fluid in the catheter and dome from the diaphragm, as shown in Figure 2.17. The pressure in the fluid in the dome is communicated to the transducer diaphragm; usually a fluid film is employed to minimize the risk of creating an air space, which would increase the volume displacement of the transducer.

Usually, the membrane in the dome is strong enough to permit unscrewing and removal of the transducer. In this way the patient can be transported or the transducer replaced. As attractive and practical as such domes are, great care must be taken to eliminate all air between the dome membrane and transducer diaphragm.

Summary

The spring-loaded piston analog for the diaphragm in a pressure transducer permits easy identification of the factors that govern the operation of such devices. Calculations with this model are in reasonable agreement with data obtained experimentally. However, there are other more important considerations that must be discussed.

Although the figure of merit of a pressure transducer is its volume displacement, other factors should be considered before deciding on the acquisition of a transducer with an extremely small volume displacement. For example, the foregoing theoretical considerations were developed assuming a stiff-walled catheter containing an incompressible fluid. Both assumptions may not be fulfilled in practice. Plastic catheters do not have stiff walls; the walls are viscoelastic, and there is the possibility of creating a second (mass–spring) resonant system, represented by the volume displacement of the catheter and the mass of fluid within it. In addition, water, which is the major component of the fluid filling the transducer and catheter, is not incompressible. For example, 1 mL of water, which is a good approximation to the volume in the transducer dome, will decrease its volume by about 6.1×10^{-6} mL by the application of 100 mm Hg pressure at room temperature. Converted to volume displacement this value is 0.006 mm^3/100 mm Hg. Therefore, the volume displacement of a transducer is the sum of that of the catheter, that of the compressibility of the fluid filling it, and that of the transducer itself. It is obvious that the high-fidelity capabilities of a pressure transducer can only be realized with a stiff-walled short catheter which does not contain even the tiniest air bubble, the compressibility of which can completely dominate the volume displacement of the transducer and catheter.

Electrical Safety Considerations

In the first blood-pressure transducers, the elastic membrane was of metal and often provided an electrical connection with the recording apparatus. Thus there was a direct connection via the vascular system to ground. Although the resistance of a fluid-filled catheter was high, an unintentional ground was placed on the subject. If the subject came into contact with a ground-referred voltage, leakage current could flow with the hazard of precipating ventricular fibrillation. Soon, however, the metallic elastic member was isolated from the electronic sensing system, thereby eliminating the conductive ground path. With the increased use of defibrillators, the breakdown voltage of the capacitive path to ground was increased. Today, a typical pressure transducer can withstand 5000–10,000 V without breakdown. However, there is still a capacitive path that offers a low impedance for high-frequency current, such as electrosurgical or diathermy current. Care must therefore be exercised when using these modalities to ensure that high-frequency leakage current does not flow in the vascular system through the fluid-filled catheter to the

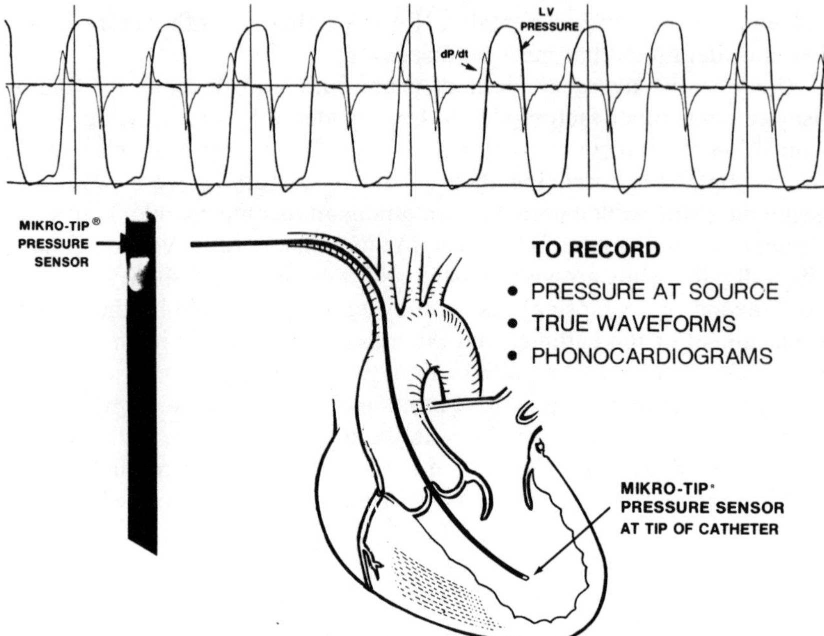

FIGURE 2.18. The Millar Mikro-Tip® pressure transducer. (Courtesy Millar Instruments, Houston, Texas.)

transducer and to ground. In such circumstances it is wise to disconnect the transducer from the electronic recorder and also to ensure that the connector does not accidentally come into contact with ground.

Catheter-Tip Transducers

In the catheter-type transducer, blood pressure is communicated to the elastic member via a fluid-filled catheter; consequently, the transducer is outside of the body. Providing that the catheter length and diameter are chosen appropriately to satisfy the requirements of the transducer, faithful pressure recordings can be obtained. With the catheter-tip transducer, the elastic member (and the electrical-detecting system affixed to it) is palced in a blood vessel; thus, the elastic member is in direct contact with the blood. This arrangement avoids the damping and resonance often encountered with catheter-type systems and guarantees the highest fidelity for converting pressure to an electrical signal.

One of the most popular of the catheter-tip transducers is the Millar Mikro-Tip® unit, which is shown in Figure 2.18. In this device, there are two strain-gauge elements attached to an elastic member, which is on the side of the catheter at the tip. The back of the elastic member communicates with the environment via the lumen of the catheter, which carries the leads from the strain-gauge elements to the connector. The application of pressure increases the resistance of one and decreases the resistance of the other strain-gauge element. These two elements constitute one-half of a Wheatstone bridge; the other half is formed by two resistors mounted within the electrical connector. Thus, the device contains two active strain-gauge elements, which are arranged so that changes in temperature do not affect the zero baseline or sensitivity. A very attractive feature of the Mikro-Tip® transducer is its high output. For example, an output of 25 mV is produced in response to the application of a pressure of 300 mm Hg with 3.5 V of excitation. The response time is so short that heart-valve and blood-flow sounds (murmurs) can be reproduced.

The Mikro-Tip® transducer is available in a variety of configurations. Some models have a side port for withdrawal of blood or the injection of fluid at the site of pressure measurement. Transducers with as many as six pressure sensors and models with electromagnetic flow sensors have also been fabricated.

Rate of Pressure Change (*dp/dt*)

An index of vigor of contraction of the heart is expressed by the rate of change of pressure, designated by the first-order differential *dp/dt*, which is merely the slope of (or the tangent to) the pressure wave at a given point. Figure 2.19 illustrates an arterial pressure wave and the meaning of *dp/dt*. Note that the slope changes throughout the wave. Figure 2.20 illustrates this point and displays the pressure wave and its derivative *dp/dt* recorded continuously. Since the nature of a differentiating system

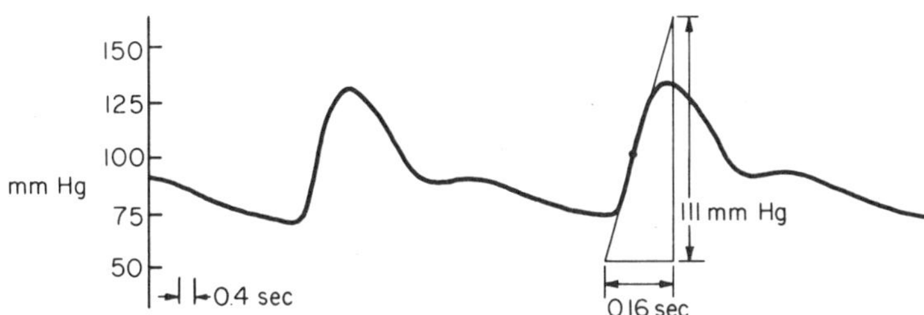

FIGURE 2.19. A typical arterial pressure record and the rate of change of pressure on the rising phase; dp/dt = 111 mm Hg/0.16 sec = 694 mm Hg/sec.

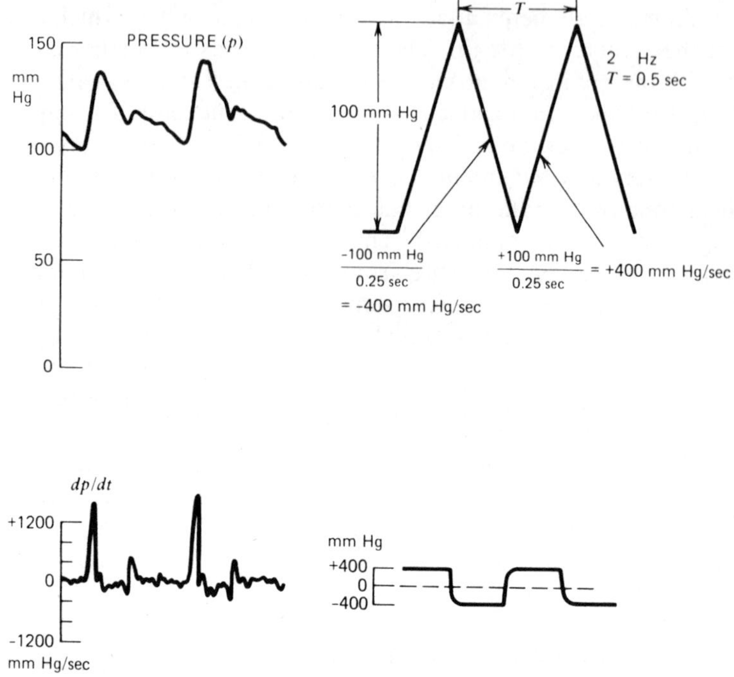

FIGURE 2.20. Arterial pressure and its derivative and the triangular-wave method used for calibration.

favors reproduction of high-frequency components, any high-frequency components and any high-frequency noise in the pressure channel will be enhanced by differentiation.

In cardiovascular studies, the maximum rate of change of left or right ventricular or aortic pressure is often used as an indicator of myocardial contractility. In such a case, the value listed is dp/dt_{max}. It was thought that there would be a normal range of values which would permit defining normal and abnormal cardiac dynamics. Unfortunately, this hope was not realized because there is a large variation in the maximum value of dp/dt among subjects. However, dp/dt still has value in monitored subjects, because a decrease may indicate diminished myocardial dynamics.

It is of considerable importance to understand the nature of a derivative-recording channel and know how it is calibrated; Figure 2.21 provides important information on this subject. Note that when a square wave of pressure ($+p$) is applied to a pressure-recording system (A_1), the same pressure wave is reproduced. However, with a differentiator (dp/dt) is inserted in a similar recording channel (A_2) as shown, an output is

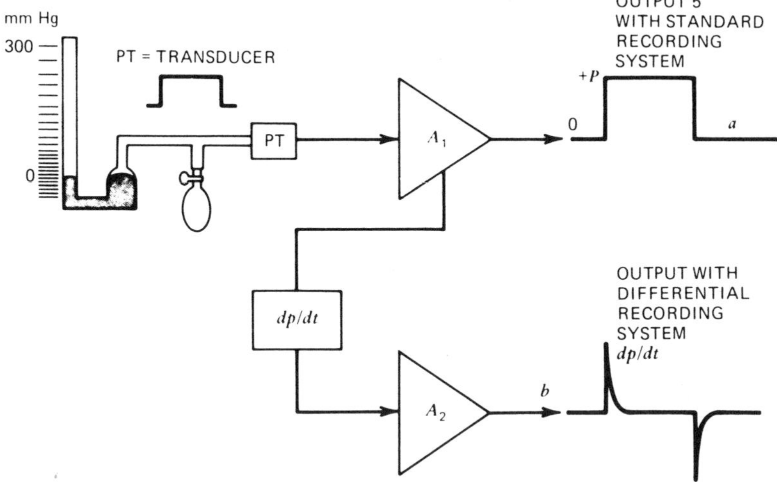

FIGURE 2.21. The characteristics of a differentiation (dp/dt) circuit. When a square-wave pressure pulse is applied to a recording system (A_1), it is reproduced as shown ($0 + p$). When this signal is passed through the differentiator (dp/dt), only the rapidly changing portions of the pressure wave are reproduced, dp/dt. PT is the pressure transducer.

obtained only when the pressure is changing. The amplitude displayed by the dp/dt channel is proportional only to the rate of change of pressure presented to it.

Obviously the ideal way to calibrate a dp/dt channel would be to connect a hydraulic generator, which provides a known and constant rate of change of pressure to the transducer. However, hydraulic pressure generators are not generally available, and other means must be sought to calibrate the dp/dt channel. There are two convenient methods used at present: one employs a triangular-wave generator and the other uses a sine-wave generator. In both cases the frequency employed is a few hertz to calibrate a typical dp/dt channel.

Triangular-Wave Calibration

The first step in calibrating a dp/dt channel consists of setting up the recording system to obtain a pressure recording and a dp/dt recording of a satisfactory amplitude as shown in Figure 2.20. Then, without altering any controls in the recording channels, known pressures are applied to calibrate the pressure recording. The pressure transducer and its processing circuitry are then disconnected and a low-frequency (e.g., 2 Hz) triangular-wave signal is fed into the pressure-recording channel. The amplitude of this new input signal is increased so that a suitably large amplitude recording is obtained, for example, a peak-to-peak amplitude equivalent to 100 mm Hg, as shown in Figure 2.20. Note that the *dp/dt* channel produces a square wave because the slope of a triangular wave is constant. In Figure 2.20, the peak-to-peak pressure is 100 mm Hg and the frequency of the triangular wave is 2 Hz. This means that the rate of pressure rise is 100 mm Hg in 0.25 seconds or + 400 mm Hg/sec. Similarly, the rate of pressure fall is − 100 mm Hg/0.25 sec = − 400 mm Hg/sec. Thus the *dp/dt* channel rises to + 400 and falls to − 400 mm Hg/sec as shown, and the zero level for *dp/dt* is midway between these two values. It is noteworthy that this recorded triangular-wave signal, although not derived from a pressure source, can be used to simulate a changing pressure signal.

Sine-Wave Calibration

Frequently a triangular-wave generator is not available and a sine-wave generator is used. The first step is as before, namely the pressure and *dp/dt* channels are first adjusted to provide recordings of adequate amplitude. Then the pressure channel is calibrated with known pressures. Without altering any controls, the pressure transducer is disconnected and a low-frequency (e.g., 4 Hz) sine-wave generator is connected to the pressure-recording channel. The peak-to-peak output of the sine-wave generator is adjusted to obtain a satisfactorily large-amplitude pressure wave, for example, 100 mm Hg as shown in Figure 2.22. When this is done, the *dp/dt* channel records a cosine wave, the peak-to-peak amplitude allows calibration of the *dp/dt* channel.

Consider a sine wave of pressure having a frequency f and a peak value p_m; mathematically this wave is expressed as $p_m \sin 2\pi ft$, where t is time. The derivative of $p_m \sin 2\pi ft$ is as follows:

$$\frac{d}{dt}(p_m \sin 2\pi ft) = 2\pi f p_m (\cos 2\pi ft)$$

Therefore the peak amplitude of the derivative (*dp/dt*) channel is $2\pi f$ times the peak amplitude of the pressure channel.

The method of using this information to calibrate the *dp/dt* channel is shown in Figure 2.22. The calibrating 4-Hz sine-wave amplitude was adjusted to 100 mm Hg peak-to-peak. This means that the pressure channel oscillated between ± 50 mm Hg. The positive amplitude of the derivative

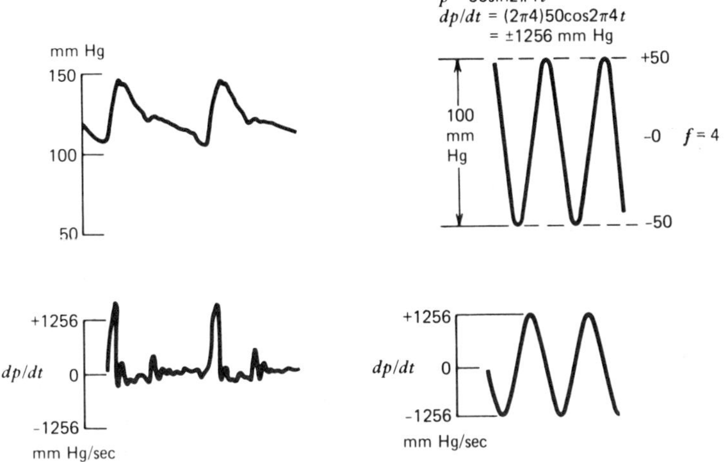

FIGURE 2.22. Calibration of a *dp/dt* channel with a sine wave.

channel is $50(2\pi \times 4) = 400\,\pi$ or 1256 mm Hg/sec. Similarly, the *dp/dt* channel has a negative amplitude of 1256 mm Hg as shown in Figure 2.22.

HISTORICAL POSTSCRIPT

The first direct measurement of blood pressure was reported by the Reverend Stephen Hales who, in 1733, wrote:

> In December I caused a mare to be tied down alive on her back; she was fourteen hands high, and about fourteen years of age, had a fistula on her withers, was neither very lean, nor yet lusty: Having laid open the left crural* artery about three inches from her belly, I inserted into it a brass pipe, whose bore was one sixth of an inch in diameter; and to that, by means of another brass pipe which was fitly adapted to it, I fixed a glass tube, of nearly the same diameter, which was nine feet in length: Then untying the ligature on the artery, the blood rose in the tube eight feet, three inches perpendicular above the level of the left ventricle of the heart.

Figure 2.23 is an artist's sketch of Hales' experiment. (Note that 8 ft 3 in. ≡ 190 mm Hg.)

*Crural = femoral.

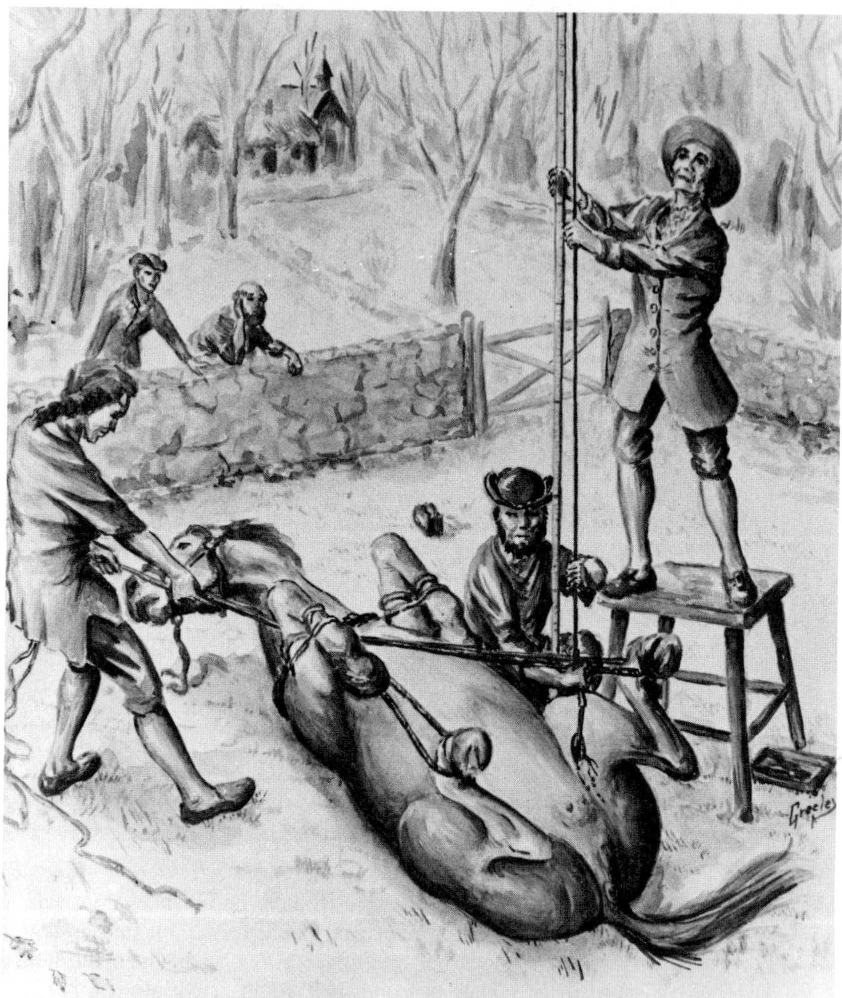

FIGURE 2.23. Artist's concept drawn from Hales' account of the first direct measurement of arterial pressure in 1733.

Hales, of course, measured mean blood pressure, noting small cardiac and respiratory variations in the height of the blood column.

The next step in measuring blood pressure provided the present-day units, mm Hg. In 1828 Poiseuille, while a medical student, employed the mercury-filled U-tube manometer to indicate mean blood pressure in the dog. It seems somewhat surprising that this advance took almost a century, in view of the fact that Hales knew of the U-tube manometer and used one to measure the pressure of sap in plants. In addition, mercury-filled barometers were in use well before Hales conducted his pioneering study.

Poiseuille left the practice of medicine and became interested in the flow of fluids. His research in this field gave us what is now known as Poiseuille's law, the hydraulic analog of Ohm's law. Poiseuille showed that fluid flow depended directly on pressure and on the radius of the tube in which flow occurred, and inversely with the viscosity and length of the tube. Poiseuille's investigations laid the foundation for rheology, the study of the flow of all matter.

Carl Ludwig, a physician–physiologist, made it possible to record pressure by placing a float on the mercury in the U-tube manometer. The float was connected to a writing lever which scratched soot from a sooted paper wrapped around a cylinder caused to rotate slowly; Figure 2.24*a* illustrates Ludwig's instrument and Figure 2.24*b* presents one of his records. Thus, analog recording was given to physiology, and changes in pressure could document themselves. The graphic record became the universal language of physiologists for some time.

From 1847 until the 1860s, only mean blood pressure and its changes were recordable because the speed of response of the mercury manometer was too slow to reproduce rapidly changing portions of the blood-pressure wave. Fick in 1864 used the Bourdon (C-spring) tube to drive a writing lever applied to a kymograph (Figure 2.25). In 1883, he developed an improved recorder consisting of an elastic membrane which was coupled to a writing lever applied to a kymograph (Figure 2.26). Fick's first manometer (Figure 2.25) indicated a much larger pulse pressure than was seen with the mercury manometer, although there was no evidence of a dicrotic notch. His second instrument (Figure 2.26) portrayed the dicrotic notch with small amplitude.

Some of the instruments of that era showed a very prominent dicrotic notch, and many displayed no notch. There arose a considerable controversy over the validity of this notch. Some thought it to be an artifact of the recording instrument; others believed that it was a genuine physiological event.

An interesting demonstration of the dicrotic wave, displayed without a manometer, was presented by Landois (1874). He used a kymograph and inserted a small-bore needle into the femoral artery of a dog, directing the jet of blood to the recording surface. There, displayed with remarkable clarity, was the blood-pressure wave with a clear dicrotic notch (Figure 2.27).

The race was then on to reduce mass and increase stiffness in recording systems to obtain a short response time. The ultimate in reducing mass

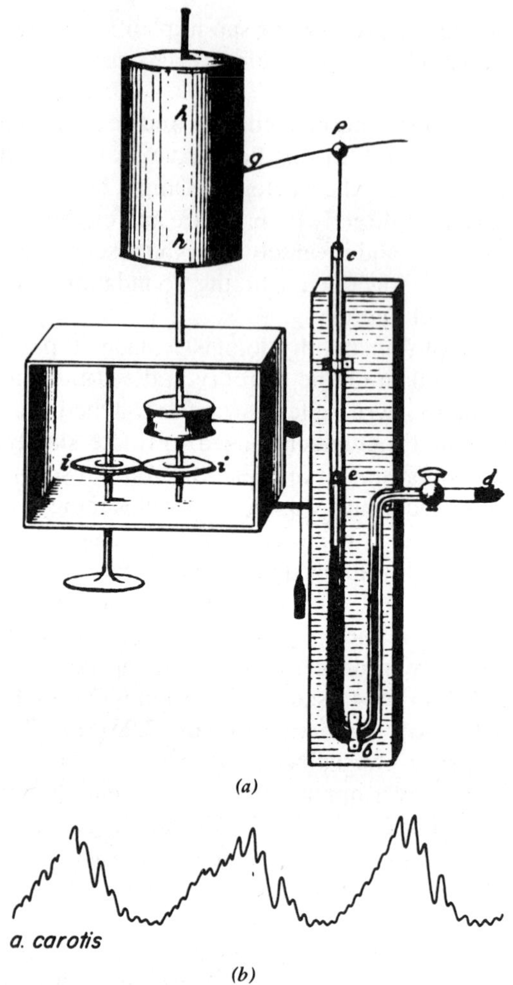

(a)

(b)

FIGURE 2.24. (*a*) Ludwig's smoked-drum kymograph (1847). (*b*) A recording of canine aortic pressure obtained with the kymograph. The large amplitude oscillations are due to respiration; the smaller oscillations represent the arterial pulse.

was achieved by Marey, a physician–physiologist in France. He recognized that the fluid-filled manometers used up to that time possessed considerable inertia and viscous damping. Accordingly, he developed air-filled systems for pressure recording. The pressure sensor consisted of a small cylindrical metal cage over which a thin rubber tube was placed. The cage was affixed to a long, thin metal tube, which in turn was connected to the display device, a recording tambour (which he also devel-

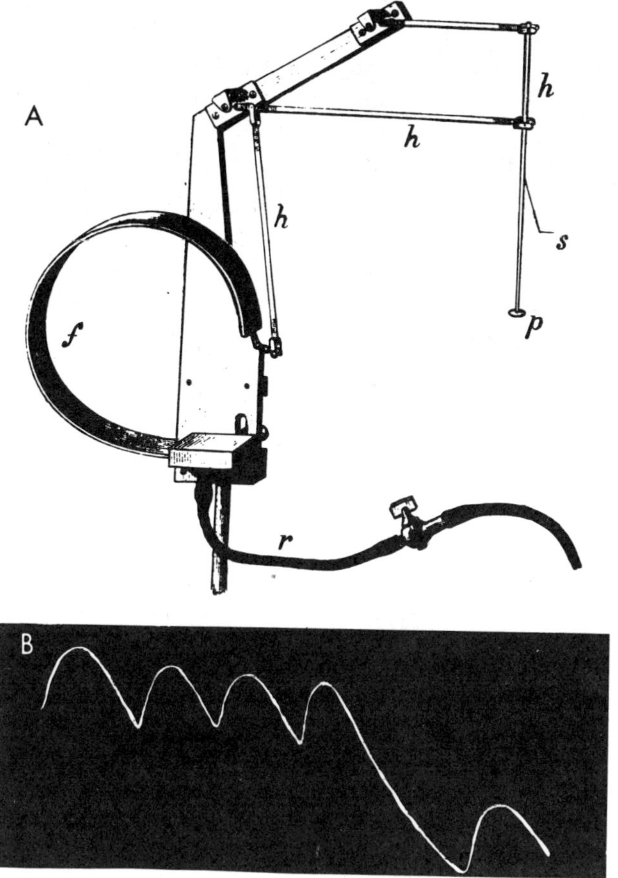

FIGURE 2.25. (*a*) Fick's C-spring pressure-recording instrument and (*b*) a typical recording obtained with it (from Fick, 1864).

oped). The tambour was a shallow cylinder covered by a thin rubber membrane coupled to a writing lever. Pressure in the environment of the metal cage squeezed the thin rubber membrane over the cylindrical cage, increasing the pressure in the tube connected to the tambour, causing the tambour lever to rise. Figure 2.28 illustrates Marey's pneumatic recording system described in 1881.

With the air-filled system just described, Marey presented excellent records of right and left ventricular pressure, right arterial pressure, and aortic pressure in the horse. This feat was indeed the first cardiac catheterization for pressure. The records (Figure 2.29) are of remarkable

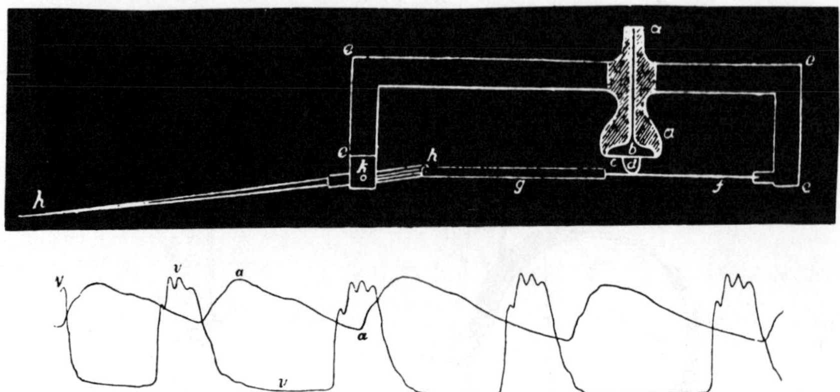

FIGURE 2.26. Fick's straight-spring direct pressure recorder and a record of left ventricular (v) and aortic (a) pressure (from Fick, 1883).

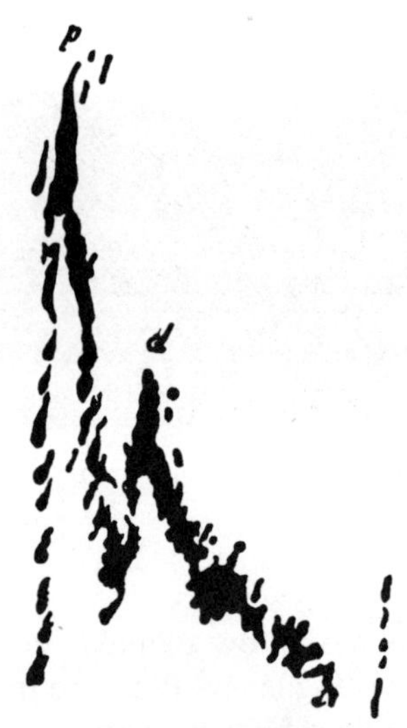

FIGURE 2.27. Landois' hemautogram, a record of blood pressure made by directing a fine jet of arterial blood against a moving chart. Clearly displayed is the dicrotic notch [from *Pfluger's Archiv.* (1874), **9**, 71].

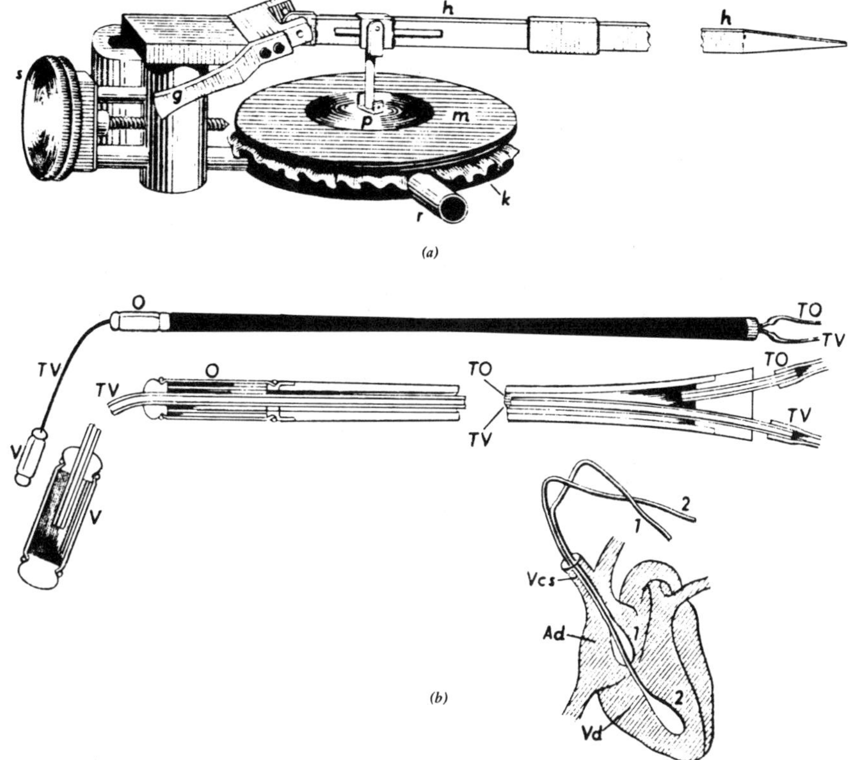

FIGURE 2.28. The air-filled pressure-recording system developed by Marey (ca. 1870): (*a*) the recording tambour and (*b*) the cardiac catheters.

clarity and were calibrated by lowering the catheter tips into different depths of water.

Marey, along with his veterinary colleague Chauveau, carried out some very remarkable studies in cardiology. An outstanding example is their discovery of the reciprocal relationship between an increase in blood pressure and a decrease in heart rate. This phenomenon later became known as Marey's law. Its discovery is illustrated in Figure 2.30. With the Marey pneumatic pressure-recording system applied to an unanesthetized standing horse, Chauveau passed his hand and arm into the dorsal colon of the horse as shown in Figure 2.30. Chauveau suddenly occluded the aorta, thereby suddenly increasing peripheral resistance and causing blood pressure to rise as shown by the sketch alongside the pressure transducer (P). Immediately, the heart rate decreased and the blood pressure fell quickly.

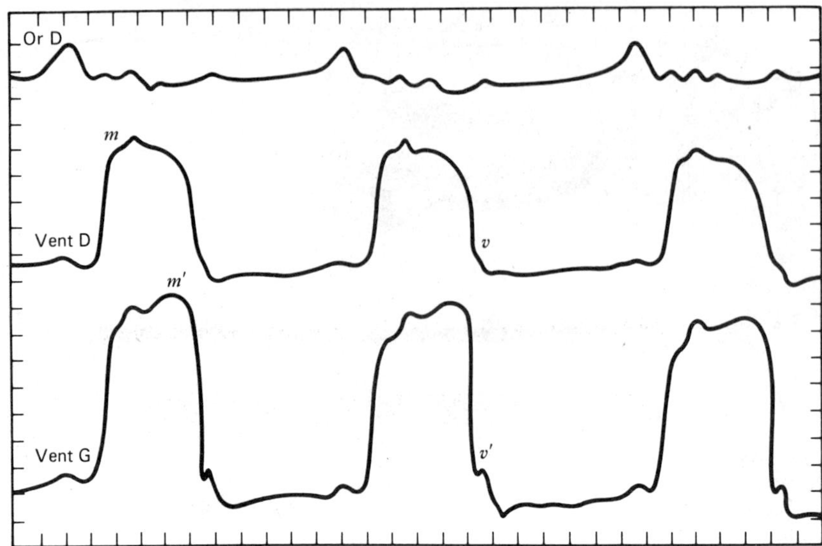

FIGURE 2.29. A record of right atrial pressure (0_v D), right-ventricular pressure (Vent. D), and left ventricular pressure (Vent. G) obtained by Marey with his pneumatic recording system.

The technique of sudden aortic clamping, which became known as the Chauveau–Marey maneuver, clearly demonstrated the regulating capabilities of the circulatory system. The underlying mechanisms (carotid–sinus and aortic–arch reflexes) were not elucidated until several decades later.

By the late 1800s, all possible reduction in the mass of writing levers had been accomplished. The next quantum leap in progress was made by Frank (1903) who solved the differential equation that underlies operation of all pressure-recording systems. He recognized that writing levers had excessive mass and eliminated them by using a light beam reflected from a mirror on the elastic member exposed to blood pressure. Thus was born the use of photographic-recording systems for blood pressure. The elastic membrane exposed to the pressure could be made stiff, resulting in short response time. The loss of sensitivity was recovered by placing the photographic surface at some distance (meters) from the mirror on the membrane. Figure 2.31 illustrates Frank's optical-recording manometer.

Many followed Frank's lead and built optically based pressure-recording systems. The characteristics of these devices were excellent and high-fidelity recordings of cardiovascular pressures were possible. Such systems were used routinely until the late 1940s.

At the dawn of the 20th century, when the optical systems were being created, the first attempts at converting pressure to an electrical signal

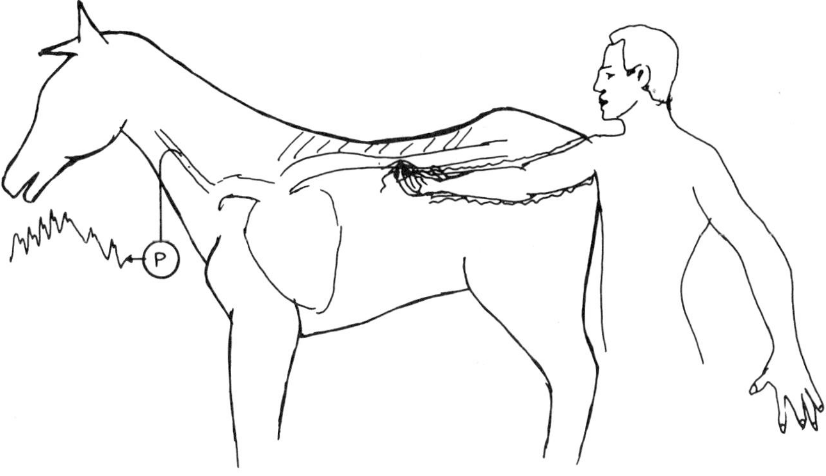

FIGURE 2.30. The Chauveau–Marey maneuver, consisting of suddenly cross clamping the aorta, causing a sudden rise in blood pressure and a reflex slowing of the heart rate.

were underway. One of the first electrical blood-pressure transducers was a catheter-tip unit, devised by Grunbaum in 1898. His device is illustrated in Figure 2.32 and consisted of a tiny capsule at the end of a catheter. On one side of the capsule was a window covered by a rubber membrane which carried an electrode. Opposite this electrode on the inner wall of the capsule was another electrode. The intervening space was filled with an electrolyte. Pressure applied to the rubber membrane decreased the

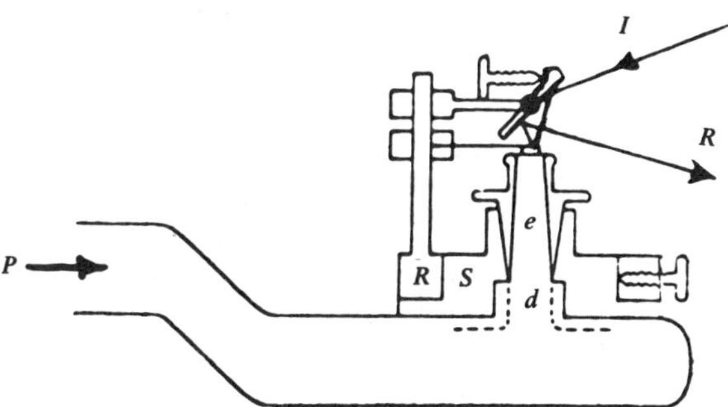

FIGURE 2.31. Frank's optical-recording manometer in which the deflection of an elastic member exposed to blood pressure (*e*) caused a mirror to deflect a light beam (*I*, *R*). [Redrawn from Frank (1924).]

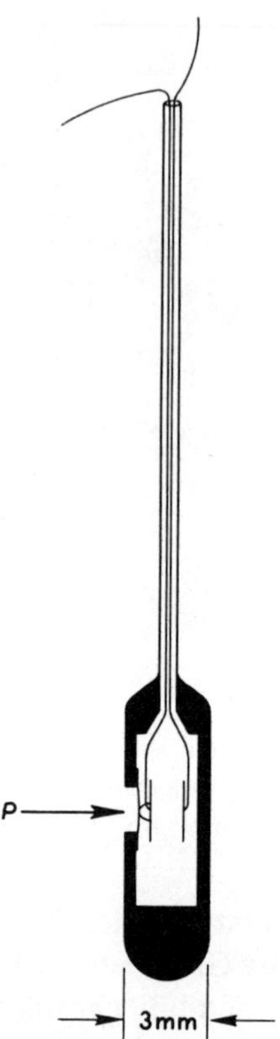

FIGURE 2.32. Grunbaum's catheter-tip electrolytic pressure transducer. [Redrawn from Grunbaum (1898).]

interelectrode distance and thereby reduced the resistance measured between the two electrodes. The resistance change was recorded by a capillary electrometer.

Grunbaum used his catheter-tip pressure transducer to record the right ventricular pressure of a rabbit. Unfortunately, no record of this remarkable feat was published.

Following Grunbaum's lead, many electrolytic pressure transducers were constructed, none of which were of the catheter-tip type. Other electrical methods were also used to detect the deflection of an elastic diaphragm exposed to blood pressure. Capacitance and inductance changes were widely used. Finally, the strain-gauge transducer was developed by Statham, and its use and characteristics were described by Lambert and Wood (1947). It is interesting to note that it was known since

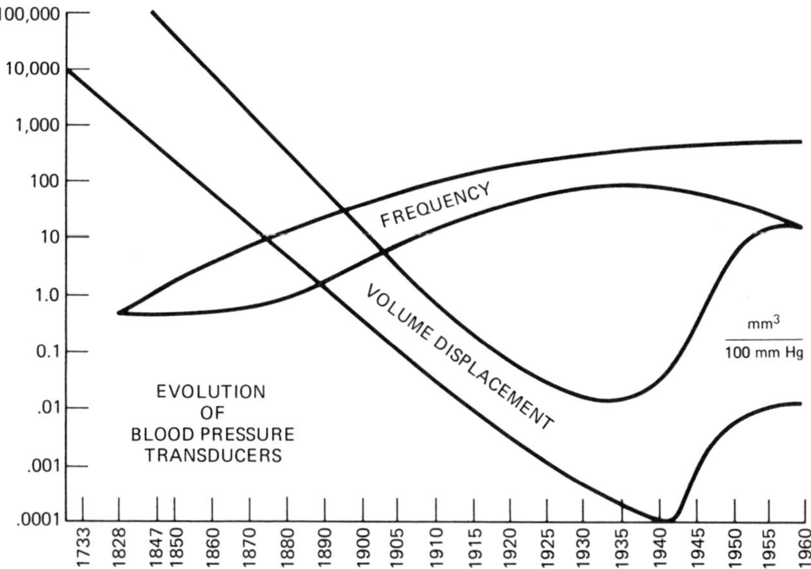

FIGURE 2.33. Historical perspective of natural frequency and volume displacement of catheter-tip-type transducers.

1876 that an increase in resistance accompanies the elongation of a wire. Why this phenomenon was not used earlier is difficult to understand.

As excellent as the fluid-filled strain-gauge transducer was, it required the use of a long fluid-filled catheter to communicate arterial pressure to the transducer. In some circumstances with long, small-bore catheters, the pressure waveform is distorted, and there were those who wanted to measure pressure at the site of its genesis. Therefore, work was started by Gauer and Gienapp (1950) to make a miniature electrical pressure transducer mounted to the tip of a catheter. Their device consisted of a linear variable differential transformer, the core of which was affixed to the tiny elastic member at the tip of the catheter. This device functioned extremely well, but did not see commercial development, although it was used extensively in aeromedical research.

Returning to the catheter-type transducer, it was stated that its two most important characteristics are the natural resonant frequency and the volume displacement. Figure 2.33 presents an historical review of typical values for these two quantities from Hales' time to 1960. This survey does not include catheter-tip types in which volume displacement is not a pertinent quantity. It is clear that volume displacements smaller than now available have been attained.

REFERENCES

Bourland, J. D. (1978). Personal communication.

Fick, A. (1864). Ein neuer Blutwellenzeichner. Reichertś u du Bors-Reymond's *Arch. Anat. Physiol.* **S583,** 543–548.

Fick, A. (1883). Ein verbesserung des Blutwellenzeichner. *Arch. ges. Physiol.* **S592,** 608–612.

Frank, O. (1903). Kritik der elastichen Manometer. *Z. Biol.* **44,** 445–613; (1912–13) **59,** 526–530; (1924) **82,** 49–65.

Gauer, O. H. and Gienapp, E. A. (1950). Miniature pressure recording device. *Science* **112,** 404–405.

Geddes, L. A. (1970). *The Direct and Indirect Measurement of Blood Pressure,* Year Book Publishers, Chicago.

Grunbaum, O. F. (1897–98). On a new method of recording alterations of pressure. *J. Physiol.* **22,** XLIX–LII.

Hales, S. (1740). *Statickal Essays. Haemastaticks,* 2nd ed., W. Innys and R. Manby, London, 361 pp.

Lambert, E. H. and Wood, E. H. (1947). The use of a resistance wire strain gauge manometer to measure intraarterial pressure. *Proc. Soc. Exp. Biol. Med.* **64,** 186–190.

Landois, L. (1874). *Pfluger's Archiv.,* **9,** 71.

Ludwig, C. (1847). Beitrage zur Kenntniss des Einflusses der Respirations bewegungen auf den Blutlauf den Aortensysteme. *Muller's Archiv. Anat.,* 240–302.

Marey, E. J. (1876). Pression et vitesse du rang. *Physiologie Experimentale,* Ecole Pratique des Hautes Etudes (Lab. de M. Marey), Paris, chap. VIII.

Piemme, T. E. (1963). Pressure measurement. *Prog. Cardiovasc. Dis.,* **5,** 574–594.

Poiseuille, J. L. M. (1828). Recherches sur la porce du coeur aortique. *Archiv. Gen. Med.* **18,** 550–555.

CHAPTER 3

Blood Pressure: Noninvasive Measurement

FUNCTIONAL DESCRIPTION

Devices that provide a quantitative measure of one or more of the three arterial blood pressures (systolic, diastolic, and mean), without requiring penetration of the skin, are designated noninvasive or indirect pressure-measuring instruments. At present all such devices are occlusive, that is, they require occlusion of an artery and employ some type of indicator to identify events occurring during gradual removal of the occlusion to indicate one or more of the three blood pressures. The combination of an air-inflated occlusive device and a pressure indicator is called a sphygmomanometer (*sphygmos* meaning pulse).

BLOOD PRESSURE

Blood pressure results from the rhythmic pumping of the heart. The term "blood pressure" usually refers to arterial pressure; however, it is to be noted that there are other blood pressures, that is, venous, cardiac chamber, capillary, etc. Figure 2.1 illustrates an arterial pressure wave and identifies systolic, diastolic, and mean pressures. All three of these pressures can be measured noninvasively. Figure 3.1 illustrates the range of systolic and diastolic pressures in males and females (Master et al., 1952) with advancing age.

OCCLUSIVE DEVICES

The most familiar occlusive device is the member-encircling cuff, which contains an air-inflatable rubber bladder in an unyielding sleeve. In older instruments, a long bandage was used to hold the cuff on the member; newer cuffs use Velcro® locking fabric or a fastener to secure the ends of the cuff. The bladder in the cuff is equipped with two tubes: one is used for inflation and deflation and the other is used to measure the pressure within the bladder. Figure 3.2 illustrates a typical cuff and its application to the upper arm. When inflated, the pressure in the bladder is transmitted through the tissues to an underlying artery, which can be occluded completely with an adequately high pressure in the bladder. It is during a reduction in this occlusive pressure that signs are sought which identify the passage of cuff pressure through systolic, mean, and diastolic pressure levels. An important consideration in the application of such an occlusive device is the relationship between its size with respect to the member to which it is applied. A complete discussion of this point will be presented subsequently. Table 3.1 lists the cuff sizes available.

At present, there are five methods of measuring one or more of the three (systolic, mean, and diastolic) arterial pressures. These methods are (1) the palpatory, (2) the oscillometric, (3) the auscultatory, (4) the ultrasonic, and (5) the flush. Table 3.2 summarizes the methods and the pressures that they measure. Complete descriptions of these methods will now be presented.

The Palpatory Method

The term "to palpate" means to feel with the hand. The palpatory method employs the finger (or an instrument) to detect the arterial pulse at a site beyond the occluding device. Figure 3.3*a* illustrates the palpatory method using a cuff applied to the biceps and connected to a mercury manometer and to a valved squeeze bulb for inflation. Two fingers are used to palpate the radial artery. Prior to inflating the cuff, the radial pulse is detected with the second and third fingers. Then the cuff is pumped up quickly to a pressure above the point of disappearance of the radial pulse. Then cuff pressure is reduced slowly (about 3 mm Hg per heart beat). At the instant when cuff pressure falls below systolic pressure, the radial pulse can be

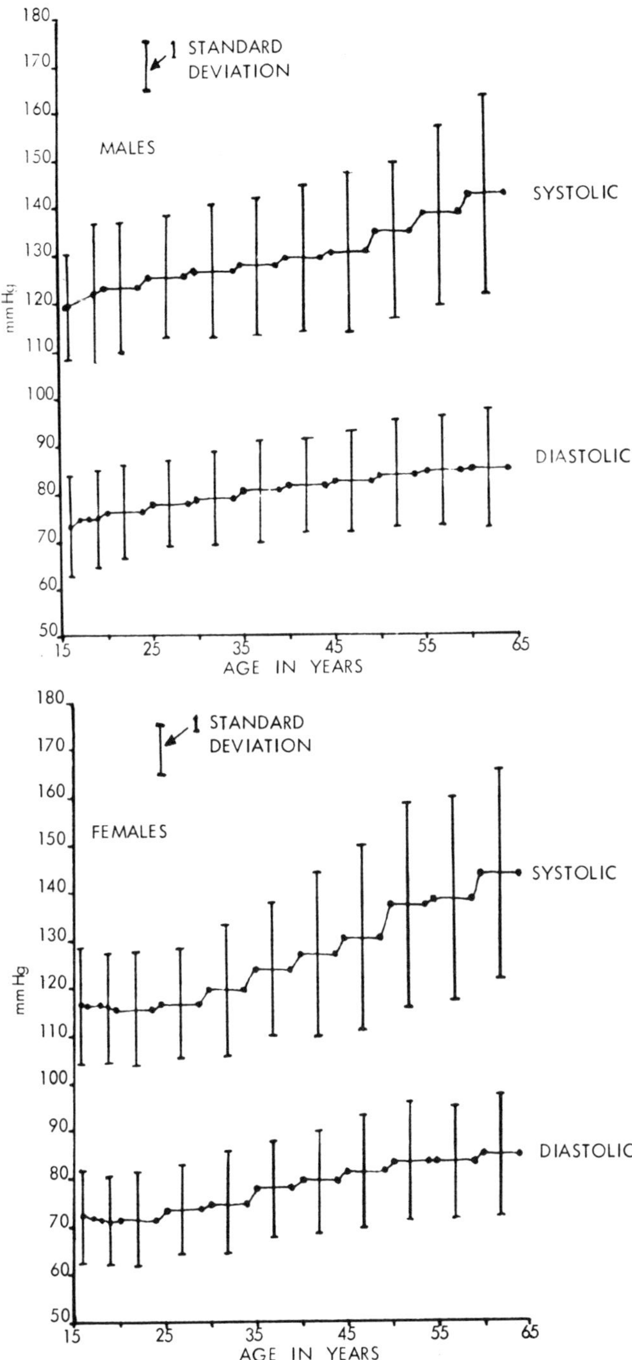

FIGURE 3.1. Systolic and diastolic arterial pressure in males and females (mean and standard deviation). Compiled from data published by Master et al. (1952).

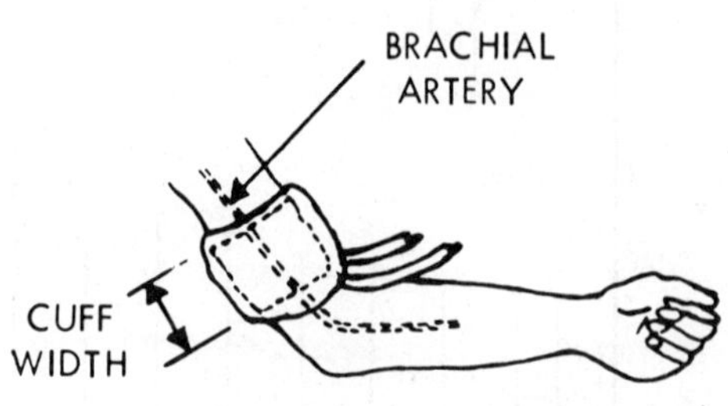

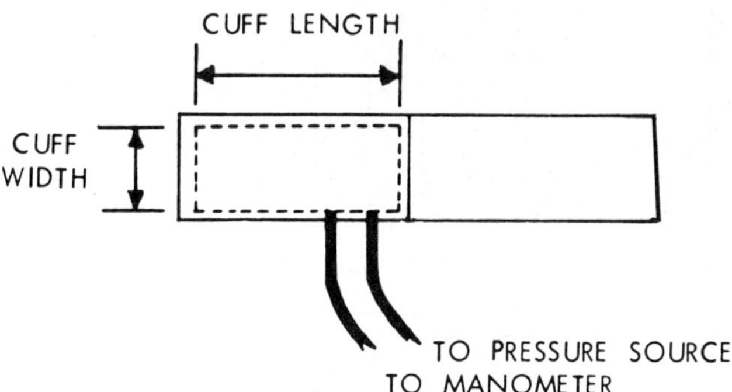

FIGURE 3.2. The blood-pressure cuff.

TABLE 3.1. Cuff Sizes Available

Cuff Designation	Width, W (cm)	Length, L (cm)	Aspect Ratio (L/W)
Newborn	2.3	6.0	2.6
	2.5	5.0	2.0
	3.0	6.8	2.3
	3.5	10.5	3.0
	3.7	7.6	2.1
Infant	4.5	11.5	2.6
	5.6	11.6	2.1
Child	8.3	15.7	1.9
	9.4	21.3	2.3
Adult	11.9	21.9	1.8
	12.4	25.9	2.1
Large adult	15.2	32.1	2.1
	15.5	31.3	2.0
Thigh	18.0	36.0	2.0
	18.6	40.2	2.2

TABLE 3.2. The Indirect Methods of Measuring Blood Pressure and the Pressures That They Measure

Method	Systolic	Mean	Diastolic
Palpatory	Yes	No	No
Oscillometric	Yes[a]	Yes	Yes[a]
Auscultatory	Yes	No	Yes
Ultrasonic (A)	Yes	No	Yes
Ultrasonic (B)	Yes	No	No
Flush	Yes	No	No

[a] Derived.

detected, and the mercury manometer reading is taken as systolic pressure. Cuff pressure is then quickly reduced to zero. For higher accuracy, the technique is repeated by inflating the cuff and noting the cuff pressure where the radial pulse disappears. Then the cuff pressure is reduced and the cuff pressure for reappearance of the pulse is noted. Systolic pressure can be taken as the average of the disappearance and reappearance pressures.

When the correct size cuff is used, the palpatory method underestimates systolic pressure by about 5–10 mm Hg. Figure 3.3*b* documents the method by showing a record of cuff pressure and the distal pulse. The palpatory method does not provide values for mean or diastolic pressure.

The Oscillometric Method

With the oscillometric method, the amplitude of oscillations that appears on the cuff-pressure indicator is used to identify transitions as cuff pressure passes systolic and mean pressures. Because the amplitude of cuff-pressure oscillations is so small, it is necessary to employ some form of amplification to allow witnessing their change in amplitude as cuff pressure is reduced.

Cuff pressure is raised quickly to well above systolic pressure; this point can be identified by noting the disappearance of the radial pulse. With suprasystolic pressure in the cuff, the underlying artery is completely occluded throughout the cardiac cycle. However, under the upper edge of the cuff, the artery pulsates with blood pressure. This pulsation is communicated to the upper edge of the cuff via the intervening tissues, and small-amplitude oscillations appear on the cuff-pressure indicator. Cuff pressure is reduced slowly (e.g., 3 mm Hg per beat), and when it is just below systolic pressure, a spurt of blood flows in the artery under the

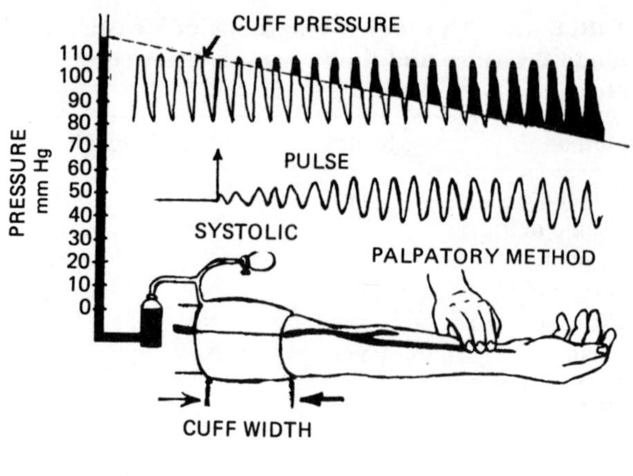

(a)

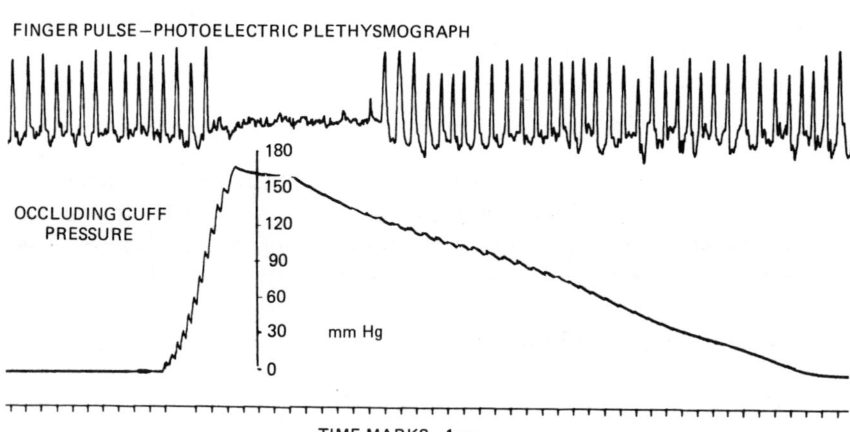

(b)

FIGURE 3.3. The palpatory method.

cuff and the cuff-pressure oscillations become larger, as shown by *S* in Figure 3.4*a*. This transition from small-amplitude oscillations (above systolic pressure) to increasing amplitude is a criterion for reading cuff pressure to obtain a pressure slightly above systolic pressure. With continued deflation of the cuff, the oscillations increase, reach a maximum, and then decrease as shown in Figure 3.4*b*. The point of maximum oscillations (*M*) in cuff pressure is very close to true mean arterial pressure. There is no indication for the instant when cuff pressure passes diastolic pressure.

The oscillometric method provides a good value for mean arterial pressures. That the point of maximal oscillations is expected to reflect mean

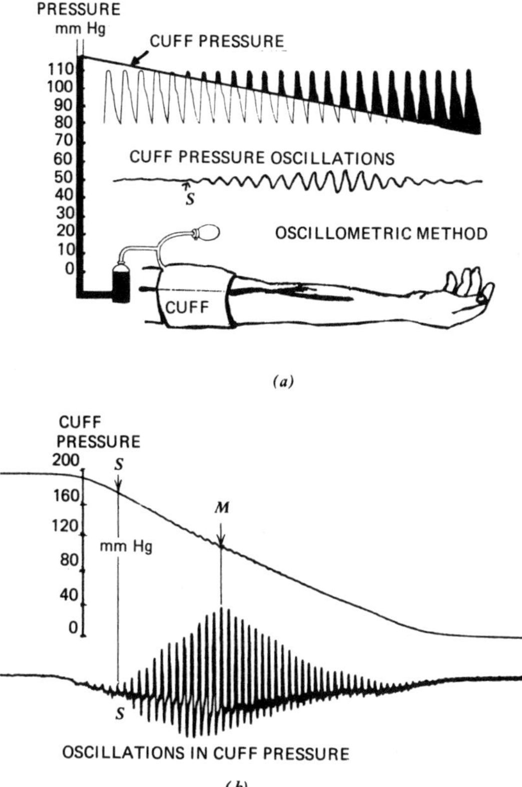

FIGURE 3.4. The oscillometric method.

arterial pressure was shown by Posey et al. (1969) in studies which used an exteriorized artery in a compression chamber. Blood from a dog flowed through the artery during these studies. Mauck et al. (1980) reported theoretical and experimental studies that support the mean pressure endpoint. It is, however, possible to derive values for systolic and diastolic pressures, as will be described.

There are commercially available electronic instruments that identify the point of maximal oscillation in cuff pressure and present this value on a digital indicator. Verification studies for mean blood pressure carried out to date in the human by Ramsey (1979) and Yelderman and Ream (1979) indicate that there is a high correlation between indirectly and directly measured mean blood pressure. Figure 3.5 presents the data obtained by Ramsey (1979). A similar study was reported by Kimble et al. (1981) who compared indirect mean (Dynamap) arterial pressure with

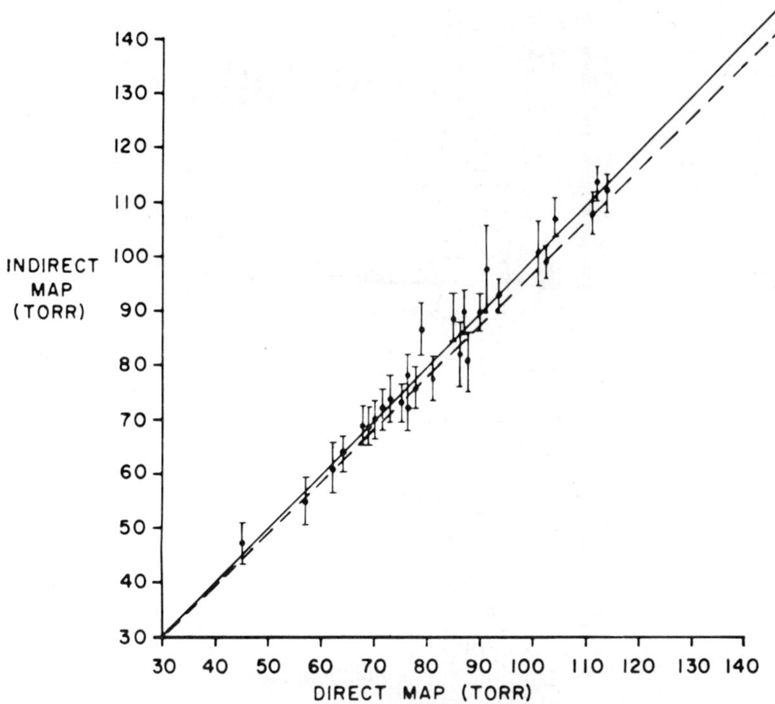

FIGURE 3.5. Indirect mean arterial pressure (MAP) versus direct mean arterial pressure in human subjects obtained using the oscillometric method. The solid line is a line of equal values and the dashed line is the regression line IND = 0.822 DIR + 7.48. The correlation coefficient is 0.98. The vertical lines represent ± 1SD. [From Ramsey, M. (1979) *Med. Biol. Eng. & Comput.*, **17**, 11–18, by permission.]

direct umbilical artery mean pressure in 17 newborn infants ranging in weight from 700 to 3600 g. The ratio of cuff width to arm circumference was between 0.45 and 0.70. The indirect (IND) mean pressure was related to the direct mean pressure (DIR) by the relationship IND = 0.822 DIR + 7.48, with a correlation coefficient of 0.853. The pressure range over which data were acquired was 20–65 mm Hg (mean).

There are also oscillometric instruments that indicate systolic, mean, and diastolic pressure. The systolic criterion will be discussed subsequently. That diastolic pressure is indicated may be surprising in view of the fact that there is no obvious transition in the oscillation amplitude as cuff pressure passes diastolic pressure. The manner by which diastolic pressure is identified requires an explanation.

During cuff deflation, the sudden increase in cuff-pressure oscillations is slightly above systolic pressure, and the point of maximal oscillations is the criterion for reading cuff pressure to obtain mean pressure. The sudden increase in cuff-pressure oscillations is slightly above systolic pressure in humans. In some oscillometric instruments another criterion is used for identifying systolic pressure; the criterion is the point where the oscillation amplitude attains a selected ratio of the maximum oscillation amplitude, usually about 50%.

Since there is no consistent transition in oscillation amplitude to identify diastolic pressure, some have selected cuff pressure when the oscillations attain a preselected ratio of the maximum amplitude, usually around 0.8.

To investigate potential systolic and diastolic criteria, the author (Geddes et al., 1983) carried out studies in adult human subjects using the auscultatory method as the reference. A standard (12-cm) cuff containing a tiny contact microphone within the bladder (Geddes et al., 1968) was applied to the upper arm of 23 subjects. Cuff pressure along with the Korotkoff sounds and amplified cuff-pressure oscillations were recorded. The auscultatory sounds were monitored aurally and the first (phase I) sound and the point of silence (phase V) were identified on the record to indicate systolic and diastolic pressure. Data were obtained at normal and elevated blood pressure produced by exercise, followed by isometric contraction of the leg muscles to maintain a high peripheral resistance.

Figure 3.6 illustrates a typical record and reveals several important features. For example, cuff pressure for systolic oscillometric pressure (S_o), as signaled by the sudden increase in cuff-pressure oscillations, was consistently above cuff pressure using the first Korotkoff sound, which identifies auscultatory systolic pressure that is known to be slightly below intraarterial systolic pressure. At normal systolic pressure (120 mm Hg), the oscillometric criterion overestimated systolic pressure by 8%.

In the same subjects, the amplitude of cuff-pressure oscillations (A_s) corresponding to auscultatory systolic pressure was measured and expressed as a ratio of the maximum amplitude (A_m), which occurs at mean pressure. For 23 subjects, the ratio A_s/A_m decreased from 0.57 to 0.45 over the systolic pressure range of 100 to 190 mm Hg. At normal systolic pressure (120 mm Hg), the ratio was 0.55.

The oscillation amplitude (A_d) corresponding to auscultatory diastolic pressure was measured and expressed as a ratio of the maximum amplitude (A_m), which occurs at mean pressure. In the 23 subjects, the ratio A_d/A_m decreased from 0.82 to 0.74 over the diastolic pressure range of 55 to 115 mm Hg. At normal diastolic pressure (80 mm Hg), the ratio was 0.82.

There are commercially available instruments that use the oscil-

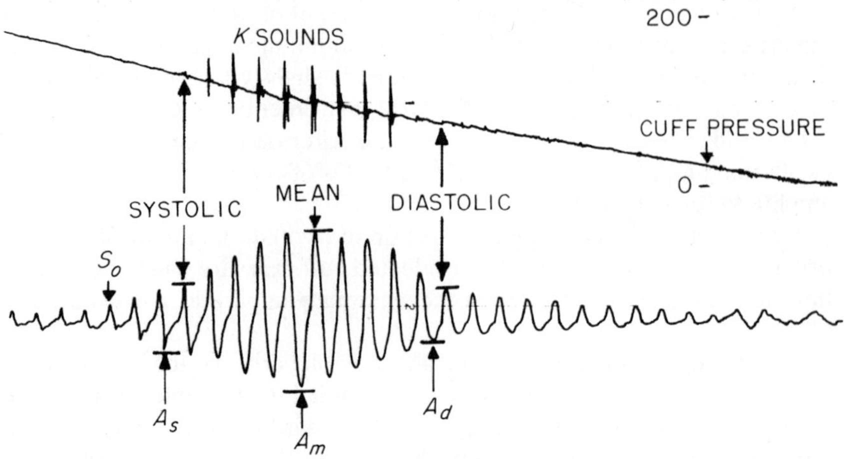

FIGURE 3.6. Cuff pressure with superimposed Korotkoff sounds and amplified cuff pressure oscillations. S_o is the point where cuff-pressure oscillations start to increase. A_s is the amplitude corresponding to auscultatory systolic pressure and A_d is the amplitude corresponding to auscultatory diastolic pressure. A_m is the maximum oscillation amplitude, which signals mean pressure.

lometric method to indicate systolic and diastolic pressure. The criteria used to identify these pressures are considered proprietary. Nonetheless, most manufacturers have carried out verification studies to their own satisfaction.

Verification of the algorithms used in the Dinamap (Critikon, Tampa, Florida), were reported by Friesen and Lichter (1981) who compared systolic and diastolic oscillometric pressures with direct arterial pressures (radial, brachial, and umbilical) in premature infants, neonates, and term babies. Cuff width was chosen on the basis of arm circumference. For systolic pressure, the relationship was IND = 0.94DIR + 3.53, where IND is the DINAMAP reading and DIR is the direct pressure. For diastolic pressure IND = 0.98DIR + 1.70. These results indicate an excellent agreement between indirect and direct pressures in a patient population in which it is difficult to obtain indirect blood pressure.

One of the considerable advantages of the oscillometric method is that only one device (the cuff) need be applied to the subject. Another advantage is that it can be used on animals (Geddes et al., 1977, 1980 and Latshaw et al., 1979) and children and infants in whom the auscultatory method usually fails. It can also be used successfully in situation of low blood pressure (hypotension).

The Auscultatory Method

Auscultation refers to listening to sounds that occur within the body. The auscultatory method employs the sounds produced by blood flowing in an artery being relieved of compression to indicate the instant when cuff pressure should be read to obtain systolic and diastolic pressures. The arterial sounds are called the Korotkoff sounds in honor of the Russian physician who first proposed the method in 1905.

To obtain systolic and diastolic pressure with the auscultatory method, the brachial artery is located just beyond the cuff and the receiver of a stethoscope is placed over this point (Figure 3.7). Cuff pressure is raised quickly to a point well above the suspected systolic pressure. Cuff pressure is then reduced slowly (e.g., 3 mm Hg per beat) while the observer listens to the sequence of arterial sounds that evolves. As cuff pressure falls below systolic pressure, a spurt of blood passes under the cuff and a sound is heard in the stethoscope, directing the operator to read cuff pressure to identify systolic pressure. As cuff pressure continues to fall, the sounds become louder, then softer, then very loud, acquiring a thumping character, after which they suddenly become muffled and usually disappear. This orderly sequence of sounds has been divided into five phases (Figure 3.8) for descriptive purposes. Systolic pressure is read at the point of appearance of sound (phase I). Most clinicians take the point of disappearance of sound (phase V) as diastolic pressure. However, because in some persons the sounds persist all the way to zero cuff pressure, it has been recommended that phase IV, the point of muffling (which appears in all subjects), be accepted as the diastolic criterion. Ordinarily, the cuff pressure difference between phases IV and V is small (Figure 3.8). Many clinicians use phase IV if the sounds persist to an abnormally low pressure. Some list phases IV and V pressures for diastolic, thereby aiding future observers. Over the years, various AHA committees have recommended phase IV or V, and there still appears to be disagreement. Surely listing the pressures for all three phases would diminish the controversy. Thus blood pressure would be designated by three numbers corresponding to appearance/muffling-silence.

For the correct cuff size, in relation to the member to which it is applied, the accuracy of systolic pressure is fairly well established. Indirect systolic pressure is, on the average, about 4 mm Hg below arterial systolic pressure. Diastolic pressure correlations are not so well established. Using phase IV (muffling), indirect diastolic pressure is about 4–8 mm Hg above arterial diastolic pressure. If phase V (silence) is used, indirect diastolic pressure is often closer to arterial diastolic pressure.

The auscultatory method is the standard in adult clinical medicine. The

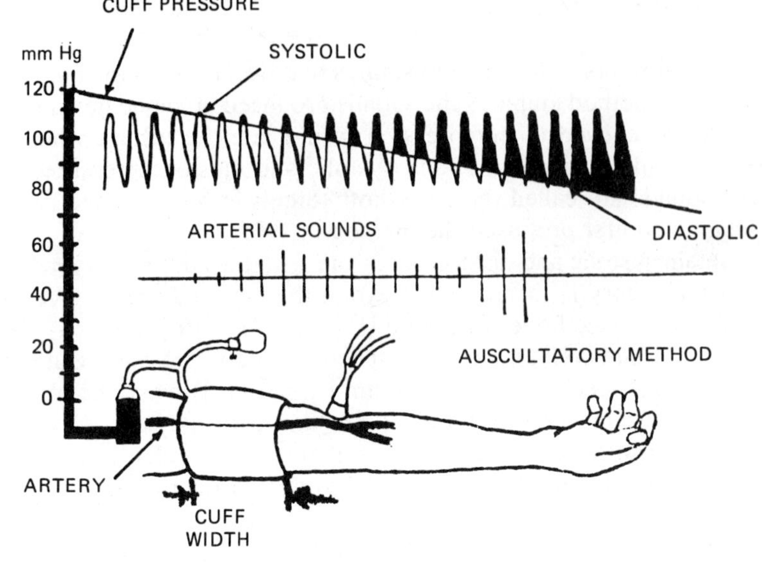

(a)

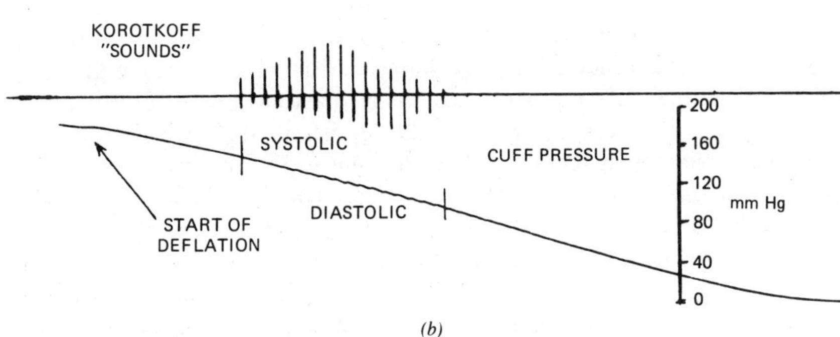

(b)

FIGURE 3.7. The auscultatory method.

method often fails in small children because the frequency spectrum of the arterial sounds is below that for human audition. For the same reason it fails in adult subjects with low blood pressure. It usually fails when applied to most animals because the arterial sounds cannot be heard consistently.

The Ultrasonic Method

Ultrasound is used in two ways to measure blood pressure indirectly. With one method, arterial-wall motion is sensed and with the other

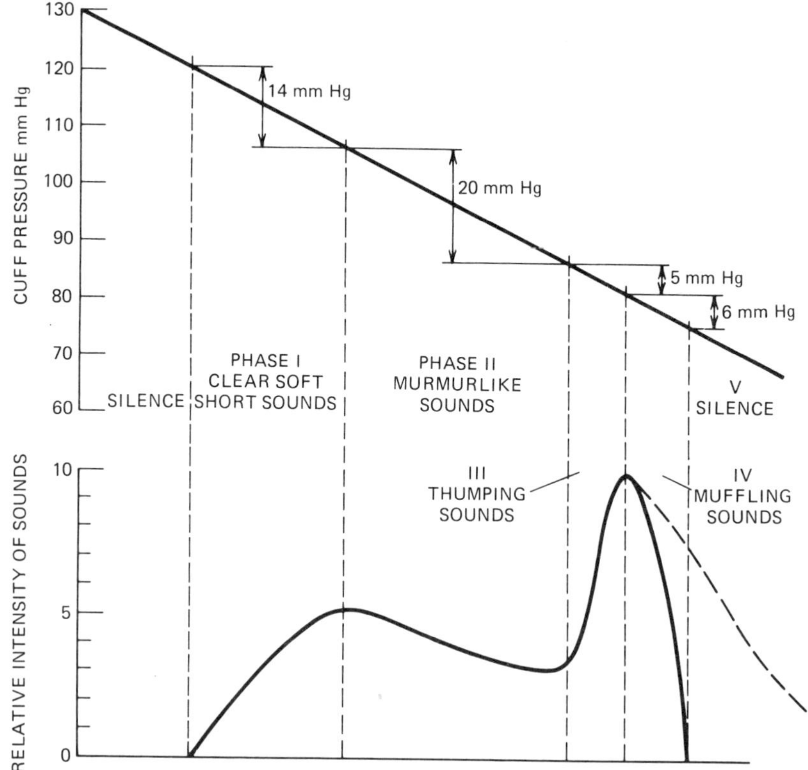

FIGURE 3.8. The sound phases of the auscultatory method.

method, blood flow is measured using the transcutaneous Doppler blood flowmeter. Both methods employ the standard member-encircling air-inflated cuff.

Because the walls of the artery beneath an occluding cuff experience a characteristic motion during cuff deflation, Ware and Laenger (1967) showed that it is possible using ultrasound to identify these movements. The principle is implemented with two small piezoelectric elements: one emits ultrasound and the other detects the ultrasonic echo reflected from the underlying artery. Both piezoelectric elements are placed on the member beneath the cuff and are coupled to the skin acoustically with a light oil.

With the ultrasonic-detection method, vessel-wall velocity is used to characterize the events during cuff deflation. There are characteristic transitions in the ultrasonic signal as cuff pressure passes systolic and

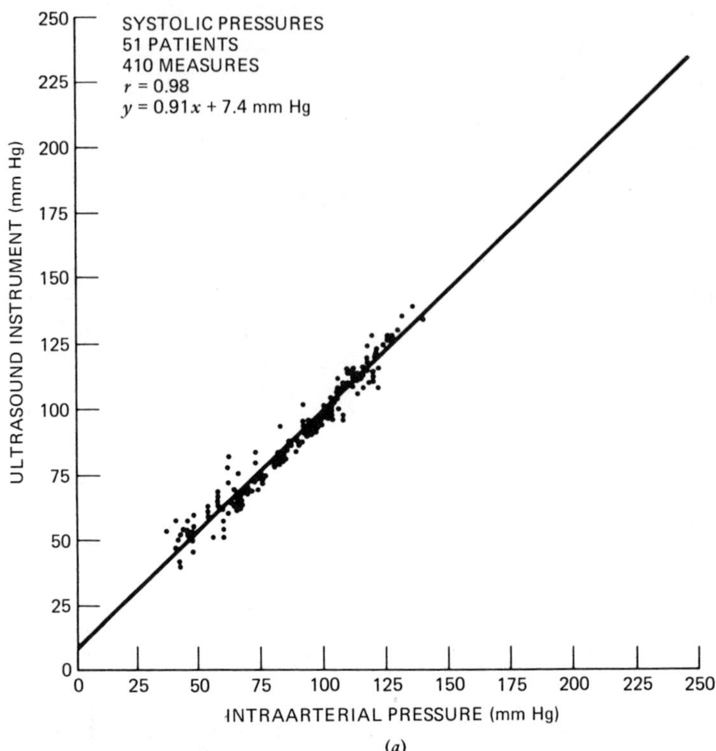

FIGURE 3.9a. (*a*) Systolic pressures obtained with the ultrasound instrument were compared to intraarterial pressures in 51 patients. The 410 comparisons ranged from 40 to 140 mm Hg and showed a correlation coefficient of 0.98. The equation of the regression line is $y = 0.91x + 7.4$ mm Hg.

diastolic pressure. In comparative tests, the ultrasonically derived pressures are close to those obtained with the auscultatory method. Excellent reviews of the technique were reported by Hochberg et al. (1971). Figure 3.9 presents correlation data obtained on human subjects and reported by Hochberg et al. (1971). It is clear that the ultrasonic method provides values for systolic and diastolic pressures that are close to intraarterial values.

With the other ultrasonic method, the Doppler blood-flow transducer is placed on the skin over an artery distal to the cuff. A light acoustic coupling oil is employed. When the artery is open, the familiar pulsatile Doppler flow signal is heard or recorded graphically. When the artery is occluded by the cuff, the flow signal disappears. During cuff deflation, the first appearance of flow is the signal to read cuff pressure to identify systolic pressure.

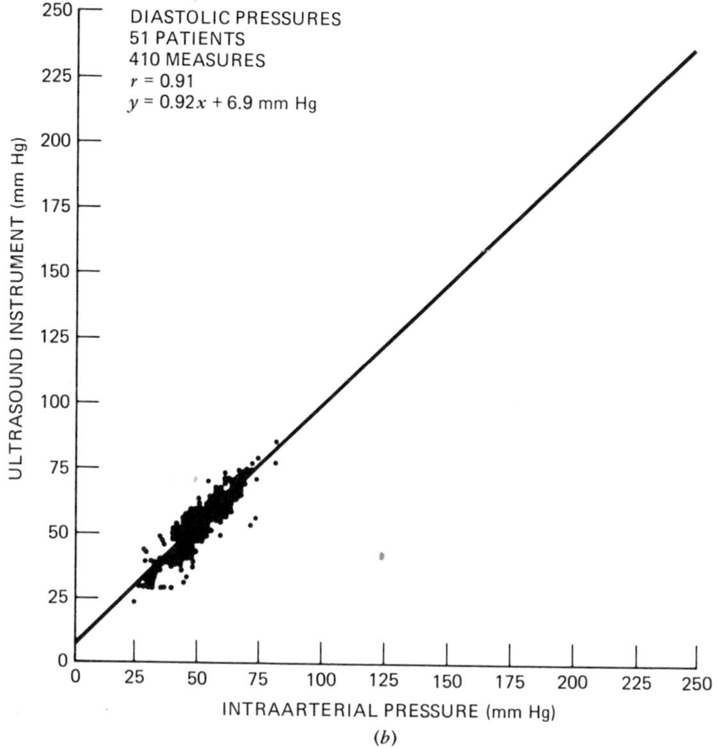

FIGURE 3.9b. (*b*) Diastolic pressures obtained with the ultrasound instrument (BPI) were compared to intraarterial pressures in 51 patients. The 410 comparisons ranged from 25 to 87 mm Hg and showed a correlation coefficient of 0.91. The equation of the regression line is $y = 0.92x + 6.9$ mm Hg. [Redrawn from Hochberg et al. (1971).]

The Flush Method

With the flush method, an elastic bandage and the conventional member-encircling cuff are used to determine systolic pressure. The technique consists of tightly wrapping a member with an elastic bandage, starting from the tip of the extremity and progressing to the trunk. This procedure squeezes all of the blood out of the member. Then the cuff is applied just above the trunk end of the elastic bandage and inflated to a high pressure to prevent blood from entering the member. Then the bandage is removed. The opposite member is then placed beside the blanched member; both are examined in a bright light. Cuff pressure is then reduced slowly, and as it passes systolic pressure, blood enters the member and it flushes red. Cuff pressure is read as systolic at this instant. Usually the subject feels a sensation of heat at the same time. There is no indication for the instant when cuff pressure passes mean or diastolic pressures.

Although the flush method is cumbersome to apply, it is often the only technique that can be used when all others fail. The flush method sees most service in pediatrics.

Summary

To summarize, with the known end points, there is no single indirect method for measuring all three blood pressures. None of the indirect cuff-based methods allows continuous measurement of any arterial pressure. With all methods, the accuracy attainable depends on use of the correct cuff size in relation to the member to which it is applied. This subject will be discussed subsequently; however, at present, the recommended cuff width for man is about 40% of the member circumference. The characteristics of the three most popular methods—the auscultatory, the oscillometric, and the palpatory—are summarized in Figure 3.10. To make this record, cuff pressure, its amplified oscillations, the Korotkoff sounds, and the distal pulse were recorded simultaneously. Cuff pressure was raised quickly to 190 mm Hg and reduced to zero slowly. Note that the amplitude of cuff-pressure oscillations increased at 164 mm Hg, just above the appearance of the first Korotkoff sound at 157 mm Hg. Very slightly below this cuff pressure, the radial pulse appeared. With continued deflation of the cuff, the Korotkoff sounds changed slightly in character. The amplitude of the oscillations in cuff pressure increased, reached a maximum, then decreased. The point of maximal oscillations (108 mm Hg) is close to estimated mean arterial pressure for this subject. As cuff pressure continued to fall, the Korotkoff sounds disappeared at 92 mm Hg, indicating diastolic pressure. There are no transitions in cuff-pressure oscillations or in the radial pulse pressure to indicate diastolic pressure.

Cuff Size

Mention was made earlier about the importance of using a cuff having dimensions that are appropriate for the member to which it is applied. At present there is a standard series of cuff sizes designed to accommodate the arms and legs of adults and children. Table 3.1 provides a listing of the sizes that are presently available. Note that the aspect ratio (length-to-width) of the bladders is in the vicinity of 2. The width of the bladder is the dimension that is used to describe cuff size and is that dimension measured along the member (see Figure 3.2). Some advocate the use of a longer bladder to distribute the cuff pressure more evenly.

It is well known clinically that it is necessary to use the correct cuff

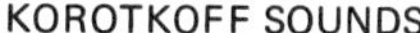

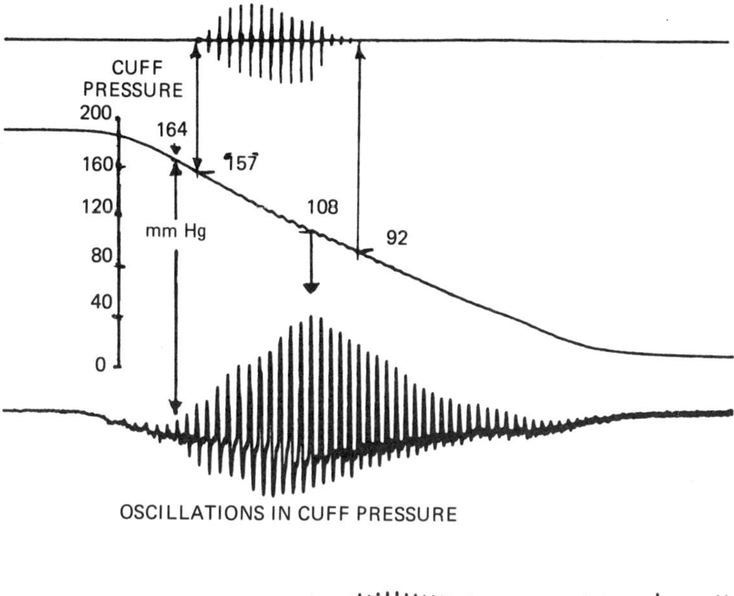

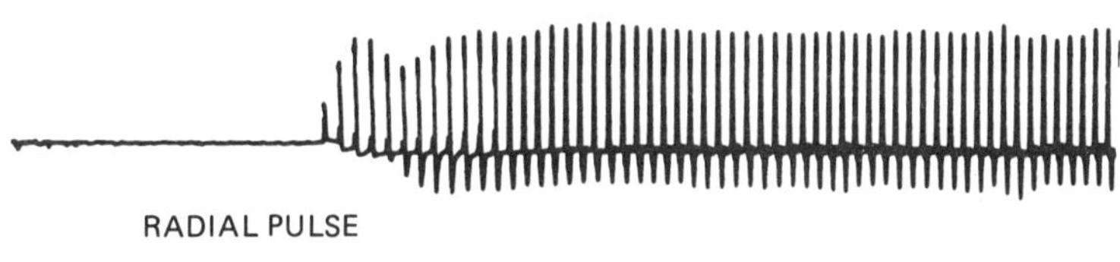

FIGURE 3.10. The auscultatory, oscillometric, and palpatory methods of measuring blood pressure indirectly.

width to obtain reliable blood-pressure readings. The American Heart Association recommends a cuff width that is 1.2 times the diameter of the member to which it is applied. Because the diameter of a member is difficult to measure, this recommendation can be restated as cuff width should be $1.2/\pi$ or about 40% of the member circumference. It is well known clinically that use of a cuff that is too narrow provides values for systolic, mean, and diastolic pressures that are falsely high. The use of a cuff that is too wide provides values for indirect pressure that are slightly low; although no explanation exists for the latter nor is there agreement on this point. For example, Burch and DePasquale (1962), Kirkendal et al. (1967), Park et al. (1976), Geddes and Whistler (1978), and Kimble et al. (1981) have shown that a cuff that is too wide gives slightly low values for blood pressure in humans. Conversely, Alexander et al. (1977), using a static elastic model for the arm, reported that a cuff that is too wide does not provide falsely low values for indirect blood pressure. It is for the future to resolve this issue.

Conclusions

Since all of the occlusive methods just described employ a member-encircling arterial-occluding cuff, there is perhaps no better way to conclude this section than to provide guidelines for those who plan to use the cuff method. The following recommendations, drawn from the author's experience, should alert the user to several important features of the indirect measurement of blood pressure.

1. Use the correct size cuff which, for a human, has a width equal to 40% of the member circumference. The use of a cuff that is narrow gives falsely high values for systolic, diastolic, and mean pressures. The use of a cuff that is too wide gives slightly low values.
2. Use a cuff with two tubes, one for inflating and deflating the cuff and the other for measurement of pressure in the cuff. The use of a cuff with one tube invites error due to the pressure drop along the tube. The indicated pressure will be lower than the cuff pressure by virtue of the flow-dependent pressure drop along the tube. If cuff pressure is lowered incrementally, and the pressure is measured when there is no flow in the tube, this source of error is removed. This practice is not recommended if the cuff is deflated very slowly.
3. Apply the cuff snugly. A cuff that is applied loosely will give slightly high values for indirect blood pressure. Do not apply the cuff over clothing.
4. Place the arm so that the cuff is at heart level. A vertical difference of 5.5 in. is equivalent to a 10 mm Hg difference in pressure. If the cuff is above heart level, the measured pressure is lower, if below the heart level, the measured pressure is higher.
5. Inflate the cuff quickly to the point of disappearance of the distal pulse. Then deflate the cuff quickly. This maneuver seats the cuff on the member and allows more even transmission of the pressure to the member. Failure to seat the cuff usually results in a falsely high first measurement of indirect pressure.
6. Inflate the cuff quickly and deflate it slowly at a rate of about 3 mm Hg per heart beat. Indirect blood pressure measurement is a

sampling technique, and a rate of deflation that is based on time will provide poorer resolution with low heart rates.

7. Be sure that the underlying muscles are relaxed. If the muscles are not relaxed, a higher cuff pressure will be needed to occlude the underlying artery and the indirect pressures will be falsely high.
8. With the auscultatory method, systolic pressure is read at the first appearance of the Korotkoff sounds. Diastolic pressure is read in two ways: at the point of muffling and at the instant of the expected occurrence of a sound after the last Korotkoff sound. Three numbers should be used to identify blood pressure, that is, cuff pressure for appearance/muffling—silence. In practice the point of silence is usually taken as diastolic pressure. Listing both diastolic criteria avoids misinforming a subsequent observer about the diastolic pressure.
9. Do not reinflate the cuff during deflation to obtain a better reading for systolic and diastolic pressure. Reinflation causes congestion in the arm distal to the cuff and alters the sounds and may produce an auscultatory gap.
10. During cuff deflation with the auscultatory method, the sounds sometimes appear, disappear, reappear, and disappear. The cuff pressure between the first disappearance and reappearance is called the auscultatory gap, the cause of which is unknown. The auscultatory gap can often be eliminated by raising the arm above the head (with the cuff deflated) to drain the arm venous reservoir. The cuff can then be inflated to above suspected systolic pressure and the arm is lowered. When cuff pressure is reduced slowly, the auscultatory gap is usually eliminated. This technique may be used to enhance the Korotkoff sounds if they are very faint.
11. Be aware of the fact that blood pressure is not a fixed quantity; there are normal respiratory variations, as well as emotionally induced changes. Moreover, in some pathological states there can be very low frequency (a few per minute) vasomotor variations. Respiratory variations amount from a few to more than 10 mm Hg, depending on the type of breathing. Slow deep breathing produces large-amplitude variations, shallow rapid breathing produces much smaller variations in blood pressure. If the heart rate is not constant, systolic and diastolic pressure will not be constant. There is a small variation in heart rate with respiration in normal subjects, this is called sinus arrhythmia. With an irregular ventricular rate, as in untreated atrial fibrillation, systolic and

diastolic pressure vary widely from beat to beat. Vasomotor (Traube–Hering) waves may be as large as the pulse pressure. In this situation the respiratory variations are superimposed on the slowly changing vasomotor waves. Emotionally induced changes in blood pressure can amount to more than 20 mm Hg. In fact, such changes are used in polygraphic examinations to identify stressful questions.

12. Take care of the equipment. Be sure that the mercury reservoir is filled and that the mercury and manometer tubing are clean. Check the calibration of aneroid-type gauges frequently with a mercury manometer.
13. Have a full range of cuff sizes for children, adults, and obese adults, and for the thigh and leg.

CONTINUOUS MEASUREMENT OF INDIRECT ARTERIAL PRESSURE

Cuff Method

In psychophysiological studies and in polygraphic examinations for the detection of deception, a continuous record of relative blood pressure is obtained. During interviews, which involve stressful questions (which are answered with a simple yes or no), blood pressure and heart rate usually increase. The technique employed to detect these changes is a variant of the oscillometric method described previously.

To record relative blood pressure changes, an arm cuff is inflated to a pressure that is usually near diastolic pressure, for example, 80 mm Hg. The pressure in the cuff is recorded continuously with a high-gain, suppressed-zero recording system. Thus, the recording pen indicates cuff-pressure oscillations riding on the cuff-pressure baseline. When the subject is stressed, blood pressure increases, thereby raising the cuff pressure slightly, which is displayed by a rise in the baseline of the recording (Figure 3.11a). The oscillations in cuff pressure decrease in amplitude because the rise in blood pressure has moved the point of maximal cuff-pressure oscillations away from cuff pressure. If, however, the cuff pressure had been set to a point just above that for maximum oscillations, an increase in blood pressure results in an increase in cuff-pressure oscillations (Figure 3.11*b*), as well as a rise in the baseline of the recording. This response (Geddes and Newberg, 1977) occurs because blood pressure has moved toward the cuff pressure for maximal oscillations. Thus, while

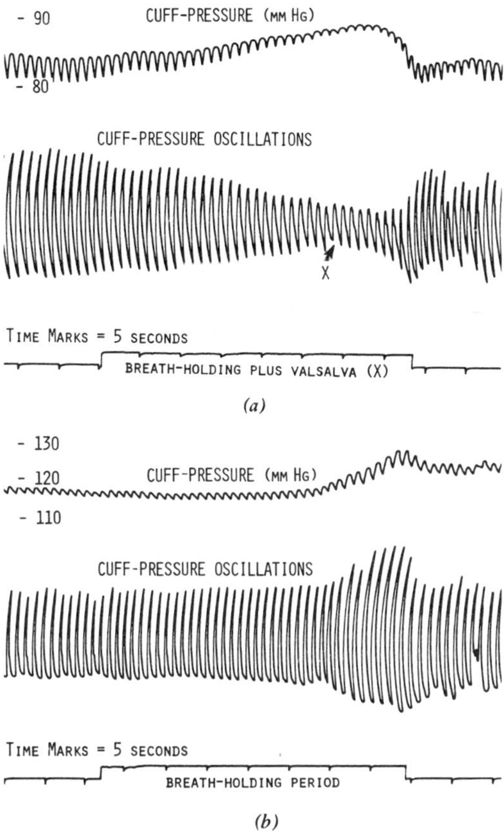

FIGURE 3.11. The "cardiac channel" record of relative blood pressure in polygraphic examination: (*a*) cuff pressure below mean arterial pressure; (*b*) cuff pressure above mean arterial pressure.

recording relative blood pressure with an inflated member-encircling cuff, an increase in blood pressure causes the baseline of the recorder to rise. Whether the amplitude of the oscillations decreases or increases depends on the initial setting of the cuff pressure. If it is set below the point for maximal oscillations, the oscillation amplitude will decrease. If cuff pressure is set just above the point of maximal oscillations in cuff pressure, an increase in blood pressure will cause a rise in the baseline and an increase in amplitude of the oscillations. These two distinctly different responses are shown in Figure 3.11. To date, it has not been shown that the rise in baseline cuff pressure is equal to the rise in diastolic or mean blood pressure. It is expected that the rise in cuff pressure may be somewhat less than the rise in blood pressure. Despite the lack of quantification, this

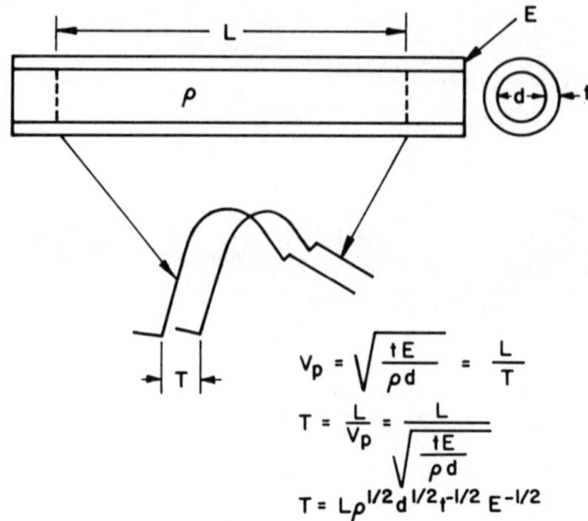

FIGURE 3.12. The propagation time (T) of a pulse along a tube depends on the diameter (d), thickness (t), and modulus of elasticity (E) of the tube. It also depends on the density of (ρ) of the fluid therein and the length (L) of the tube. V_p is pulse-wave velocity (L/T).

change is both reproducible and measurable. It should be obvious, however, that this method can be used for only short periods of time owing to the discomfort of a partially inflated cuff.

Pulse-Transit Time Method

It has long been known that the velocity of propagation of the pulse wave from the left ventricle to a peripheral artery is dependent on the dimensions and stiffness (modulus of elasticity) of the intervening vessels. Pulse-wave velocity is defined as the distance that the pulse wave travels in 1 sec. Pulse-wave velocity is determined by measuring the transit time between passage of the pressure pulse wave at two different sites along an artery. Figure 3.12 illlustrates the method.

The velocity of propagation of a pulse wave injected into a thin-walled elastic tube is given by the Moens–Korteweg equation:

$$V_p = \sqrt{\frac{tE}{\rho d}} = \frac{L}{T}$$

In this expression V_p is the pulse-wave velocity, t and d are the thickness and diameter of the tube, ρ is the density of the fluid within it, and E is the modulus of elasticity of the material from which the tube is made. The modulus of elasticity of a specimen of material is defined as the ratio of

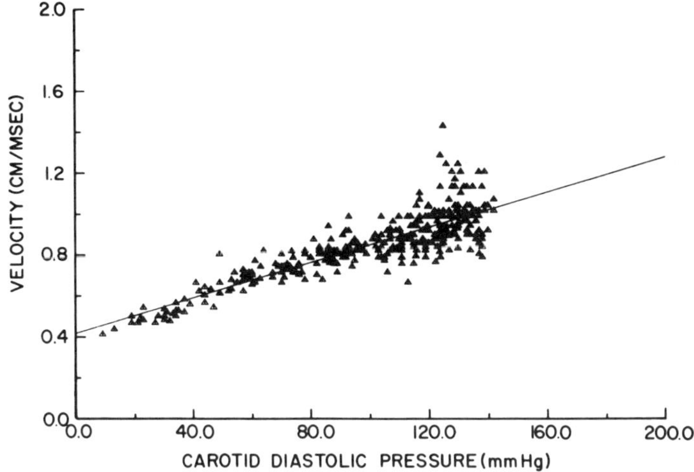

FIGURE 3.13. The relationship between pulse-wave velocity (V_p) and diastolic (D) pressure in the canine aorta, $V_p = 4.27 \times 10^{-3} D + 0.419$, with a correlation coefficient of 0.85. [From Geddes et al. (1981), by permission.]

stress (deforming force per unit area) to strain (extension per unit length). From the Moens–Korteweg equation it can be seen that the velocity of propagation will depend on pressure if any of the quantities (d, t, E) depend on pressure. The diameter d increases and the wall thickness t decreases with increasing pressure. Hughes et al. (1979) showed that the modulus of elasticity (E) increases exponentially with increasing pressure. The degree to which pulse-wave velocity varies with pressure depends on the way in which d, t, and E vary with pressure. In practice it is found that the increase in E is larger than the decrease in t and increase in d, with increasing pressure. Geddes et al. (1981) showed that the pulse-wave velocity in the dog aorta increased linearly with increasing pressure. Figure 3.13 illustrates this point.

In a practical situation, the measurement of pulse-wave velocity requires division of the distance between the two arterial pulse detectors (L) by the difference in time (T) between the start of the upstrokes of both pressure pulses (see Figure 3.12). The pulse-wave velocity obtained in this manner is the diastolic pulse-wave velocity. To use pulse-wave velocity as an indicator of change in arterial pressure, it is more convenient to measure the change in pulse-transit time, because the distance between the arterial pulse detectors remains constant. Since pulse-wave velocity increases linearly with blood pressure, and since velocity is distance divided by time, the pulse-transit time is inversely related to an increase in blood pressure. In other words, an increase in blood pressure will de-

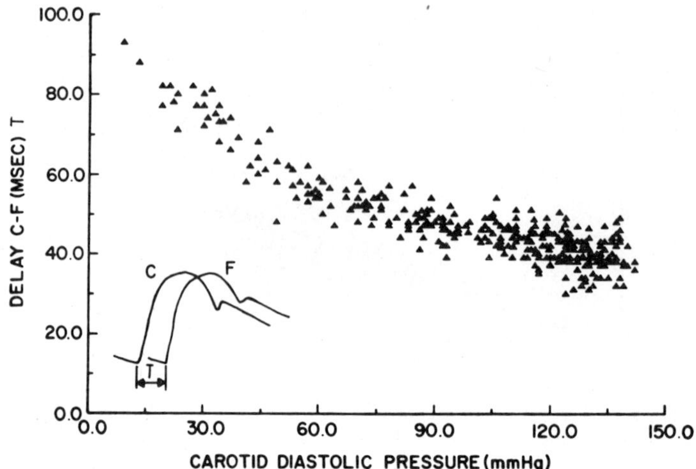

FIGURE 3.14. The relationship between pulse-transit time (τ) and carotid diastolic blood pressure [From Geddes et al.)1981), by permission.]

crease the pulse-transit time. Figure 3.14 illustrates the relationship between pulse-transit time and diastolic pressure.

Measurement of Pulse-Transit Time

As shown previously, pulse-transit time decreases with an increase in blood pressure. Therefore, to use this physical phenomenon optimally, it is necessary to employ two arterial pulse detectors. Many different arterial pulse pickups have been developed [see review by Geddes and Baker (1975)]. The most popular pulse detector employs a piezoelectric element, which is applied directly to the skin above an artery. Despite the high efficiency of the piezoelectric and other force transducers, there is often difficulty in coupling them to detect the pulse in a superficial artery. Even when well applied, it is often difficult to have them remain in place for a prolonged period. A simple solution employs a small, partially inflated bladder applied to a member, with the pressure pulses within it displayed graphically. Such a technique can be used to detect the brachial, radial, and dorsal pedis artery pulses by using bladders of a convenient size applied to the skin over the artery with masking tape.

It is sometimes expedient to use the *R* wave of the electrocardiogram (ECG) as a timing signal for pulse-transit-time measurements. Figure 3.15 illustrates the relationship between the *R* wave and the aortic and radial artery pulses. Note that the apex of the *R* wave occurs well before ven-

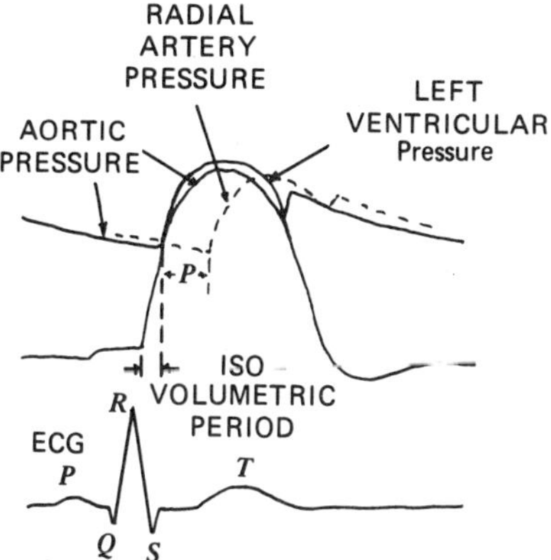

FIGURE 3.15. Aortic, left ventricular, and radial artery pressure in relation to the ECG. *P* is the pulse-transit time from the aortic valve to the radial artery.

tricular rejection, which is preceded by the period of isovolumetric contraction.

The author conducted a series of pulse-transit-time studies in dogs to examine the validity of using the *R* wave of the ECG as a timing reference. Figure 3.16 presents the relationship between *R*-carotid pulse-transit time and diastolic pressure. Figure 3.17 presents the relationship between *R*-femoral pulse-transit time and carotid diastolic pressure and Figure 3.14 presents the true carotid–femoral pulse-transit time and carotid diastolic pressure in the same animal. The poorest correlation between transit time and pressure was obtained with the *R*-carotid measurement. A better correlation was found with the *R*-femoral transit time, and the best correlation was found between the true pulse-transit time (carotid–femoral) and carotid diastolic pressure (Figure 3.14). As predicted by the Moens–Korteweg equation and by the manner in which its components vary with pressure, an increase in blood pressure produces a decrease in pulse-transit time.

The relationship between pulse-wave velocity and calculated mean arterial pressure in human subjects was investigated by Gribbin et al. (1976). Pulse pickups were placed over the brachial and radial arteries and the pulse-transit time was measured. In order to vary the effective blood pressure, the arm was placed in a box to which negative and positive air pressure could be applied. With this technique the arterial distending pressure could be changed ±80 mm Hg. At each pressure level the pulse-wave velocity was measured, and it was demonstrated that pulse-wave velocity increases with an increase in the calculated mean arterial pressure.

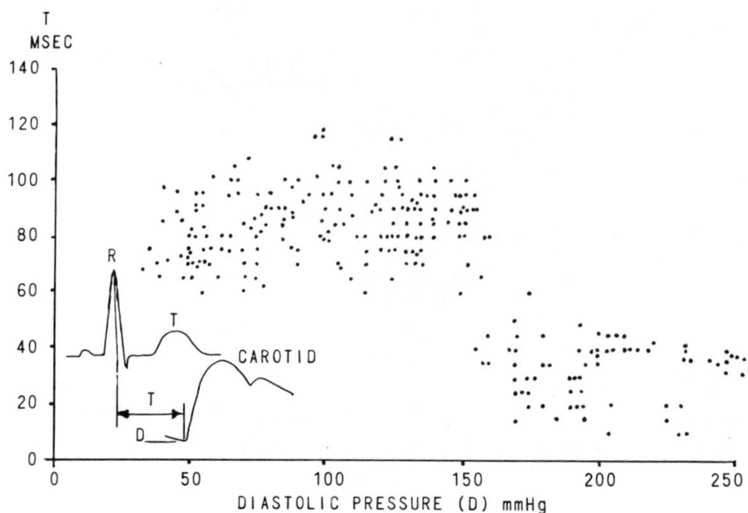

FIGURE 3.16. The relationship between the delay (T) between the R wave of the ECG and the onset of the carotid pulse versus carotid diastolic pressure in the dog. [From Geddes et al. (1981), by permission.]

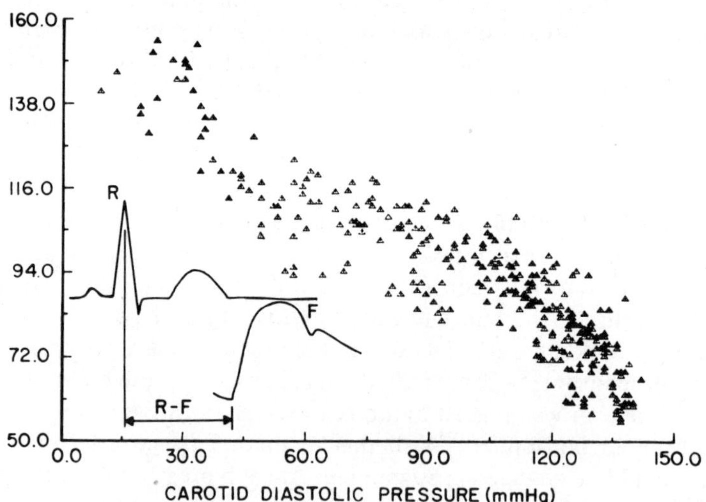

FIGURE 3.17. The relationship between the R wave of the ECG and the onset of the femoral pulse and carotid diastolic pressure in the dog. [From Geddes et al. (1981), by permission.]

The decrease in pulse-transit time, as measured between the *R* wave of the ECG and the onset of the radial pulse, was measured as a function of blood pressure in humans by Steptoe et al. (1976). Arterial pressure was changed by physiologic and pharmacologic maneuvers. It was found that an increase in mean arterial pressure reduced the transit time as measured from the *R* wave of the ECG to the radial pulse. The data obtained on all subjects were similar, except when amyl nitrite was administered to lower the blood pressure. This drug shortens the duration of the isovolumetric period, while a reduction in blood pressure decreases pulse-wave velocity and thus prolongs the pulse-transit time. Therefore, caution must be exercised in interpreting transit-time changes when the *R* wave of the ECG is used as a substitute for a pulse detector.

There is some controversy over which of the three blood pressures (diastolic, mean, or systolic) is tracked by pulse-transit time. From the theory of pulse propagation in elastic tubes, the pulse is propagated by its introduction at the prevailing (i.e., diastolic) pressure. However, as the literature shows, pulse-transit time has been correlated with changes in all three pressures.

AUTOMATED MEASUREMENT OF INDIRECT BLOOD PRESSURE

For mass screening and for home use, many automated and semiautomated indirect blood-pressure-measuring devices have been developed and are now available in retail stores. Each employs one of the principles described in this chapter. However, it is important to recognize that virtually all of the epidemiological data on blood pressure have been acquired with the auscultatory method. It is for this reason that the performance of a device should be compared with data obtained with the auscultatory, as well as with direct measurements.

Many of the automated and semiautomated devices employ the auscultatory method. Usually, a small contact microphone is incorporated into the lower third of the cuff to detect the Korotkoff sounds. The ultrasonic method, which detects the vessel-wall movements, is also popular. One instrument employs the oscillometric method and indicates systolic, mean, and diastolic pressure, along with heart rate. The accuracy of these devices depends on the built-in criteria used to identify the three pressures. In other words, with the auscultatory method, although phase I is used for systolic pressure, phase IV or V may be used for diastolic pressure in different instruments. Likewise, with the ultrasonic method, although the systolic point is easily identified, the diastolic point can be made to correspond to Phase IV or V of the auscultatory method. With the oscillometric method, the sudden increase in pulse amplitude or a ratio of oscillation amplitude can be used for systolic pressure; the point of maximal oscillations is used to identify mean pressure. However, the endpoint for diastolic pressure is not universally accepted. Often cuff pressure for a specified amplitude of oscillations, in relation to the maximum amplitude, is used.

Several important points should be noted about automatic and semiautomatic devices for measuring blood pressure indirectly. The Task Force on High Blood Pressure of the National Institutes of Health (Bethesda, MD) issued a report (1974) on such devices. The report called attention to the widely differing uses (e.g., mass screening or home use) for such devices. For example, if mass screening is desired, the number of measurements per hour (throughput) is a consideration, with less emphasis on cost. If home use is the goal, the cost becomes a primary consideration, with less concern over the time taken to make a measurement. If field screening is the goal, the throughput rate and portability are important considerations, with less emphasis on cost.

The Task Force recognized that there were more than 20 manufacturers of automated and semiautomated devices at that time (1974). The report tabulated the performance data provided by these manufacturers, listing the major operating and performance characteristics. The data contained in the report's tables are both voluminous and useful for those contemplating routine use of such devices.

Studies are underway on the accuracy of the many automated and semiautomated devices. Some studies make comparisons with direct blood pressure; others use the auscultatory method as a reference. Informative as these studies will be, the single most important feature about an instrument is that the reading that it provides is based on an electronically specified and implemented algorithm; that is, the detector, whatever it is, is instrumented to read the same thing every time a measurement is made. Therefore, with a well-designed and constructed instrument, a high precision (i.e., reproducibility) is expected. It should be remembered that a high precision is not necessarily synonymous with high accuracy, which is the condition for the measurement to be very close to the true value. A device that has high precision can be useful for indicating changes, although it may provide an error in its reading.

Finally, the issue of cuff width should be kept in mind. Screening devices which use the same size cuff for large and small arms will produce erroneous data, in proportion to the inappropriateness of a cuff width for the arm.

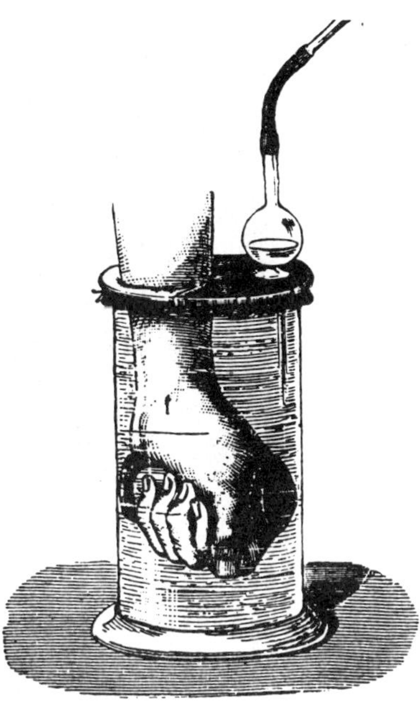

FIGURE 3.18. Marey's experiment in which hydraulic counterpressure applied to the hand forced blood out of the hand and thereby demonstrated the concept of counterpressure to measure blood pressure indirectly.

HISTORICAL POSTSCRIPT

In the early 1800s many attempts were made to measure blood pressure indirectly by placing weights on the skin over a superficial artery. The goal was to determine the force that would occlude the artery and thereby cause the pulse to disappear distally. The first demonstration that a counterpressure could be used to determine blood pressure was presented by Marey around 1876. His experiment consisted of placing a hand and forearm in a water-filled chamber to which pressure could be applied with a suitable seal around the forearm, as shown in Figure 3.18. Marey noted that during pressurization, the hand and forearm blanched. Obviously the counterpressure exceeded arterial systolic pressure. Very likely Marey noted oscillations on the manometer used to indicate the counterpressure and in one of his subsequent studies placed the hand and forearm in the cylindrical water-filled metal chamber with a viewing window, as shown in Figure 3.19. The fluid pressure surrounding the arm was increased by raising a water-filled reservoir. The pressure in the chamber was recorded on a kymograph as shown.

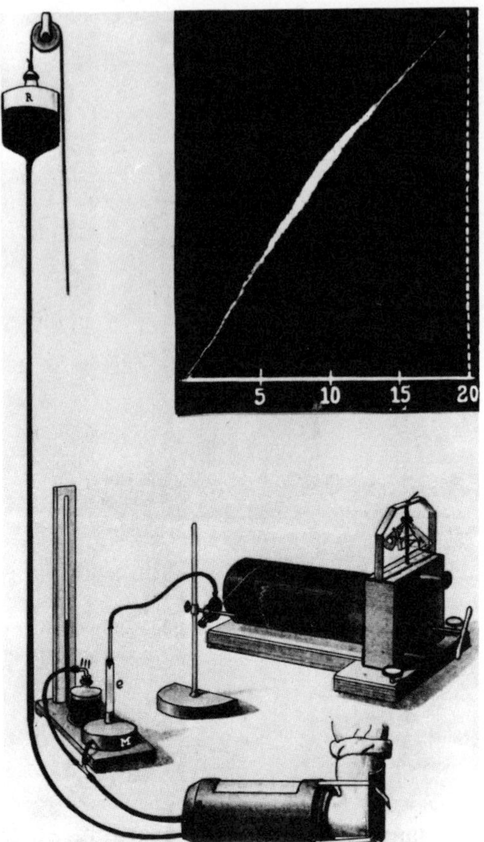

FIGURE 3.19. Marey's method of applying counterpressure to the hand and forearm to measure blood pressure. [From Marey, E. J. (1876). Pression et Vitesse du Sang. Physiologie Experimentalle Paris. Ecole Pratique des Hautes Etudes Lab. de M. Marey.]

In Marey's recording, shown in Figure 3.19, as the counterpressure was increased, the oscillations in pressure started to increase, reached a maximum, and decreased gradually, finally diminishing markedly in amplitude. Marey believed that with the counterpressure for maximal oscillations, the arterial wall was relieved of tension throughout the cardiac cycle, and blood pressure was communicated directly to the water in the compression chamber.

Numerous fluid-filled and air-filled compression chambers were made for the arm and digits. However, little clinical use was made of these instruments. Nonetheless, the concept of applying a counterpressure to measure blood pressure indirectly had taken root. The first air-filled, arm-

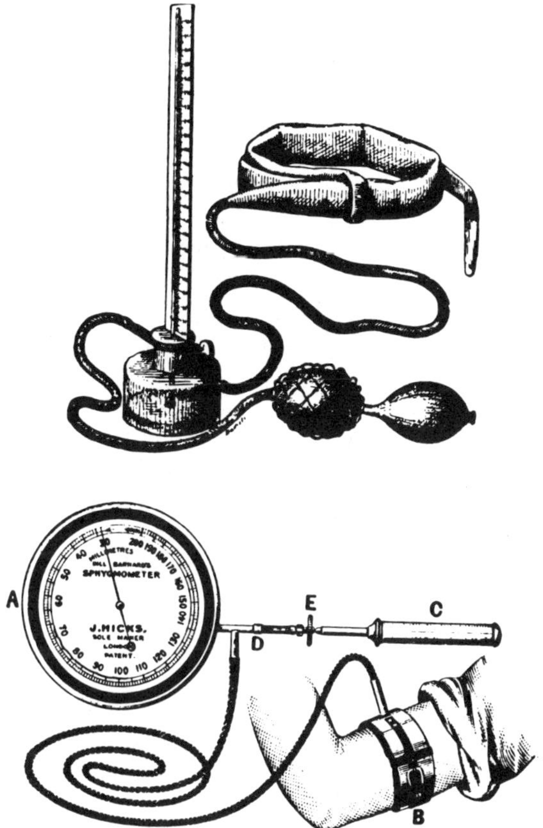

FIGURE 3.20. The first pneumatic arterial occluding cuffs reported by Riva-Rocci (1896) upper, and Hill and Barnard (1897), lower.

encircling cuffs were reported by Riva-Rocci (1896) in Italy and Hill and Barnard (1897) in England. Figure 3.20 illustrates these devices. At last, clinically usable instruments were at hand, and it became possible to determine systolic pressure by noting the counterpressure for disappearance of the radial pulse. However, the first cuffs were found to be too narrow, and it was Von Recklinghausen (1901, 1906) who introduced use of a wider cuff.

It was noted that there was an orderly sequence of oscillations appearing on the indicator used to measure cuff pressure. In fact, this sequence was that described by Marey who applied counterpressure to an arm in a water-filled chamber (Figure 3.19). With suprasystolic pressure in the cuff applied to the arm, small-amplitude oscillations were evident. As cuff pressure was reduced slowly, the oscillations suddenly started to increase as cuff pressure dropped below systolic pressure. The amplitude of the oscillations continued to increase, reached a maximum, then decreased gradually. At first clinicians used the point of sudden increase in amplitude as the systolic criterion. The point of maximal oscillations was taken as the diastolic criterion. This end point was proven to be above diastolic pressure and probably caused abandonment of the oscillometric method. Coincidentally, the auscultatory method was gaining acceptance. Moreover, in some situations, there was not a distinct cuff pressure for maximal oscillations. For all of these reasons, the oscillometric method fell into disuse until being revived only recently for animal and human use.

Korotkoff, a Russian physician, knew about vascular sounds and pointed out that they could be used to identify systolic and diastolic pressures. He stated that when a Riva–Rocci blood-pressure cuff was placed on the arm, inflated quickly, and deflated slowly, there could be heard an orderly sequence of sounds in a stethoscope placed over the antecubital fossa. There are no better words than his own, which are (trans. by Geddes et al., 1966):

> On the basis of his observations, this reporter has arrived at the conclusion that a completely compressed artery in a normal condition does not produce any sound. Taking advantage of this situation the reporter proposes the sound method for determining the blood pressure in humans. The sleeve (cuff) of Riva-Rocci is placed on the middle ⅓ of the arm toward the shoulder. The pressure in the sleeve is raised quickly until it stops the circulation of the blood beyond the sleeve. Thereupon, permitting the mercury manometer to drop, a child's stethoscope is used to listen to the artery directly beyond the sleeve. At first no audible sound is heard at all. As the mercury manometer falls to a certain height the first short tones appear, the appearance of which indicates the passage of part of the pulse wave under the sleeve. Consequently, the manometer reading at which the first tones appear corresponds to the maximum pressure. With a further fall of the mercury in the manometer, systolic pressure murmurs are heard which change again to a sound (secondary). Finally, all sounds disappear. The time at which the sounds disappear indicates a free passage of the pulse wave; in other words, at the moment the sounds disappear, the minimum blood pressure in the artery exceeds the pressure of the sleeve. Consequently, the reading of the manometer at this time corresponds to the minimum blood pressure. Experiments on animals gave positive results. The first sound-tones appear (10–12 mm Hg) sooner than the pulse, for the perception of which (art. radialis) the breakthrough of a greater part of the pulse wave is required.

As clear as this concept is, not all who heard Korotkoff's presentation were enthusiastic. One in the audience stated that these were familiar vascular sounds heard by pressing any stethoscope down on the skin over an artery. Another stated that Korotkoff was hearing heart sounds communicated along the arterial system. Korotkoff pointed out quite correctly that if this were true, they should be heard best when the cuff pressure was low and the artery is open; but this did not occur. The sounds were only present when cuff pressure fell below systolic and was above diastolic pressure.

Clinical acceptance of the Korotkoff sounds to measure blood pressure in humans was slow. A paper by Gittings (1910) urged physicians to use it. There were numerous papers comparing the auscultatory method (as it became known) with the oscillometric method. There were very few studies in which direct arterial pressure in humans was compared to values obtained with the cuff and stethoscope, principally because of a lack of pressure transducers and because of the infrequency of opening arteries. By the late 1930s, such studies were reported, and the correlation data were analyzed by committees which recommended the best technique and the accuracy expected. The first committee presented its report in 1939 which represented the opinions of the American Heart Association (AHA) and the Cardiac Society of Great Britain and Ireland (1939). Since then, the AHA has presented two other reports on this subject (1951 and 1967). The best cuff size and deflation technique have been defined, and although systolic pressure is not in doubt, there is still some controversy over the best indicator (i.e., phase IV or V) for diastolic pressure. As stated previously, the author recommends listing cuff pressure for both diastolic endpoints.

Automatic Devices

Automated blood-pressure-measuring devices were by no means unknown in the 1930s. Many devices were built that automatically inflated the cuff to hunt for obliteration of the radial pulse and thereby track systolic pressure. Others employed the oscillometric method and tracked systolic pressure and cuff pressure for maximal oscillations, which, at that time, were believed to indicate diastolic pressure.

The most interesting automatic blood-pressure-measuring devices employed the auscultatory method. The first to automate this method was Omberg (1936). His self-cycling instrument used the standard occluding cuff connected to a compressed-air line controlled by a solenoid valve. The information to actuate the solenoid valve was derived from a microphone which detected the appearance of the Korotkoff sounds. The sounds were amplified and the circuitry arranged so that the solenoid could be activated either by the appearance or by the disappearance of the sound. Thus the cuff pressure could be cycled to track systolic or diastolic pressure.

Gilson et al. (1941) and Gilson (1942) described an instrument that used the auscultatory method to register systolic and diastolic pressure at any preselected time. Gilson's instrument consisted of a device that was programmable to inflate the occluding cuff to a predetermined pressure in 3 sec, then release the pressure slowly for 22 sec. A stethophone detected the Korotkoff sounds and an amplifier increased these signals, which were recorded graphically, thereby enabling the identification of systolic and diastolic pressures.

An elegant use of the auscultatory method to indicate blood pressure was due to Gilford and Broida (1954) of the National Bureau of Standards. Their instrument consisted of an electronically controlled occluding cuff, an amplifier to increase the Korotkoff sounds, and an interlocking timing mechanism which programmed the sequence of events. The program started with a gradual rise in the occluding cuff pressure. As diastolic pressure was reached, sounds (phase IV) appeared and caused a pressure gauge to sample and hold the reading of the pressure in the cuff. As cuff pressure continued to rise, the sounds passed through phases III, II, and, finally, I. After phase I was reached the sounds disappeared and another pressure gauge sampled and held the reading for systolic pressure. Thus systolic and diastolic pressure were read on two panel pressure-indicating instruments. Sampling of the blood pressure was usually carried out every minute, and since systolic and diastolic pressure readings were available as electrical signals, they were recorded graphically on a calibrated chart, along with other physiological variables such as heart rate and respiration.

Gilford and Broida's instrument was turned over to the Mt. Alto Veterans Hospital for clinical trials. It was used on some 20 patients for varying periods up to 21 hr. The clinical results were encouraging and were published by Rose et al. (1953). Blood-pressure records during normal sleep and under anesthesia were clear and easily readable. Continuous records were made during transfusion, which produced a dramatic increase in blood pressure shortly after the transfusion was begun. Recordings on hypertensive patients, undergoing hexamethonium therapy, showed a marked drop in blood pressure when the drug was administered.

Since the 1950s, and particularly now with the advent of microprocessors, numerous automated devices have been developed for measuring blood pressure indirectly. There are now coin-operated devices in public places that allow anyone to measure his or her blood pressure. It should be recognized, however, that such devices assume that the subject has an adult-sized arm.

REFERENCES

Alexander, H. (1977). Criteria in the choice of an occluding cuff for the indirect measurement of blood pressure. *Med. Biol. Eng. Comput.* **15**, 2–10.

American Heart Association (1939). Joint Recommendations of the American Heart Association and the Cardiac Society of Great Britain and Ireland. Standardization of blood pressure readings. *Amer. Heart Journ.* **18**, 95–101.

American Heart Association (1951). Recommendations for human blood-pressure determination by sphygmomanometers. *Circulation* **4**, 503–509.

American Heart Association (1967). Recommendations for human blood-pressure determination by sphygmomanometers. *Circulation* **36**, 980–988.

Burch, G. E. and DePasquale, N. P. (1962). *Primer of Clinical Measurement of Blood Pressure.* C. V. Mosby Co., St. Louis.

Friesen, R. H., and Lichter, I. L. (1981). Indirect measurement of blood pressure in neonates and infants utilizing an automatic noninvasive oscillometric monitor. *Anesth. Analg.* **10**, 742–745.

Geddes, L. A. and Baker, L. E. (1975). *Principles of Applied Biomedical Instrumentation,* 2nd ed., Wiley, New York.

Geddes, L. A., Chaffee, V., Whistler, S. J., Bourland, J. D., and Tacker, W. A. (1977). Indirect mean blood pressure in the anesthetized pony. *Am. J. Vet. Res.* **38**, 2055–2057.

Geddes, L. A., and Newberg, D. C. (1977). Cuff pressure oscillation in the measurement of relative blood pressure. *Psychophysiology,* **14**, 198–202.

Geddes, L. A., and Whistler, S. W. (1978). The error in indirect blood pressure measurement with the incorrect size of cuff. *American Heart Journal* **96**, 4–8.

Geddes, L. A., Hoff, H. E., and Badger, A. S. (1966). Introduction of the auscultatory method of measuring blood pressure. *Cardiovasc. Res. Ctr. Bull.* **5**, 57–74.

Geddes, L. A., Hughes, D. J., and Babbs, C. F. (1979). Pulse wave velocity as a continuous indicator of diastolic blood pressure. *Proc. AAMI 14th Annual Meeting* **14**, 89.

Geddes, L. A., Combs, W., Denton, W., et al. (1980). Indirect mean blood pressure in the dog. *Amer. J. Physiol. (Heart Circ.)* **7**, H663–H666.

Geddes, L. A., Voelz, M., Babbs, C. F., Bourland, J. D., and Tacker, W. A. (1981). Pulse transit time as an indicator of arterial blood pressure. *Psychophysiology* **18**(1), 71–74.

Geddes, L. A., Voelz, M., Combs, C., Reiner, D., and Babbs, C. F. (1983). Characterization of the oscillometric method for the indirect measurement of blood pressure. *Ann. Biomed Eng.* **10**(6), 271–280.

Gilford, S. R. and Broida, H. P. (1954). Physiological monitoring equipment for anesthesia and other uses. Natl. Bureau of Standards Report 3301, Project 1204-20-5512, May 15.

Gilson, W. E., Goldberg, H., and Slocum, H. (1941). An automatic device for periodically determining and recording both systolic and diastolic blood pressure in man. *Science,* **94**, 194.

Gilson, W. E. (1942). Automatic blood pressure recorder. *Electronics,* **15**, 54–56.

Gittings, J. C. (1910). Auscultatory blood pressure determinations. *Arch. Int. Med.* **6,** 196–204.

Gribbin, B., Steptoe, A., and Sleight, P. (1976). Pulse wave velocity as a measure of blood pressure change. *Psychophysiology* **13,** 86–90.

Hill, L. and Barnard, H. (1897). A simple and accurate form of sphygmomanometer or arterial pressure gauge contrived for clinical use. *Brit. Med. J.* **2,** 904.

Hochberg, H. M., et al. (1971). Accuracy of an automated ultrasound blood pressure monitor. *Curr. Therap. Res.* **13,** 129–138; **13,** 473–481; **13,** 482–488.

Hughes, D. J., Babbs, C. F., Geddes, L. A., and Bourland, J. D. (1979). Measurement of Young's modulus of elasticity of the canine aorta with ultrasound. *Ultrasonic Imaging* **1,** 356–367.

Karvonen, M. J. (1962). Effect of sphygmomanometer cuff size on blood pressure measurement. *Bull. World Health Organization* **27,** 805–808.

Kirkendal, W. M., Burton, A. C., Epstein, F. H., and Freis, E. D. (1967). Recommendations for human blood pressure determinations by sphygmomanometer. *Circulation (American Heart Association)* **86,** 980.

Kimble, K. J., Darnall, R. A., Yelderman, M. et al. (1981). An automatic oscillometric technique for estimating mean arterial pressure in critically ill neonates. *Anesthesiol.* **54,** 423–425.

Korotkoff, N. S. (1905). On the subject of measuring blood pressure. *Bull. Imp. Military Med. Acad. St. Petersburg* **11,** 365–367.

Korteweg, D. J. (1878). Ueber die Fortpflanzungsgeschwindigkeit die Schaller in elstischen Rohen. *Ann. Phys. Chem.* **5,** 525–542.

Latshaw, J. T., Whistler, S. J., Fessler, J. F., and Geddes, L. A. (1979). Indirect measurement of blood pressure in the normotensive and hypotensive horse. *Equine Vet. J.* **11,** 191–194.

Master, A. M., Garfield, C. I. and Walters, M. B. (1952). *Normal Blood Pressure and Hypertension,* Lea and Febiger, Philadelphia.

Mauck, G. B., Smith, C. R., Geddes, L. A., and Bourland, J. D. (1980). The meaning of the point of maximum oscillations in cuff pressure in the indirect measurement of blood pressure II. *J. Biomech. Eng.* 102:28–33.

Moens, A. I. (1878). *Die Pulsecurve,* E. J. Brell, Leiden.

Omberg, A. C. (1936). An apparatus for recording systolic blood pressure. *Rev. Sci. Instru.* **7,** 33–34.

Park, M. K., Kawabor, I., and Guntheroth, W. G. (1976). Need for an improved standard for blood pressure cuff size. *Clin. Pediatrics* **15,** 784–786.

Posey, J. A., Geddes, L. A., Williams, H., and Moore, A. G. (1969). The meaning of the point of maximum oscillations in cuff pressure in the indirect measurement of blood pressure. Part I. *Cardiovasc. Res. Ctr. Bull.* **8,** 15–25.

Ramsey, M. (1979). Noninvasive automatic determination of mean arterial pressure. *Med. Biol. Eng. Comput.* **17,** 11–18.

Riva-Rocci, S. S. (1896). Un nuovo sfigmanometro. *Gonz. Med. Torino* **17,** 981–996.

Rose, J. C., Gilford, S. R., Broida, H. P., Soler, A., Pattenope, E. A., and Freis, E. P. (1953). Clinical and investigative applications of a new instrument for continuous measurement of blood pressure and heart rate. *New England J. Med.* **249,** 615–617.

Steptoe, A., Smulyan, H., and Gribbin, B. (1976). Pulse wave velocity and blood pressure change: calibration and applications. *Psychophysiology* **13,** 488–493.

Task Force on High Blood Pressure (1974). *Automated Blood Pressure Measuring Devices for Mass Screening,* National Heart, Lung and Blood Institute, Bethesda, MD 20014, U.S. Department of Health, Education and Welfare, DHEW Publication N, (NIH) 76-929.

Von Recklinghausen, H. (1901). Ueber Blutdruckmessung beim Menschen. *Arch. Exp. Path. Pharm.* **46,** 78–132.

Von Recklinghausen, H. (1906). Unblutige Blutdruckmessung. *Arch. Exp. Path. Pharm.* **5,** 325–504.

Ware, R. W. and Laenger, C. J. (1967). Indirect blood pressure measurement by Doppler ultrasonic kinetoarteriography. *Proc. 20th Ann. Conf. Eng. Med. Biol.* **9,** 27–30.

Yelderman, M. and Ream, A. K. (1979). Indirect measurement of mean blood pressure in the anesthetized patient. *Anethesiol.* **50,** 253–256.

CHAPTER 4

The Measurement of Cardiac Output and Blood Flow

CARDIAC OUTPUT

The heart is a two-sided stroke pump in a double circulatory system. The right heart pumps blood through the lungs; the left heart pumps blood through the rest of the body. The output of the right heart is equal to the output of the left heart. In fact, the output of the right heart, after flowing through the lungs, is the input to the left heart. Similarly, the output of the left heart, after flowing through the arteries to the capillaries and collecting veins, is the input to the right heart. Figure 4.1 illustrates these points. Cardiac output is therefore the output of either the right or left heart. Cardiac output (*CO*) is equal to the volume of blood ejected per beat, which is called stroke volume (*SV*), multiplied by heart rate (*HR*). Thus

$$CO = SV \times HR$$

It is easy to measure heart rate, but there are very few methods for measuring stroke volume. It is for this reason that recourse is taken to methods that measure the average cardiac output, which is usually expressed in liters per minute. To compare cardiac output in large and small subjects and among different species, two methods of normalization are used. One method expresses cardiac output per unit of body weight; the

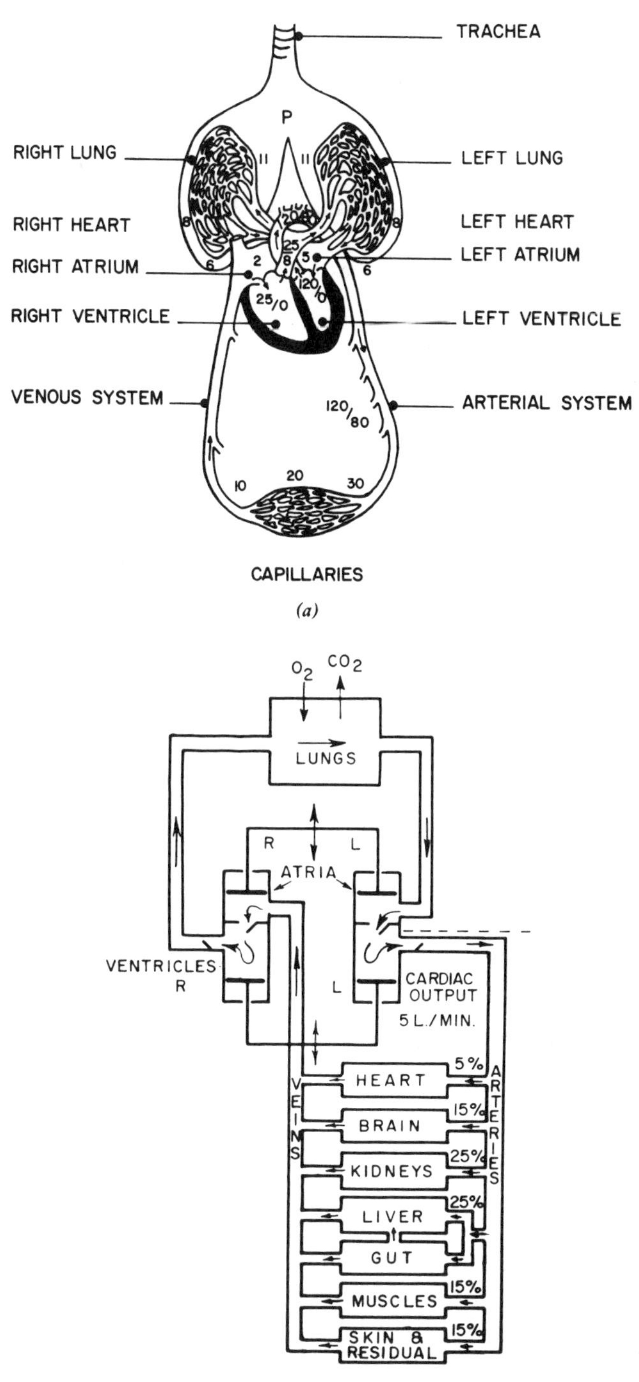

FIGURE 4.1. (*a*) The circulatory system. (*b*) Mechanical analog of the circulatory system.

TABLE 4.1. Cardiovascular Data[a]

Species	Weight (kg)	Area (m^2)	State	Cardiac Output	Cardiac Index ($L/min/m^2$)	*CO* (mL/min/kg)
Human (5 yr)	18.0	0.82	Basal	2.28	2.78	122
Human (25 yr)	68.5	1.85	Basal	5.10	2.76	74.7
Human (60 yr)	69.8	1.79	Basal	4.55	2.54	65.2
Dog	6.4	0.39	Basal	1.12	2.9	175
Goat	16.1	0.71		2.2	3.1	137
Goat	23.7	0.91	Basal	3.1	3.4	131
Horse	283	4.30	Standing	18.8	4.4	66.4

[a]Data from W. S. Spector (ed.) (1956). *Handbook of Biological Data,* Saunders, Philadelphia.

other divides it by the body surface area. Thus the units are mL/min/kg of body weight and L/min/m^2 of body surface area. The latter unit is more frequently used and is given the special name "cardiac index." Table 4.1 presents typical basal values for both quantities for a variety of species. Note the similarity of cardiac index values.

It is of some interest to note that the cardiac output for a typical 70-kg adult male subject at rest is about 5 L/min. If the heart rate is 72 beats/min, the stroke volume is 5000/72 = 69.4 mL. Such a subject would have a body surface area of about 1.85 m^2; therefore, the cardiac index is 5/1.85 = 2.7 L/min/m^2. The cardiac output per kilogram of body weight is 5000/70 = 71.4 mL/min/kg. In such a subject, if cardiac output dropped to 3 L/min, consciousness would be impaired.

Muscular exercise increases cardiac output dramatically. Table 4.2 presents typical values. Highly trained long-distance runners, when in condition, can increase their cardiac output from a resting value of 5 to 25 or 30 L/min with maximal exercise. It is interesting to note that trained athletes have a resting heart rate that is much lower than untrained subjects; the heart rate of a trained athlete is 40–50 beats/min at rest. The resting cardiac output is about the same as in other subjects of similar size; therefore, the stroke volume of an athlete is much larger than that of an untrained subject. In general, there are two major cardiovascular differences in athletes: (1) the resting heart rate is low and (2) following exercise, the heart rate returns to a resting level very rapidly. In fact, the ability of the heart to increase its output and to return quickly to a resting value after exercise are cardiovascular parameters that identify physical fitness.

The cardiac output is shared by the various organs and tissues. A typical resting distribution is shown in Table 4.3 and Figure 4.1*b*. It is

TABLE 4.2. Range of Cardiac Output in Humans

Activity	Duration (hr)	Output (L/min)	Power to Blood (W)
Dinner	1	6.37	1.41
Relaxation	3	7.17	1.59
Sleep	8	6	1.33
Dressing, etc.	1	9.03	2.00
Driving	0.5	8.32	1.85
Moderate work	4	8.6	1.91
Walking	0.25	10.5	2.33
Lunch	0.5	6.37	1.41
Walking	0.25	10.5	2.33
Moderate work	4.0	8.6	1.91
Driving	0.5	8.32	1.85
Moderate exercise	1.0	11.5	2.55
Average		7.6	1.68

interesting to note that the heart takes about one-twentieth of its output (via the coronary arteries) for its own operation. The brain requires about one-seventh of the cardiac output. These two important areas have a high priority for circulation, and there is little control over their flow rates. However, the amount of blood going to the other vascular beds is under considerable control, depending on the circumstances. Kidney, hepatic–portal, muscle, and skin blood flows can and do vary considerably depending on circumstances. Figure 3.1*b* illustrates these controls.

Table 4.3 shows the extraction of oxygen from the blood for the various circulatory regions. Note that the heart extracts the highest proportion of oxygen in comparison to other organs. It is noteworthy that venous blood contains a wide range of oxygen saturations. It is for this

TABLE 4.3. Distribution of Cardiac Output

Distribution (Human) Region	*CO* (%)	Approximate Fraction	O_2 cm^3/ 100 cm^3 A-V O_2 Difference	Venous[a] Saturation (%)
Hepatic/portal	25	1/4	3.4	83.3
Kidneys	25	1/4	1.4	93
Brain	15	1/7	6.2	69
Heart (coronaries)	5	1/20	11.4	43
Skeletal muscle	15.5	1/6	6	70
Skin and residual	14.5	1/7		

[a] Note that venous system contains blood of varying saturations.

TABLE 4.4. Blood Volumes[a]

Species	mL/kg
Human	
Male	74–85
Female	63–74
Dog	66–102
Monkey	60–75
Guinea pig	72–75
Rabbit	55–72
Rat	45–63
Cattle	52–62
Goat	57–82
Swine	61–69
Horse	71–109

[a] Altman, P. L., et al. (1960). *Handbook of Circulation,* NRC, National Academy of Science, Contract AF 33(616)-3972.

reason that the most representative sample of venous blood is found on the pulmonary artery.

BLOOD VOLUME

Before discussing the methods for measuring cardiac output, it is of value to identify the amount of blood in the body. Table 4.4 presents typical values for blood volume for different species in mL/kg of body weight. In humans, the blood volume is typically about 7% of the body weight. Often the blood volume is stated as 70 mL/kg of body weight.

The blood volume of a subject is remarkably constant; however, its distribution is of some interest. For example, 60% is found in the veins and 13% is in the arteries. The lungs accommodate 12%, the heart 8%, and, surprisingly enough, only about 7% is in the capillaries, where all of the metabolic exchange takes place. It should be clear that a very small change in the size of the venous reservoir would allow accommodation of a large volume of blood. Venous pooling of blood is a serious problem in cardiovascular shock. The spleen is a reservoir for red cells that can be delivered to the circulation following blood loss. Parenthetically, when blood is donated by human volunteers, about 500 mL are withdrawn. Such a donation amounts to about 10% of the blood volume and is relatively unnoticed by the average donor.

The volume of blood in a subject is measured with the dilution technique, which is used to measure the volume of any irregularly shaped or inaccessible container. A measured amount (m) of detectable substance (indicator) is introduced to the fluid-filled container and, after complete mixing, a sample is withdrawn. The concentration (c) of the indicator in the sample is then measured; therefore, the volume of the container $V = m/c$.

In applying the dilution principle to measure blood volume, the indicator must have special properties. For example, there must be a minimum loss of indicator through the kidneys or by trapping in an organ. For this reason, two types of indicator are used: one combines with the plasma proteins and the other becomes incorporated in the red cells. Thus what is measured is either plasma volume or red-cell volume. Blood volume is calculated by measuring the fraction of cells (by centrifugation) and scaling the result. The fraction of cells is called the packed-cell volume (PCV) and is often expressed as a percentage. Because there are so many more red cells than platelets or leukocytes, the percent red-cell volume (or hematocrit) is often used as a descriptor of the cell fraction in blood.

Evan's blue, a dye that attaches to plasma albumin, and radioiodine-labeled albumin are the most frequently used indicators. The concentration of Evan's blue is measured with a spectrophotometer (at 640 nm) and the concentration of radioiodine-labeled albumin is measured with a radioactivity detector. The technique employed consists of drawing a blood sample and centrifuging it to separate the plasma from the cells. This procedure produces a plasma sample (blank) without the indicator and allows calculation of the packed-cell volume (cell fraction).

The indicator is injected intravenously and time is allowed for mixing of the indicator. At 10, 20, and 30 min, venous blood samples are withdrawn and centrifuged, and the concentration of indicator is measured in the plasma sample. With Evan's blue, the concentration is proportional to the optical density [$\log_{10}$ (1/transmission)]. Similarly, the count-per-minute rate is proportional to the concentration of the radioiodine albumin. These concentrations are plotted on a graph, which shows the slight loss of indicator. Figure 4.2 illustrates a typical concentration–time curve which is extrapolated to zero time to identify the concentration of the indicator corresponding to zero loss. This zero-time concentration is divided into the amount of indicator injected to obtain plasma volume. As a practical matter, it is more convenient to plot the optical density or counts/minute versus time and extrapolate to obtain the zero-time value. This figure can then be converted to concentration by adding a known amount of indicator to the plasma bank and measuring it. The blood

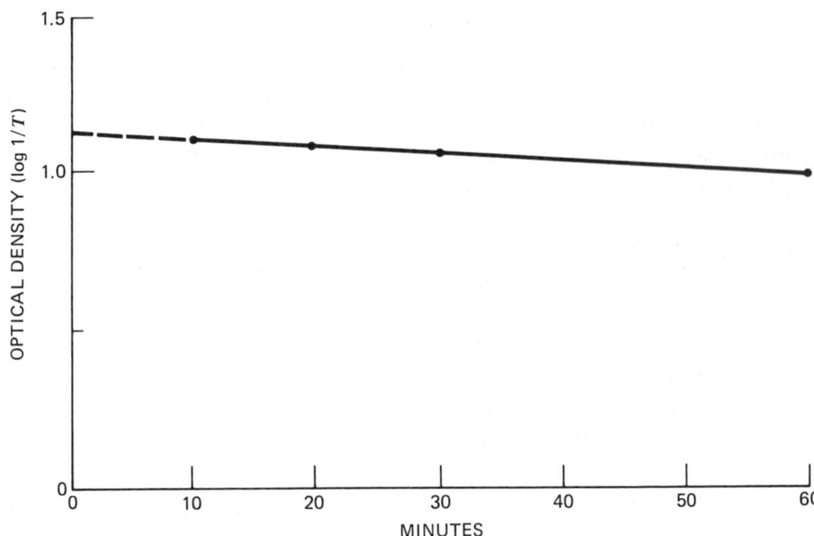

FIGURE 4.2. Calculation of blood volume by determination of the zero-time concentration of an injected indicator.

volume is the plasma volume divided by (1 − PCV), where PCV is the packed-cell fraction.

DILUTION METHODS FOR CARDIAC OUTPUT

Although there are numerous methods of measuring cardiac output, the two that are most frequently used are the Fick and the indicator–diluation methods. Both employ the dilution principle and will now be described. An indirect method which employs recording of the electrical impedance changes that appear between thoracic electrodes is also employed in some clinics; this method will also be described.

Fick Method

Venous blood flowing through the lungs from the right heart to the left heart picks up oxygen and releases carbon dioxide (Figure 4.3*a*). In 1870 Fick stated that if the amount of oxygen taken up (or the amount of carbon dioxide liberated) per minute is known and the oxygen (or carbon dioxide) concentration in the blood entering and leaving the lungs is known, it is possible to calculate blood flow through the lungs (cardiac output). A convenient way of understanding Fick's proposal is shown in Figure 4.3*b*. Consider delivery of oxygen to the blood to be equivalent to a conveyor belt in which venous blood from the right heart comes along in 100-mL beakers which pass a dispensing reservoir that delivers oxygen. Thus the (arterial) beakers that have passed the oxygen dispenser contain more oxygen. Assume that the concentration of oxygen in the venous blood is 15 mL/100 mL blood (i.e., 15 volumes percent, V%) and that the concentration of oxygen in the arterial beakers is 20 mL/100 mL blood. In this steady-state conveyor-belt system it was found that 250 mL of oxygen disappeared from the dispensing reservoir each minute. Each 100-mL beaker of blood took up 20 − 15 = 5 mL of oxygen; therefore, 250/5 = 50 beakers must have passed each minute. Cardiac output must therefore by 50 beakers × 100 mL/beaker = 5000 mL. These facts are usually expressed by the following familiar expression:

$$\text{Cardiac Output} = \frac{\text{oxygen uptake/min}}{\text{arterial} - \text{venous oxygen concentration}}$$

Using the numbers given in the conveyor-belt analog:

$$CO = \frac{250\ \text{mL/min}}{20/100 - 15/100} = \frac{250 \times 100}{5} = 5000\ \frac{\text{mL}}{\text{min}}$$

The oxygen uptake is measured using a spirometer equipped with a carbon dioxide absorber. A typical record of oxygen uptake is shown in Figure 4.4. Note that the oxygen uptake, which is the slope of the recording, must be corrected to body temperature, and saturated with water vapor by using the correction factor shown in Table 4.5. The concentration of oxygen in the arterial and venous blood is less easily measured. Two instruments, the Van Slyke manometric apparatus or the LexO_2con analyzer, are used. The former is a gasometric instrument in which the oxygen content is measured by removal of the oxygen from the blood sample. The LexO_2con is an electrochemical instrument that counts the oxygen molecules and indicates the O_2 content in the sample of blood introduced. The indication represents volume percent at 0°C and 760 mm Hg dry air. Therefore this figure must be corrected to body temperature and ambient pressure, saturated.

The Fick method is extremely reliable but requires steady-state conditions. It can be applied using carbon dioxide and, with slightly more difficulty, foreign gases. The highest accuracy is obtained when the mixed venous sample is obtained from the pulmonary artery; right ventricular blood is next best. The arterial sample can be obtained from any convenient artery.

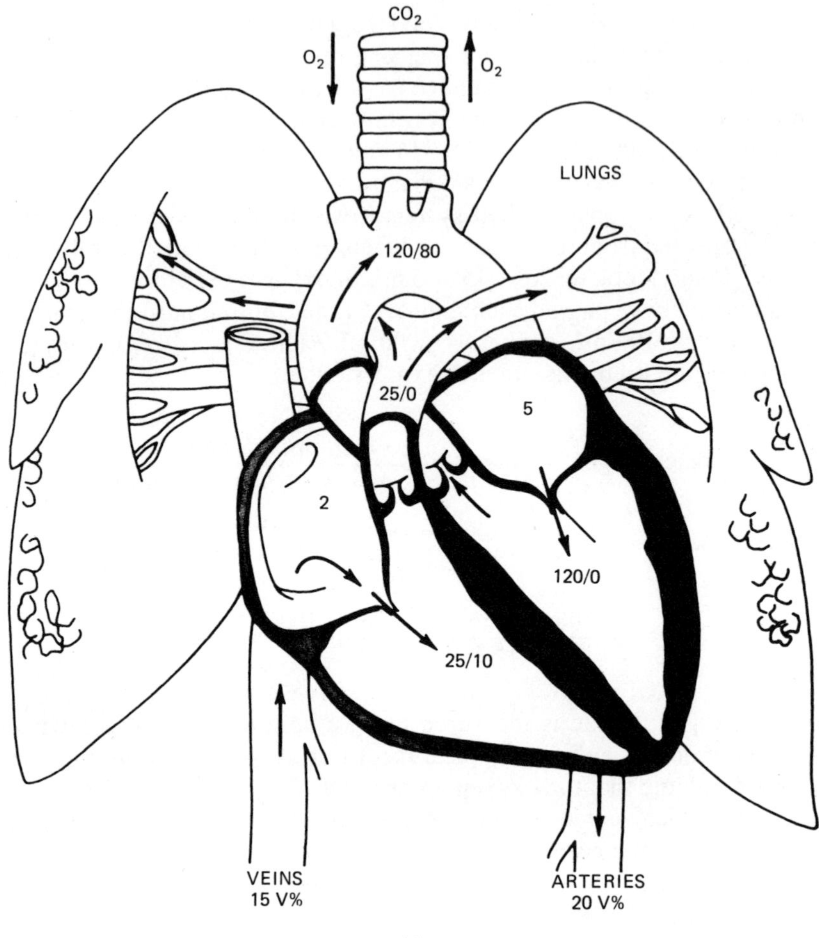

FIGURE 4.3. (*a*) The pulmonary circuit. (*b*) Principle employed in the Fick method using the conveyor-belt analog.

Indicator-Dilution Method

Stewart (1921) showed that if a known concentration of indicator is introduced into a flowing stream and the temporal concentration of the indicator is measured at a downstream point, it is possible to calculate the volume flow. To illustrate the salient points of the indicator-dilution method, consider a fluid flowing at a constant rate in a tube of cross-sectional area a, as shown in Figure 4.5. Assume that m grams of a soluble and detectable indicator are rapidly introduced to form a uniform cylinder

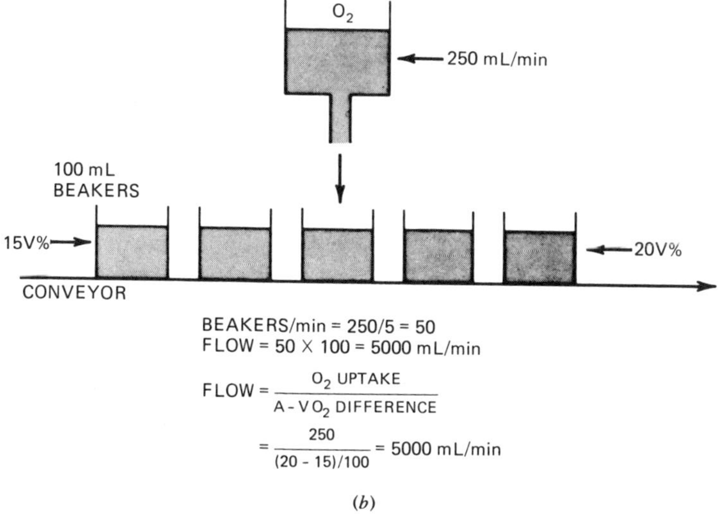

(*b*)

FIGURE 4.3 *(Continued)*

of indicator in the fluid. If a concentration detector is placed slightly downstream and its output is recorded, an idealized rectangular concentration–time curve of amplitude C will be recorded as the cylinder passes. The practical use of this idealized concentration–time curve will now be illustrated.

In a tube containing a flowing fluid, flow is equal to the velocity of flow (v) multiplied by the cross-sectional area (a); flow $\phi = va$. Velocity is distance divided by time, and in the model the cylinder of indicator moves L units of distance in t sec, the value for t being identified on the concentration–time curve; therefore, $v = L/t$. Substituting L/t for velocity, $\phi = La/t$. However, La is the volume of the cylinder (V) and, therefore, $\phi = Vt$. It is not possible to measure the volume of the cylinder, but it is possible to measure concentration (C), which is equal to m/V. Substituting this quantity gives

$$\phi = \frac{m}{Ct} = \frac{\text{mass of indicator injected}}{\text{concentration} \times \text{time}}$$

The expression just derived illustrates that in the idealized case, if m grams of indicator are injected and the calibrated downstream concentration–time curve is recorded, it is possible to calculate flow. In a practical situation, the cylinder of indicator would be spread out into a teardrop shape owing to the velocity profile in the tube. Therefore, the concentration–time curve will rise rapidly and fall slowly as shown in Figure 4.5*b*.

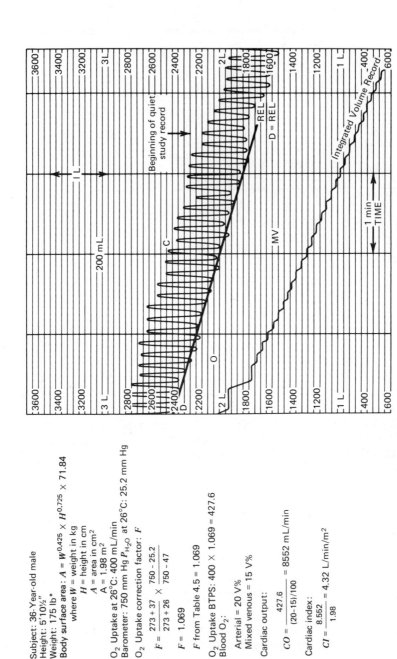

Subject: 36-Year-old male
Height: 5′10½″
Weight: 175 lb*
Body surface area: $A = W^{0.425} \times H^{0.725} \times 71.84$
where W = weight in kg
H = height in cm
A = area in cm^2
A = 1.98 m^2

O_2 Uptake at 26°C: 400 mL/min
Barometer: 750 mm Hg P_{H_2O} at 26°C: 25.2 mm Hg

O_2 Uptake correction factor: F

$$F = \frac{273 + 37}{273 + 26} \times \frac{750 - 25.2}{750 - 47}$$

F = 1.069

F from Table 4.5 = 1.069

O_2 Uptake BTPS: 400 × 1.069 = 427.6
Blood O_2:

Arterial = 20 V%
Mixed venous = 15 V%

Cardiac output:

$$CO = \frac{427.6}{(20-15)/100} = 8552 \text{ mL/min}$$

Cardiac index:

$$CI = \frac{8.552}{1.98} = 4.32 \text{ L/min/m}^2$$

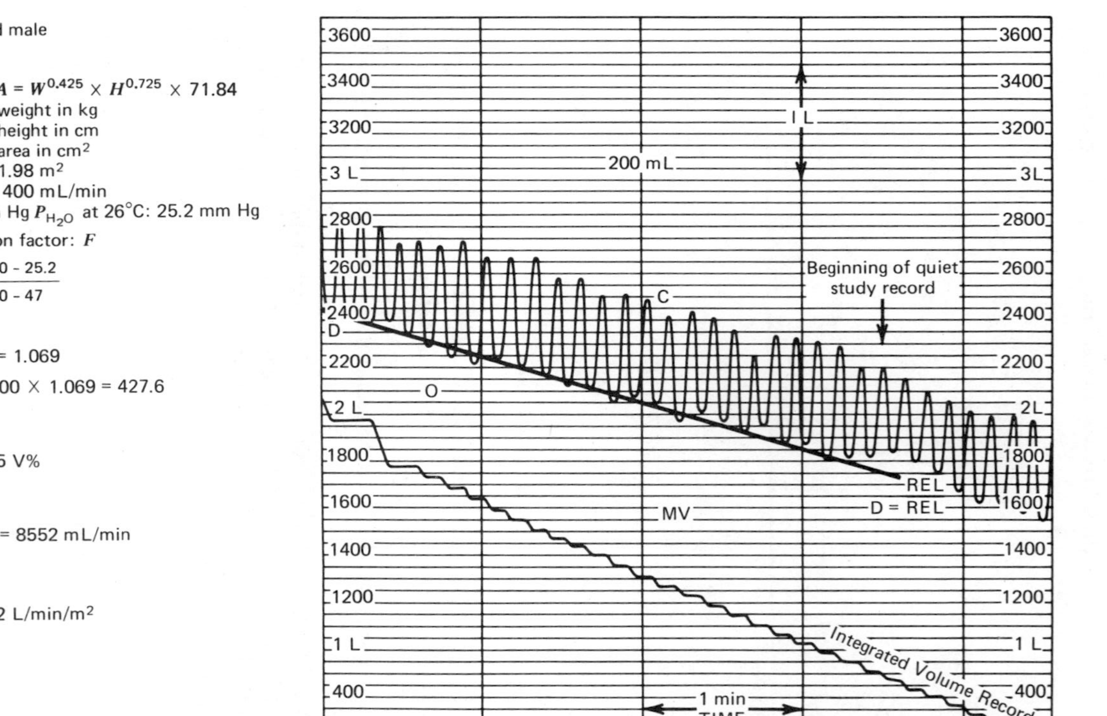

FIGURE 4.4. Measurement of oxygen uptake with a spirogram, and sample calculation of cardiac output using the Fick method.

TABLE 4.5. Correction Factor (F) for Standardization of Collected Volume[a]

Temperature (°C)/P_B	640	650	660	670	680	690	700	710	720	730	740	750	760	770	780
15	1.1388	1.1377	1.1367	1.1358	1.1348	1.1339	1.1330	1.1322	1.1314	1.1306	1.1298	1.1290	1.1283	1.1276	1.1269
16	1.1333	1.1323	1.1313	1.1304	1.1295	1.1286	1.1277	1.1269	1.1260	1.1253	1.1245	1.1238	1.1231	1.1224	1.1217
17	1.1277	1.1268	1.1266	1.1249	1.1240	1.1232	1.1224	1.1216	1.1208	1.1200	1.1193	1.1186	1.1179	1.1172	1.1165
18	1.1222	1.1212	1.1203	1.1194	1.1186	1.1178	1.1170	1.1162	1.1154	1.1147	1.1140	1.1133	1.1126	1.1120	1.1113
19	1.1165	1.1156	1.1147	1.1139	1.1131	1.1123	1.1115	1.1107	1.1100	1.1093	1.1086	1.1080	1.1073	1.1067	1.1061
20	1.1108	1.1099	1.1091	1.1083	1.1075	1.1067	1.1060	1.1052	1.1045	1.1039	1.1032	1.1026	1.1019	1.1094	1.1008
21	1.1056	1.1042	1.1034	1.1027	1.1019	1.1011	1.1004	1.0997	1.0990	1.0984	1.0978	1.0971	1.0965	1.0960	1.0954
22	1.0992	1.0984	1.0976	1.0969	1.0962	1.0964	1.0948	1.0941	1.0935	1.0929	1.0923	1.0917	1.0911	1.0905	1.0900
23	1.0932	1.0925	1.0918	1.0911	1.0904	1.0897	1.0891	1.0884	1.0878	1.0872	1.0867	1.0861	1.0856	1.0850	1.0845
24	1.0873	1.0866	1.0859	1.0852	1.0846	1.0839	1.0833	1.0827	1.0822	1.0816	1.0810	1.0805	1.0800	1.0795	1.0790
25	1.0812	1.0806	1.0799	1.0793	1.0787	1.0781	1.0775	1.0769	1.0764	1.0758	1.0753	1.0748	1.0744	1.0739	1.0734
26	1.0751	1.0710	1.0738	1.0732	1.0727	1.0721	1.0716	1.0710	1.0705	1.0700	1.0696	1.0691	1.0686	1.0682	1.0678
27	1.0688	1.0682	1.0677	1.0671	1.0666	1.0661	1.0656	1.0651	1.0640	1.0641	1.0637	1.0633	1.0629	1.0624	1.0621
28	1.0625	1.0619	1.0614	1.0609	1.0604	1.0599	1.0595	1.0591	1.0586	1.0582	1.0578	1.0574	1.0570	1.0566	1.0563
29	1.0560	1.0555	1.0550	1.0546	1.0548	1.0537	1.0533	1.0529	1.0525	1.0521	1.0518	1.0514	1.0519	1.0507	1.0504
30	1.0494	1.0496	1.0486	1.0482	1.0478	1.0474	1.0470	1.0467	1.0463	1.0460	1.0450	1.0453	1.0450	1.0447	1.0444

[a] From Kovach, J. C., Paulos, P., and Arabadjis, C. (1955). *J. Thorac. Surg.* **29,** 552–554.

$V_s = FV_c$, where V_s is the standardized condition and V_c is the collected condition.

$$V_s = \frac{(1 + 37/273)}{(1 + t°\text{C}/273)} \times \frac{(P_B - P_{H_2O})}{(P_B - 47)} V_c = FV_c$$

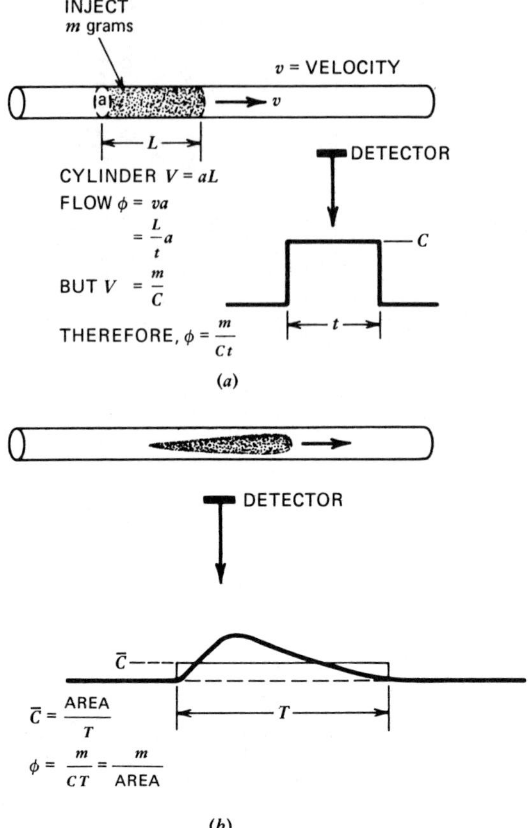

FIGURE 4.5. Genesis of the dilution curve.

However, a rectangular concentration–time curve can be obtained from this typical dilution curve by measuring the area under it and dividing by the base. Performing this operation provides a mean concentration $\bar{C}$ for the time t. Thus,

$$\phi = \frac{m}{\bar{C}t}$$

There is an extremely important subtletly about this flow expression. Note that it is only necessary to know the amount (m) of indicator injected and the downstream concentration–time curve. The concentration–time curve can be recorded from any downstream branch. The important requirement is that the indicator is injected so that it mixes with all of the

TABLE 4.6. Indicators

Material	Detector	Retention Data
Evans blue (T1824)	Photoelectric, 640 μm	50% loss in 5 days[a]
Cardiogreen	Photoelectric, 800 μm	50% loss in 10 min[b]
Coomassie blue	Photoelectric, 585–600 μm	50% loss in 15–20 min[c]
Saline (5%)	Conductivity cell	Diffusible[d]
Albumin^{131}I	Radioactive	
^{24}Na, ^{42}K, D_2O, DHO	Radioactive	Diffusible[d]
Hot–cold solutions	Thermo-detector	Diffusible[d]

[a] Connolly et al. (1954).

[b] Fox (1960); Wheeler (1958).

[c] Taylor (1959).

[d] It is estimated that there is less than 15% loss of diffusible indicators during the first pass.

flow. In the measurement of cardiac output the indicator is injected into the right atrium, right ventricle, or pulmonary artery and the dilution curve is obtained by withdrawing arterial blood (from any large artery) into the detector at a constant rate. With the thermal-dilution method, injection is into the right atrium and detection is in the pulmonary artery.

Before describing practical application of the indicator-dilution method, several important facts should be recognized, the most important of which is that cardiac output must remain constant for the duration of measurement. The characteristics of the indicator are also very important. Obviously, it must be detectable and not be a stimulant or depressant to the circulatory system. It must be retained for a period long enough to permit inscription of a dilution curve. Indicators that are lost from the circulation between the injection and measuring sites provide a falsely high value for cardiac output because $\bar{C}$ is too small and is in the denominator of the flow expression. Indicators that are rapidly cleared from the circulation allow repeated determinations without indicator buildup. Indicators that are retained in the circulation can build up to excessively high concentrations if repeated determinations are made. Since, usually, indicators are colored dyes, there is the possibility of altering skin color until the indicator is cleared.

A wide variety of indicators are used to measure cardiac output; Table 4.6 presents a typical list, along with the type of detector employed for each. However, in clinical medicine, the dye and thermal-dilution methods are perhaps the most popular.

The method of obtaining a dilution curve from which cardiac output can be calculated is shown in Figure 4.6. The site of injection for the

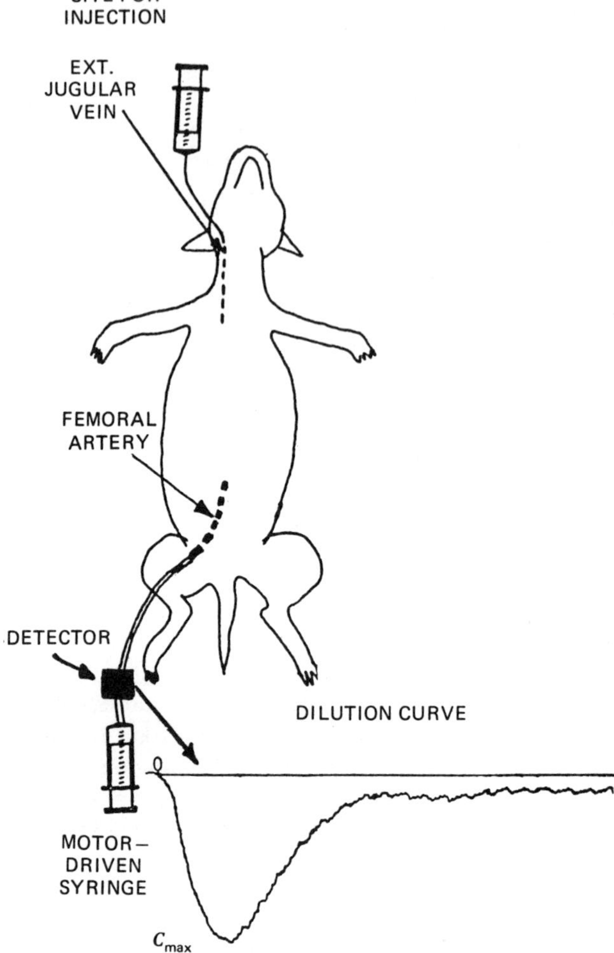

FIGURE 4.6. The indicator-dilution technique.

indicator is the right atrium, ventricle, or pulmonary artery. In the illustration, a catheter connected to the indicator-filled syringe has been advanced down the right jugular vein. In the human the basilic vein in the arm is used as the entry point.

To inscribe the dilution curve, an arterial catheter is connected to the detector for the indicator, which is in turn connected to a motor-driven withdrawal syringe as shwn in Figure 4.6. The catheter is introduced into a major artery, such as the femoral, and advanced into the aorta. The indicator is then injected rapidly and blood is drawn through the detector, the output of which is recorded to obtain the dilution curve as shown. Note that the dilution curve does not return to zero indicator concentration because of recirculation of the indicator. In order to process the dilution curve, this recirculation must be removed and the dilution curve for a single pass must be synthesized. The method of performing this correction will now be described.

Because the descending limb of the dilution curve is exponential, semilogarithmic plotting of this part of the curve provides a means of identifying the end of the first pass, which, for practical purposes, is taken as the time for the dilution curve to fall to 1% of its maximum concentration. Semilogarithmic plotting is usually performed first on the uncalibrated dilution curve so that a true single-pass curve can be synthesized and measured for area to determine the mean height for the time of one pass. Figure 4.7*a* illustrates a typical dilution curve showing recirculation on the downslope; Figure 4.7*b* presents a plot of the downslope of this curve. Note that the part of the curve reflecting recirculation departs from the linear portion of the downslope. Extrapolation of the linear portion allows identification of the time for the practical end of the dilution curve, which is taken as 1% of the maximum height (C_{max}) of the dilution curve, that is, the time corresponding to $C_{max}/100$. The dilution curve can be completed by plotting the heights for times earlier than the extrapolated end time as shown by the dashed line in Figure 4.7*a*. Then the area under the corrected dilution curve is measured and divided by its length; this gives a mean height which is converted to a mean concentration ($\bar{C}$) after calibration of the detector in terms of amplitude on the record.

Calibration of the detector is accomplished easily by obtaining a blood sample and adding a known amount of indicator to it. Then this mixed sample is drawn through the detector and the deflection is recorded. In this example, the indicator calibration amplitude corresponds to 0.43 g/L of indicator in blood. The mean concentration (area of the dilution curve divided by its base) corresponds to a mean concentration of 0.173 g/L of indicator in blood. Since the corrected dilution curve is 18.5 sec in duration, the cardiac output per minute is as follows:

$$CO = \frac{60 \times 0.15}{0.173 \times 18.5} = 2.81 \text{ L/min}$$

As stated previously, this value for cardiac output would be expressed as cardiac index, that is, cardiac output per square meter of body surface area. In this case the body weight of the dog was 12 kg. The body surface area was 0.59 m^2 (area $= 11.2W^{0.667}$, where W is body weight in grams and

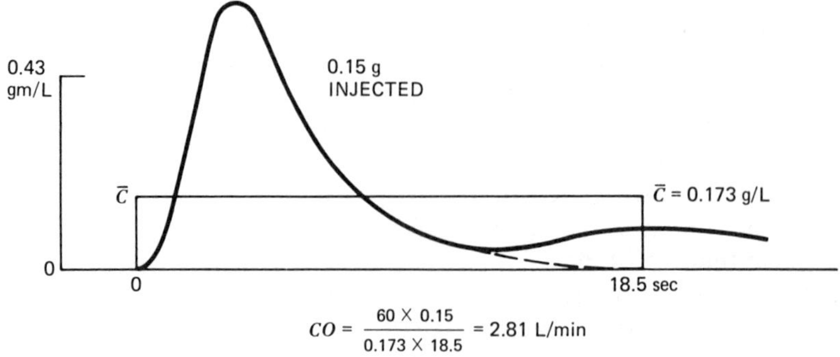

$$CO = \frac{60 \times 0.15}{0.173 \times 18.5} = 2.81 \text{ L/min}$$

FIGURE 4.7*a*. Calculation of cardiac output from the corrected dilution curve.

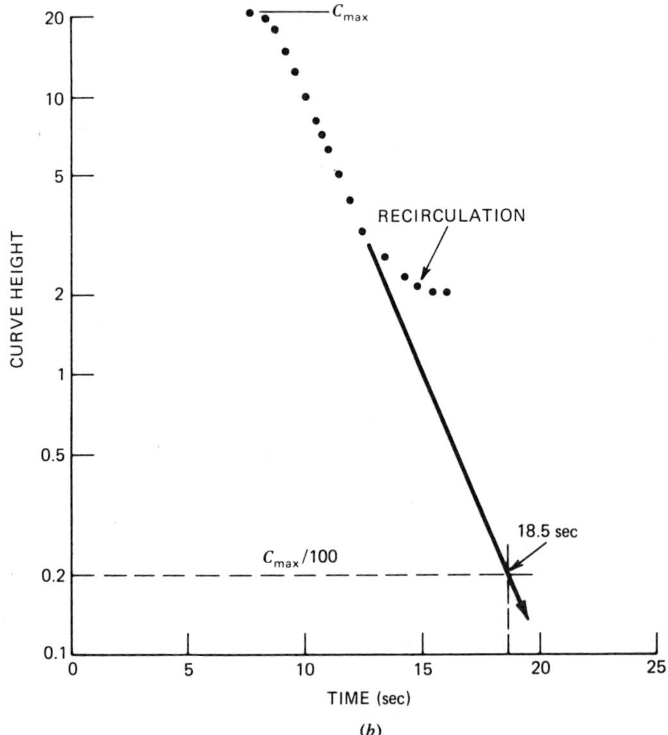

(*b*)

FIGURE 4.7*b*. Semilog plot of the downslope of the dilution curve shown in Figure 4.7*a*. Note that the portion of the downslope of the dilution curve that is exponential is linear on the semilog plot. Extrapolation of the line joining the points forming the straight line allows the acquisition of values for the dilution curve during recirculation. In practice, extrapolation is carried out to find a time corresponding to 1% of the maximum height of the dilution curve. In this example the end of the dilution curve was found to occur at 18.5 sec and the amplitudes between 12 sec (where recirculation became apparent) and 18.5 sec (the end of the curve) were used to complete the dilution curve shown in Figure 4.7*a*.

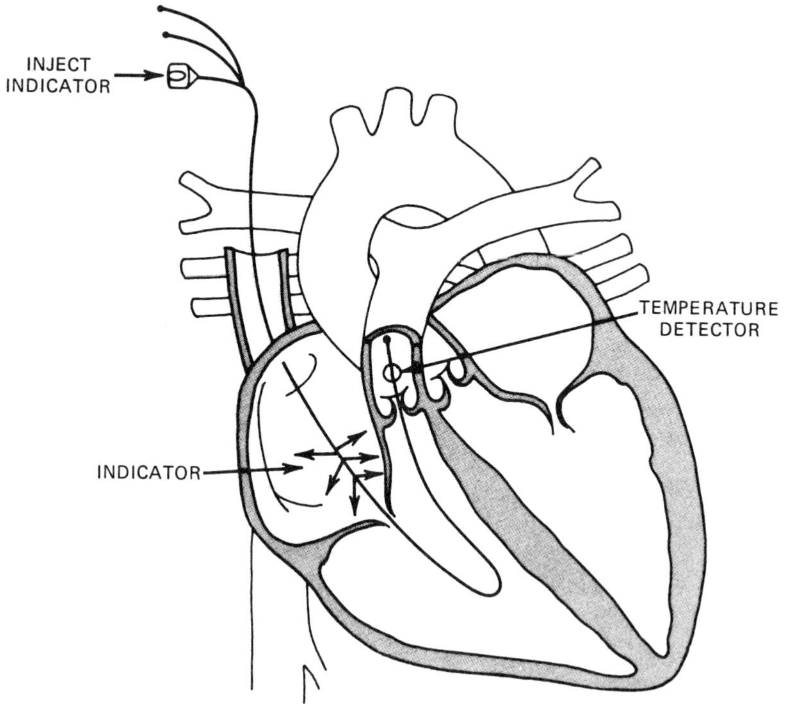

FIGURE 4.8. Method of injecting the thermal indicator into the heart.

the area is in square centimeters). Therefore, the cardiac index is 4.76 L/min/m^2; obviously, the animal was not in a basal state.

Thermal-Dilution Method

The thermal-dilution method in which the indicator is a cold liquid is a variant of the indicator-dilution method. A thermal detector is used to record the downstream decrease in temperature which, when recorded, constitutes the thermal-dilution curve. The most popular site for injection is the right atrium, and the detecting site is the pulmonary artery. A special balloon-tipped catheter (Swan et al., 1970), with a thermistor at the tip, is used to detect the temperature change. The same catheter has a side port which permits injection of the cold solution into the right atrium. Another lumen is used for pressure monitoring. Figure 4.8 illustrates the principle, and a typical thermal-dilution curve is shown in Figure 4.9.

The advantages of the thermal-dilution method are many and, in part, relate to the way it is used. Any suitable cold solution can be used as the

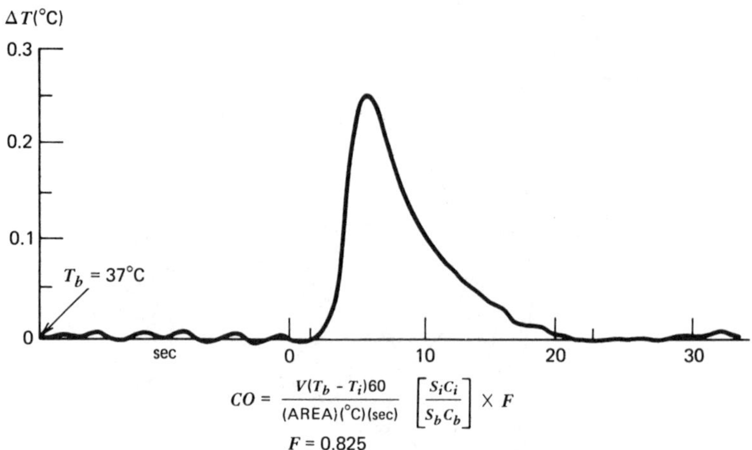

FIGURE 4.9. The thermal indicator-dilution curve.

indicator; isotonic dextrose (5%) at 0°C or at room temperature is the most popular. Because the detecting site is in the pulmonary artery and the indicator is injected into the right atrium, recirculation minimally obscures the downslope of the dilution curve. Therefore, a simple integrator can be used to determine the area under the dilution curve. Since the dilution curve is inscribed with a detector calibrated in degrees centigrade, it is not necessary to prepare calibrating solutions. Moreover, there is no indicator buildup, and dilution curves can be obtained as often as every few minutes. Diminishing these considerable advantages only slightly is the need to apply a correction factor to account for the heat transfer through the catheter and loss to the vessel walls during injection of the indicator. There is also the need to use an averaging technique to obtain the temperature of the pulmonary artery blood prior to injection of the thermoindicator. Figure 4.9 illustrates the small variations in temperature prior to appearance of the dilution curve.

The fact that a cold solution can be used as an indicator was reported by Fegler (1954) who validated the method in a model and then in dogs in which thermocouples were placed in the right ventricle and aorta. The indicator was 3–5 mL of Ringer's solution at 18°C, which was injected into the inferior vena cava. The model and the dog studies provided conclusive evidence for the accuracy of the method and the expression he developed for cardiac output. Additional corroborative data in dogs were provided by Goodyer et al. (1959), who used the dye and Fick methods as references. Two important improvements were reported in this study: (1) a thermistor was employed as the detector and (2) a correction factor was applied to compensate for heat transfer through the catheter. The method was then used in man by Ganz et al. (1971) with 5% dextrose in water at 0°C as the indicator. To reduce the need for correcting for heat loss in the catheter, a thermistor at the injection site was used to measure the temperature of the indicator as it entered the right atrium. The cardiac output values were compared with those obtained using cardiogreen dye; excellent agreement was obtained. Finally, the technique was made practical enough for bedside use by Forrester et al. (1972) who developed a balloon-tipped catheter that incorporated a thermistor at the tip. A second lumen in the catheter allowed recording pressure from the catheter tip. A third lumen communicated with an injection port 30 cm proximal from the tip of the catheter in the pulmonary artery. The catheter was introduced into an arm vein, advanced into the right atrium, where the balloon was inflated. The blood flow guided the tip into the right ventricle, and its presence there was confirmed by recording the pressure. Then the catheter was advanced into the pulmonary artery, its presence there being confirmed by the pressure recording. At this time the balloon was deflated and thermodilution curves were obtained by injection of the cold dextrose solution into the atrium via the third lumen which was in communication with the side port.

Verification Studies. After applying the correction factor for heat transfer through the #7F multilumen catheter, Forrester et al. obtained cardiac outputs on 40 critically ill patients. They validated the method with *in vitro* pump studies, and the average difference in flow amounted to about 3%. The most recent evaluation of the thermodilution method in man was presented by Weissel et al. (1975) who reported excellent agreement with values obtained with cardiogreen when a thermal correction factor was applied; Figure 4.10 presents the data.

Calculation of Cardiac Output. The expression for calculating cardiac output with the thermal-dilution method contains several terms not found in other indicator-dilution formulas because of the physical properties of the indicator and blood. The indicator is a cold solution, which abstracts calories from the blood that it contacts; thus, the indicator is negative calories. Heat-exchange calculations depend on the mass of material, its specific heat, and the temperature difference through which the material is raised or lowered. In fact, the product of these three quantities is the number of calories exchanged. For this reason the thermodilution equation must include specific heat terms. In addition, with the thermal-dilution method, a known volume (not mass) of cold liquid is injected. Volume can be converted to mass by multiplying by specific gravity.

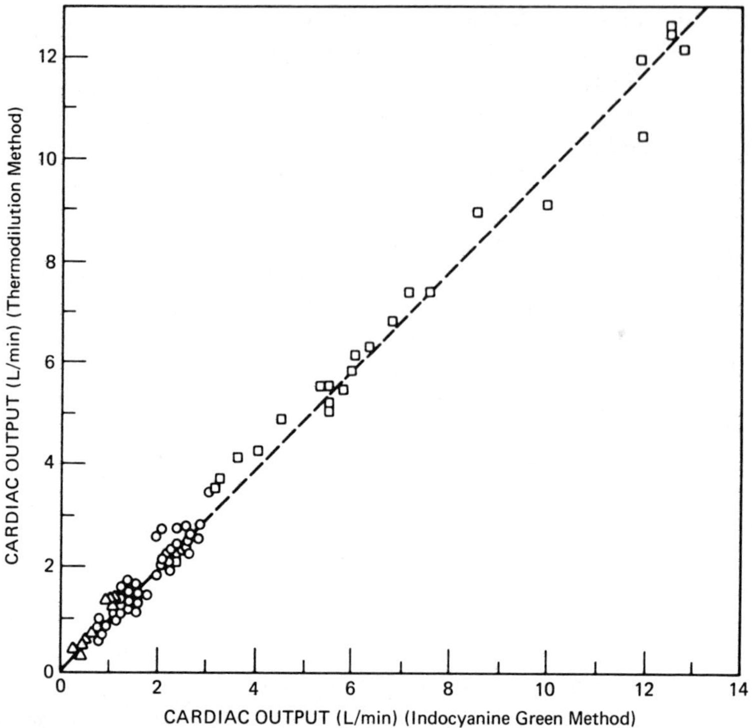

FIGURE 4.10. Eighty-three simultaneous measurements of cardiac output using thermodilution (CO_{TD}) and indocyanine green (CO_{IG}) showing close agreement [$r = 0.994 \pm 2.79$ (SEM)]. [From Weissel et al. (1975), by permission.]

Therefore, since the thermodilution method is based on heat exchange measured in calories, the flow equation must contain terms for the specific heat and the specific gravity of the indicator and blood.

The expression usually employed when a #7F thermistor-tipped catheter is employed and 5% dextrose is injected into the right atrium is as follows:

$$CO = \left(\frac{V\,(T_B - T_i)\,60}{A}\right)\left(\frac{S_i\,C_i}{S_b\,C_b}\right) F$$

where

V = Volume of indicator injected in mL

T_B = Temperature (average) of pulmonary artery blood in degrees centrigrade before injection of the indicator

T_i = Temperature of the indicator (°C)

60 = Multiplier required to convert mL/sec into mL/min
A = Area under the dilution curve in (sec) (°C)
S = Specific gravity of indicator (i) and blood (b)
C = Specific heat of indicator (i) and blood (b). The ratio $S_i C_i / S_b C_b = 1.08$ for 5% dextrose and blood of 40% packed-cell volume
F = Empiric factor employed to correct for heat transfer through the injection catheter. For a #7F catheter, $F = 0.825$ (Weissel et al. 1975).

Entering these factors into the expression gives

$$CO = \frac{V\,(T_B - T_i)\,53.46}{A}$$

where

CO = cardiac output in mL/min
53.46 = $60 \times 1.08 \times 0.825$

To illustrate how a thermodilution curve is processed, cardiac output will be calculated using the dilution curve shown in Figure 4.9:

V = 5 mL of 5% dextrose in water
T_B = 37°C
T_i = 0°C
A = 1.59°C · sec

$$CO = \frac{5\,(37 - 0)\,53.46}{1.59} = 6220 \text{ mL/min}$$

Despite the potential source of error due to heat loss through the injection catheter from which the empiric factor F is derived, the thermal-dilution method is remarkably reliable. Correlation values for cardiac output with cardiogreen dye in patients were reported by Weissel *et al.* (1975); these data are shown in Figure 4.10. The high degree of agreement using the empiric factor ($F = 0.825$) is impressive. Perhaps the most attractive feature of the thermal-dilution method is the minimal recirculation, which makes it easy to process the dilution curve by hand or a simple computer. In low-output situations, conventional dilution curves are obscured by recirculation and the endpoint is not easily determined. The lack of recirculation artifact with the thermal-dilution method makes it attractive in low-output situations. However, in very-low-output situations, there may be significant indicator heat loss to vessel walls, which will result in an overestimate of cardiac output.

Diffusible Indicators. In many instances, diffusible indicators, which leave the vascular bed via the capillaries, are used to measure cardiac output. Saline and dextrose 5% in water (D5W) are examples, and whether cardiac output is overestimated depends on the way the indicator is used. The determining factor is the presence or absence of a capillary bed between the point of indicator injection and measurement. If there is a intervening capillary bed, the indicator loss therein will result in an overestimate of cardiac output. However, if there is none, and good mixing is achieved, cardiac output will not be overestimated.

The foregoing explains why D5W, a diffusible indicator, can be used without error because injection is in the right atrium and measurement occurs in the pulmonary artery. Grubbs et al. (1983) has used saline, another diffusible indicator, to measure cardiac output without error by injecting it into the right atrium and detecting it in the pulmonary artery. Likewise we [Geddes et al. (1980)] measured left-sided output without error by injecting the saline in the left ventricle and measuring the dilution curve in the descending aorta.

If a diffusible indicator is injected into the venous system and the dilution curve recorded on the arterial side, an overestimate of 15% is typical. Chinard et al. (1962) predicted this situation, which was quantified by Grubbs et al. (1983) using saline.

IMPEDANCE CARDIOGRAPHY

The impedance cardiograph is an instrument that employs four circumferential thoracic electrodes to measure the pulsatile changes in resistance (impedance) offered to the flow of high-frequency alternating current to obtain a signal related to stroke volume. The pulsatile change in impedance is usually displayed on a graphic record, which can be processed to provide a value for stroke volume. At present, impedance cardiography is one of the very few noninvasive methods that provides a measure of stroke volume, which when multiplied by heart rate is cardiac output.

Principle

Figure 4.11 illustrates the principle employed in impedance cardiography. Low-intensity (e.g., a few milliamperes), high-frequency (e.g., 100 kHz) sinusoidal alternating current from a constant-current generator (I_k) is applied to metal-ribbon electrodes placed around the neck and abdomen

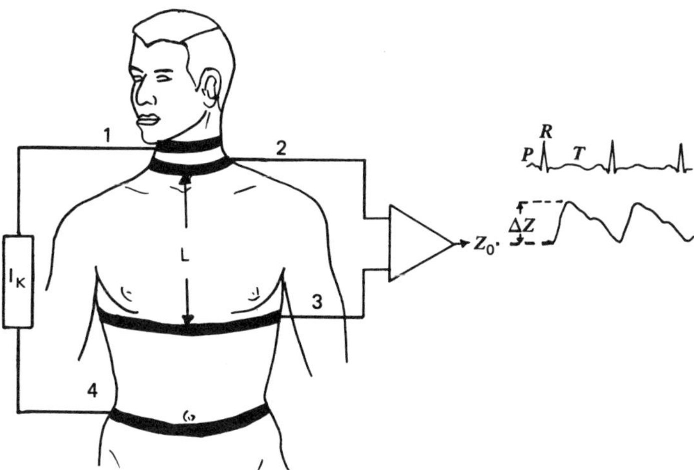

FIGURE 4.11. The tetrapolar method of recording the thoracic impedance cardiogram (Z_0 and ΔZ).

(1,4). With this arrangement, the same current flows through the subject irrespective of the subject size and electrode impedance. The flow of current through the thoracic tissues produces a potential difference detected by the two inner electrodes (2, 3), which are also metal ribbons placed around the thorax so that the heart is between them. Any variation in conducting properties of the thoracic contents will alter the potential difference between electrodes 2 and 3. Inspiration increases, and ejection of the stroke volume from the right and left ventricles decreases, the impedance between the potential-measuring electrodes. The respiratory-induced change is much larger than the cardiac-induced change. Therefore, to obtain a clear cardiac signal from electrodes 2 and 3, the subject must be breathing slowly or hold his breath for a few heart beats. Figure 4.12 illustrates the relative magnitude of the respiratory and cardiac impedance changes and Figure 4.13 illustrates typical cardiac impedance signals obtained during breath-holding.

High-frequency alternating current is used for impedance cardiography for reasons of safety. The change in thoracic impedance provides a high-frequency signal of varying amplitude appearing between electrodes 2 and 3. The varying alternating voltage is amplified and demodulated to provide an analog signal that can be recorded graphically.

Calculation of Stroke Volume

Various methods have been used to process the impedance cardiogram to obtain a value for stroke volume. The two that are presently used will be

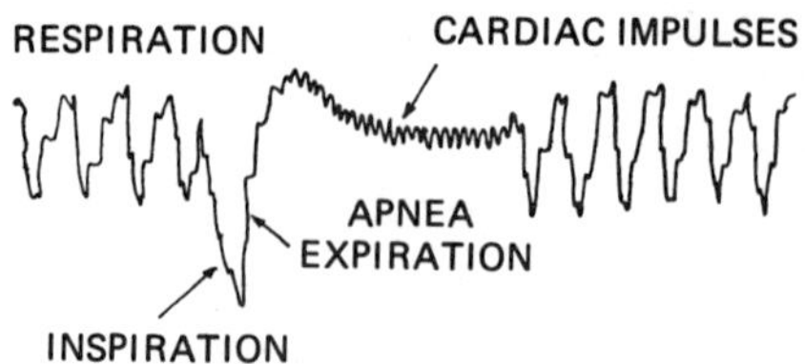

FIGURE 4.12. Respiratory and cardiac impedance changes.

described. It is important to recognize that the peak-to-peak value for ΔZ illustrated in Figure 4.11 is not the quantity used to calculate stroke volume, although it is related. The cardiac-induced impedance change reflects a change in impedance that is the difference between the inflow of blood to the thoracic vessels (from the heart) and the outflow of blood from the thoracic vessels to all other regions of the body. Therefore, to estimate the true volume change that would occur in the absence of thoracic outflow, the maximum rate of impedance change during the early ejection period is determined and used to obtain the impedance change that would have occurred with no outflow from the thoracic vessels. The rationale underlying this technique is that outflow from the thoracic vessels is minimum at the beginning of cardiac ejection. Figure 4.13 illustrates the cardiac impedance pulse and the graphical extrapolation technique used to obtain the corrected value ($\Delta Z'$) for entry in the equation developed by Kubicek et al. (1966):

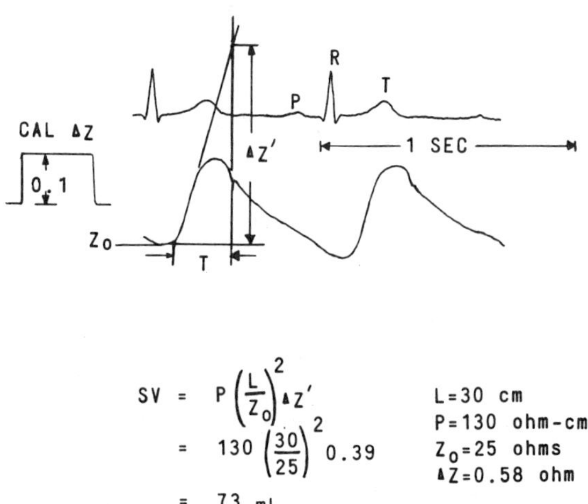

$$SV = P\left(\frac{L}{Z_0}\right)^2 \Delta Z'$$

$$= 130\left(\frac{30}{25}\right)^2 0.39$$

$$= 73 \text{ mL}$$

L = 30 cm
P = 130 ohm-cm
Z_0 = 25 ohms
ΔZ = 0.58 ohm

FIGURE 4.13. The impedance cardiogram pulse and its relation to the *R* and *T* waves of the ECG, along with a sample calculation of stroke volume.

$$SV = P\left(\frac{PL^2}{Z_0^2}\right)\left(\Delta Z'\right)$$

In this expression P is the resistivity of blood in ohm-cm at body temperature, L is the distance between the voltage-measuring electrodes (2,3) in cm, and Z_0 is the basal impedance of the thorax in ohms, which is the baseline on which the pulsatile impedance rides, and $\Delta Z'$ is the extrapolated impedance change in ohms, as shown in Figure 4.13.

Because extrapolation of the rising phase of the cardiac-induced impedance change is open to subjective error, it is often more convenient to include an electrical differentiation circuit in the impedance cardiograph. Thus two output signals are provided: one is the cardiac-induced impedance change (ΔZ) and the other is the time derivative or differential (dZ/dt) as shown in Figure 4.14. By knowing the maximum rate of change of impedance $(dZ/dt)_{max}$ and the period over which it occurs, namely, the ejection period (T), the following expression can be used to calculate stroke volume:

$$SV = P\left(\frac{L^2}{Z_0^2}\right)(T)\left(\frac{dZ}{dt}\right)_{max}$$

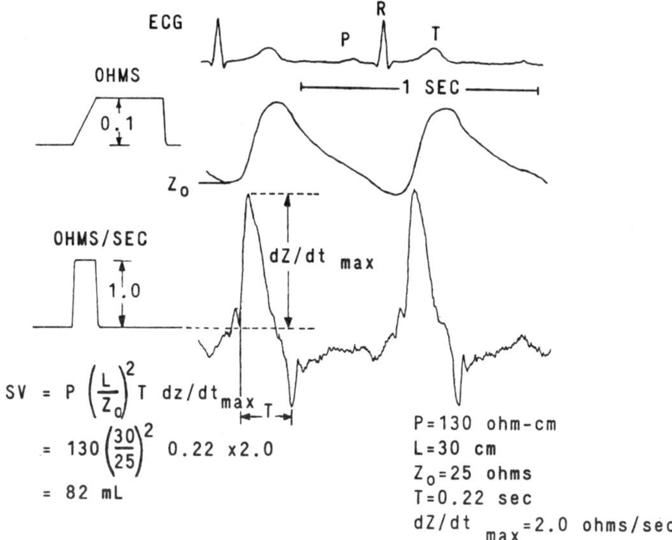

FIGURE 4.14. The impedance cardiogram and its time derivative (dZ/dt), along with a sample calculation of stroke volume.

TABLE 4.7. Resistivity of Blood at 37°C[a]

Species	Resistivity (ohm-cm)	Correlation Coefficient
Dog	$55.5e^{0.024H}$	0.98
Human	$51.6e^{0.024H}$	0.97
Babboon	$57.5e^{0.019H}$	0.99
Cow	$59.9e^{0.016H}$	0.97
Goat	$58.3e^{0.015H}$	0.99
Cat	$53.9e^{0.023H}$	0.99
Monkey	$53.7e^{0.019H}$	0.99
Sheep	$56.9e^{0.0.19H}$	0.97
Camel	$56.4e^{0.016H}$	0.98
Average for nine species	$55.2e^{0.02H}$	0.96

[a] Data obtained for packed-cell volumes (H) ranging from 0 to 50%.

Calibration signals in the impedance cardiograph allow quantification of the record to obtain Z_0 and $(dZ/dt)_{\max}$. Figure 4.14 illustrates a typical record. The value for the resistivity of blood depends on the percent packed-cell volume (H). For humans, the resistivity in ohm-cm was given by Geddes and Baker (1975) as:

$$P = 51.6e^{0.024H}$$

Often it is undesirable to draw a blood sample to measure the packed-cell volume (H) or resistivity. In such a case it is often assumed that a normal packed-cell volume of 40% exists. Therefore, the resistivity at 37°C is 130 ohm-cm. Table 4.7 presents values for a variety of species.

Verification Studies

Of particular importance is the relationship between cardiac output measured by impedance cardiography and by conventional techniques such as the indicator-dilution and Fick methods. Table 4.8 presents a summary of the validation studies to 1974. In some of these studies, the correct value for blood resistivity was used; in others an assumed value or a room-temperature value was entered into the equation. Nonetheless, it would apear that, in general, impedance cardiography provides a value for cardiac output that agrees with the true value (as obtained by an accepted method) or overestimates cardiac output by as much as about 25%. A recent comparative study by Denniston *et al.* (1976) is shown in Figure 4.15.

A large number of studies have shown that impedance cardiography tracks changes in cardiac output with good accuracy; this point was made by Denniston *et al.* (1976) in a study of normal subjects exercising on a bicycle ergometer. Figure 4.16 illustrates the ability of the impedance cardiogram to track cardiac output as determined by the indicator-dilution method using indocyanine-green dye.

Mohapatra *et al.* (1977) pointed out the important fact that the degree of overestimation of cardiac output by the impedance method is dependent on the packed-cell volume. From a study on infants and adults they developed a correction factor (F), which when multiplied by the impedance cardiac output gives true cardiac output. Thus the Kubicek stroke-volume expression becomes

$$SV = \frac{PL^2TF}{Z_0^2}\left(\frac{dZ}{dt}\right)_{\max}$$

The value for F is shown in Figure 4.17 and the mathematical expression for it is

$$F = 2.524 - 1.121 \log_{10} H$$

in which H is the packed-cell volume in percent. Note that for a packed-cell volume of 40%, the value for F is 0.83.

A practical consideration worthy of note is the value of L, the separation between the two (inner) potential-measuring electrodes. Usually this dimension measured along the sternum is different than the magnitude when measured along midaxillary lines and on the back. In this situation it is of value to determine the mean value for L by making multiple measurements (chest, back, and along midaxillary lines). This technique was advocated by Denniston et al. (1976). Because stroke volume is usually overestimated, some advocate using the minimum value for L.

In conclusion, although cardiac-output values obtained by impedance cardiography usually overestimate cardiac output, the technique is of considerable value in a variety of situations when invasive measurements cannot be made. It must be emphasized that the comparison studies made to date in humans were based on techniques (e.g., Fick and indicator-dilution) that averaged cardiac output over a minute or more, whereas the impedance method provided a value for stoke volume that was multiplied by average heart rate to obtain cardiac output. The fact that it is sometimes necessary for the subject to stop breathing for a few heart beats irritates some investigators. However, its ability to provide a value for stroke volume on a beat-by-beat basis is a highly attractive feature. Many

TABLE 4.8. Verification of Cardiac Output Values Determined by Impedance Cardiography[a]

Cardiac Output Relationship (L/min) $Z(\mathrm{CO}) = A(CO) + B$	Correlation Coefficient	Standard Error of Estimate	Subjects	Reference Method for $A(CO) + B$	ΔZ Processing Method	Principal Investigate and Year	Remarks
$0.942(CO) + 0.007$	0.959	0.026	Dog	Fick	Backslope	Allison (1966)	14–42 kg body weight
$1.124(CO) - 0.097$	0.976	0.107	Dog	Cardio-green	Backslope	Allison (1966)	14–42 kg body weight
$1.18(CO)$	—	—	Human	Cardio-green	Max derivative	Kubicek (1966)	Resting and postexercise
$0.86(CO) + 2.93$	0.680	2.33	Human	Dye	Forward slope	Harley (1967)	24 cardiac patients
$0.73(CO) + 4.91$	0.579	2.34	Human	Radioisotope	Max derivative	Judy (1969)	
$0.71(CO) + 2.06$	0.83	—	Human	Cardio-green	Max derivative	Smith (1970)	Adults—tilt table
$0.90(CO) + 0.62$	0.94	—	Human	Cardio-green	Max derivative	Smith (1970)	Adult—tilt table
$0.8(CO)$ to $1.2(CO)$	0.95	—	Human	Fick	Double slope	Kinnen (1970)	25 patients
$0.8(CO)$ to $1.2(CO)$	0.84	—	Human	Fick	Double slope	Kinnen (1970)	67 patients
$0.8(CO)$ to $4.3(CO)$	0.58	—	Human	Radioisotope	Max derivative	Baker (1971)	17 normal adults
$1.0(CO) + 0.52$	0.68	1.63	Human	Cardio-green	Max derivative	Baker (1971)	10 normal adults

$0.96(CO) + 0.56$	0.66	1.54	Human	Cardio-green	Max derivative	Baker (1971)	21 normal adults
$1.43(CO) + 1.08$	0.923	0.593	Human	Cardio-green	Max derivative	Van De Water (1971)	One subject
ca. $1.055(CO)$	—	—	Human	Cardio-green	Max derivative	Lababidi (1971)	Children (cardiac patients)
$0.91(CO) + 0.218$	0.92	—	Dog	EM flowmeter	Max derivative	Baker (1971)	Aortic blood flow
Stroke-Volume Relationship (mL) $Z(SV) = P(SV) + Q$							
$1.42(SV) + 3.5$	0.94	—	Human	Pressure gradient	Max derivative	Bache (1969)	Cardiac patient
$1.42(SV) - 5.8$	0.96	—	Human	Pressure gradient	Max derivative	Bache (1969)	Cardiac patient
$0.93(SV) + 2.0$	0.91	—	Human	Pressure gradient	Max derivative	Bache (1969)	Cardiac patient
$0.44(SV) + 5.3$	0.58	—	Human	Pressure gradient	Max derivative	Bache (1969)	Cardiac patient
$1.37(SV) + 12.4$	0.62	—	Human	Pressure gradient	Max derivative	Bache (1969)	Cardiac patient
$0.65(SV) - 1.0$	0.78	—	Human	Pressure gradient	Max derivative	Bache (1969)	Cardiac patient
$0.77(SV) + 0.4$	0.68	—	Human	Pressure gradient	Max derivative	Bache (1969)	Cardiac patient
$1.53(SV) - 5.5$	0.87	—	Human	Pressure gradient	Max derivative	Bache (1969)	Cardiac patient
$0.92(SV) + 2.3$	0.94	1.9	Dog	EM flowmeter	Max derivative	Kubicek (1970)	Aortic blood flow
$0.90(SV) + 15.2$	0.87	—	Human	Cardio-green	Max derivative	Smith (1970)	Head up (8 subjects)
$1.01(SV) + 0.82$	0.96	—	Human	Cardio-green	Max derivative	Smith (1970)	Head up (8 subjects)

[a] Geddes and Baker (1975).

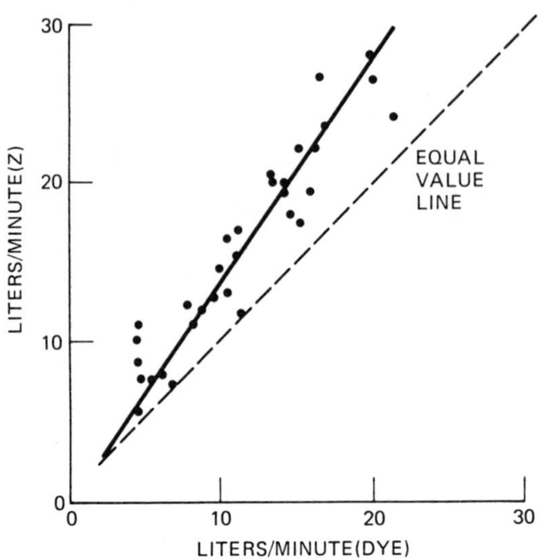

FIGURE 4.15. The relationship between impedance cardiac output (solid line) and dye-cardiac output in exercising subjects. [Redrawn from Denniston et al. (1976). By permission.]

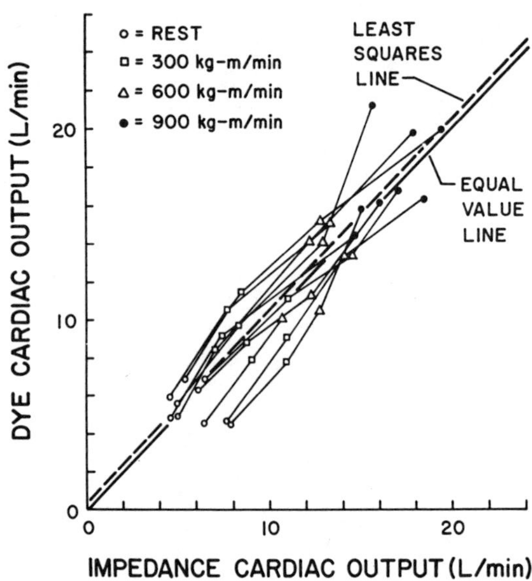

FIGURE 4.16. The relationship between dye-cardiac output and impedance cardiac output (corrected) in subjects exercising on a bicycle ergometer. [Redrawn from Denniston et al. (1976). By permission.]

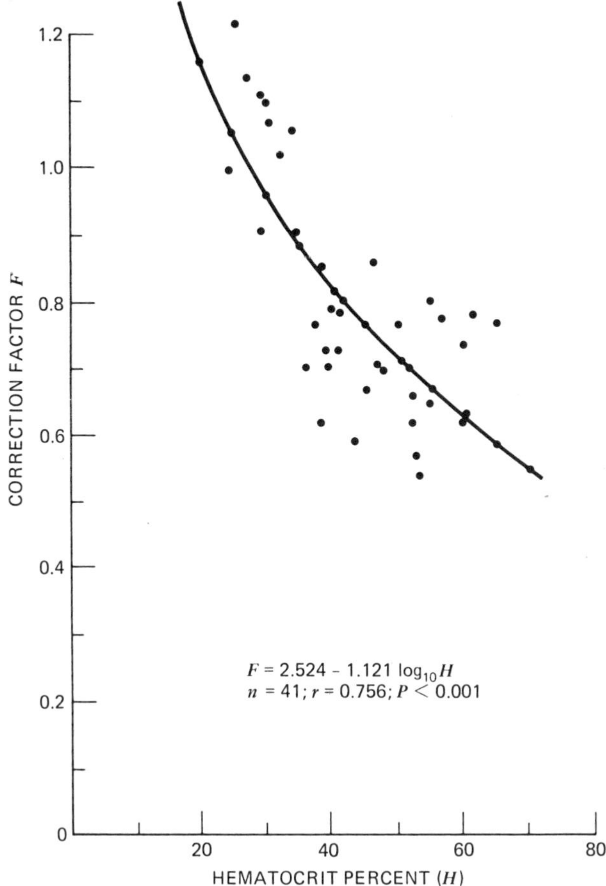

FIGURE 4.17. The correction factor (F) reported by Mohapatra *et al.* (1977) for correcting impedance cardiac output values.

newer instruments incorporate processing circuitry so that graphic recording is not needed and cardiac output is indicated on a digital display.

VENOUS-OCCLUSION PLETHYSMOGRAPHY

The ability of the venous system to drain a body segment is evaluated by measuring the segmental volume change that occurs when an occlusion is removed from the venous outflow. Devices that provide such volume changes can be air or water-filled chambers (plethysmographs) that sur-round a body segment. Recordings of such volume changes are called plethysmograms (*plethore* meaning fullness).

Whenever blood flows very slowly or becomes stagnant, there is an ever-present danger of clot formation. This situation is always present in the venous system, which is characterized by low flow velocities. In some subjects, blood clots (thrombi) form in the venous system and block venous return. Although collateral veins often open to provide a return path, there is always a danger of the thrombus breaking loose, that is, becoming an embolus, and being carried through a right heart and lodging in the lung vessels, plugging a branch of the pulmonary artery. When this occurs, the alveoli served by the plugged vessel can no longer transport oxygen into the blood and remove carbon dioxide from it. Therefore, there will be an overall reduction in gas-transport capability of the lungs.

The ability to detect a venous obstruction early is obviously highly desirable because anticoagulant therapy can be applied to reduce the likelihood of development of additional thrombi. Just how much anticoagulant therapy dissolves existing clots is controversial. It should be noted, however, that anticoagulant therapy reduces clot formation everywhere. Therefore, the therapy must be applied with great care to avoid excessive bleeding from superficial skin wounds.

Although air and water-filled plethysmographs have been used with success to measure venous drainage (Andrews and Wheeler, 1979), the electrical impedance method introduced by Wheeler et al. (1973, 1974) appears to be the most practical clinically. This method has become known as venous-occlusion impedance plethysmography or venous-occlusion phlebography (VOP); the technique is illustrated in Figure 4.18. Four metal-ribbon electrodes are placed around the body segment (arm or leg) in which venous drainage is to be evaluated. Central (toward the heart) to the four electrodes is placed a blood-pressure cuff, which is used to arrest venous outflow but not arterial flow into the segment. This is accomplished by suddenly inflating the cuff, typically to between 30–60 mm Hg. The procedure will be described subsequently. The impedance recorder is connected to the four electrodes on the member. The two outer electrodes provide a constant, low-level (100–4000 μA) alternating current (25–100 kHz). The two inner electrodes (2,3) detect the voltage that is dependent on the applied current, the spacing between the electrodes, and the impedance of the intervening tissue. The impedance is inversely related to the volume of the tissue between the two inner electrodes (2,3), which may be 10 cm apart. The voltage detected by the two inner electrodes is processed to provide a recordable signal, which identifies the limb segment volume and any changes that it experiences.

Prior to cuff inflation, the impedance record shows a steady baseline

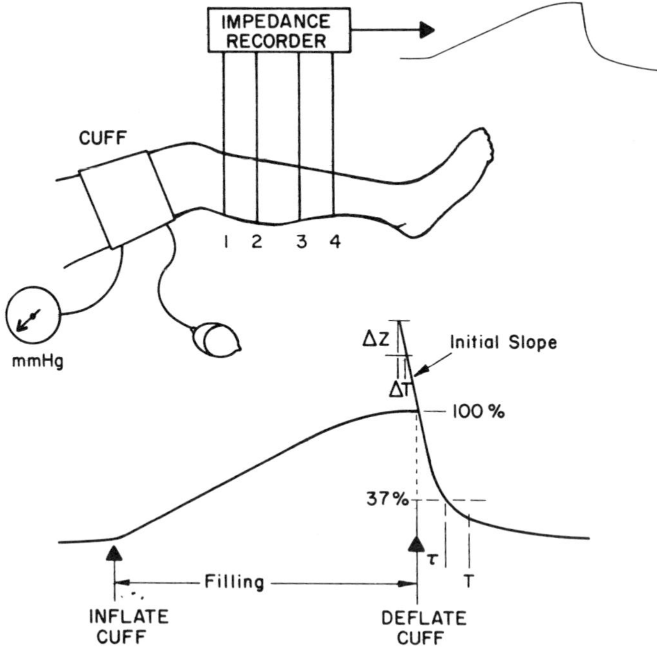

FIGURE 4.18. Principle employed in venous-occlusion plethysmography using electrical impedance to indicate segmented volume changes.

because arterial inflow and venous outflow are equal. Venous occlusion is accomplished by suddenly inflating the cuff to about 40 mm Hg and blood starts to accumulate in the body segment and the impedance decreases slowly, being displayed as a gradual rise in the recording (phlebogram) as shown in Figure 4.18. As venous pressure increases, the rate of rise in the recording decreases and typically reaches a plateau in about a minute in normal subjects. Sometimes the occlusion period is shorter, that is, 30–45 sec. The cuff is then deflated quickly (by 90% in 0.2 sec or less) and the venous system drains the engorged segment. The normal impedance phlebogram displays a rapid exponentiallike fall as shown in Figure 4.18. Several different measurements are made on the release portion of the impedance phlebogram. Since the outflow after cuff deflation approximates an exponential curve, the time constant τ (time to 37% amplitude) after deflation is measured. Another measurement is the initial slope ($\Delta Z/\Delta T$) at the instant of cuff deflation. The fall to V_0 (Figure 4.19) at a specified time T (e.g., 30 or 45 sec) is also a descriptor of the rapidity of venous drainage. Impaired venous drainage increases the time constant, decreases the initial deflation slope, and produces less fall to V_0 for the T sec value.

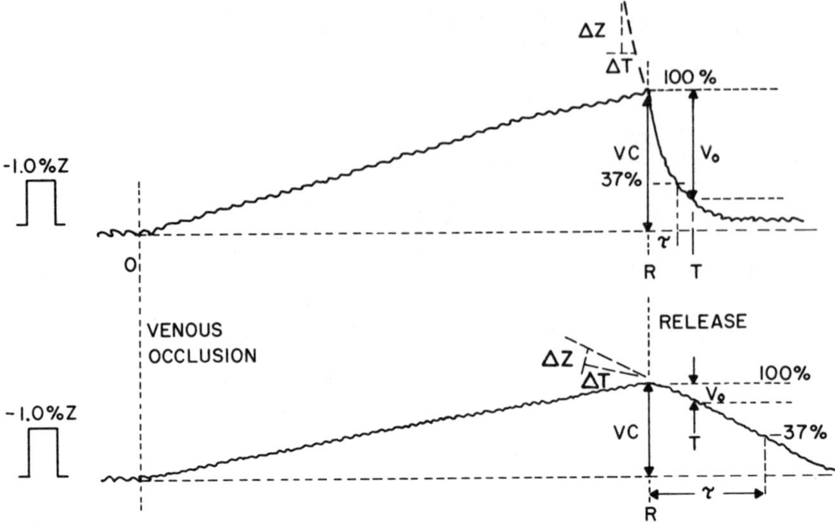

FIGURE 4.19. Venous-occlusion phlebogram for a normal subject (upper) and a subject with venous occlusive disease (lower). Note the differences in postocclusion slope $\Delta Z/\Delta T$, time constant (τ), and timed (T) impedance change V_o. [Redrawn from Andrews and Wheeler (1979).]

In a subject with impaired venous outflow the post cuff-deflation outflow time is increased as shown in Figure 4.19. This figure illustrates how the time constant (τ), initial slope ($\Delta Z/\Delta T$) and fall to V_0 in time T are altered. In venous-occlusive disease Andrews and Wheeler (1979) reported on the relative merits of each of these factors to identify venous offlusion; their data are shown in Table 4.9.

At present, venous-occlusion phlebography is one of the simplest methods for identifying deep venous occlusion. The technique is easily applied, is nonhazardous, and requires minimal cooperation from the patient. Its place in clinical medicine is, however, yet to be established.

TABLE 4.9. Evaluation of Methods for Analyzing Impedance Phlebograms[a]

Method	Accuracy (%)
Time constant	88
Outflow slope	91
3-sec Amplitude	95

[a] From Andrews and Wheeler (1979).

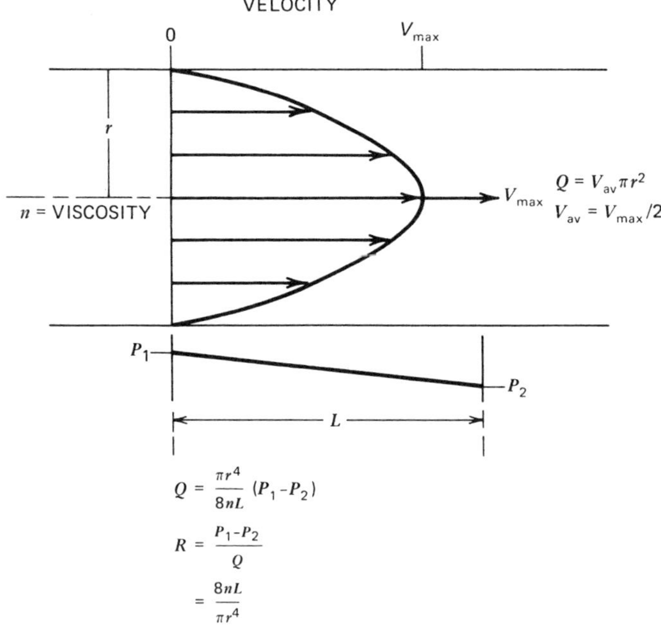

FIGURE 4.20. Poiseuille's law and laminar flow in a tube. With laminar flow, the velocity profile is parabolic and the maximum velocity (V_{max}) is twice the average velocity (V_{av}). The flow (Q) is equal to the cross-sectional area (πr^2) multiplied by the average velocity. The flow (Q) is also given by Poiseuille's law, which relates the pressure drop ($P_1 - P_2$), radius (r), viscosity (n), and length (L) of tubing between which the two pressures (P_1,P_2) are measured. The resistance (R) to flow is the pressure drop ($P_1 - P_2$) divided by flow (Q).

RESISTANCE TO BLOOD FLOW

Poiseuille's Law

Resistance is defined as pressure divided by flow. Poiseuille's law relates pressure, flow, and resistance in an hydraulic circuit in the same way that Ohm's law relates voltage, current, and resistance in an electrical circuit.

A simple illustration of Poiseuille's law is presented in Figure 4.20, which identifies the driving pressure or pressure drop ($P_1 - P_2$), measured between the ends of a tube of length L and inner radius r, in which a fluid of viscosity n is flowing. The flow Q is given by Poiseuille's law, which stated mathematically is

$$Q = \frac{\pi r^4 (P_1 - P_2)}{8n\, L}$$

In this expression, the radius (r) and length (L) are in cm, the pressure difference ($P_1 - P_2$) is in dyn/cm^2, and the viscosity (n) is in poise.

The viscosity of a fluid is the internal frictional force that opposes flow. For example, molasses, which has a high viscosity, flows less easily than water, which has a low viscosity. The unit of viscosity is the dyne per cm/cm per sec, or dyn-sec/cm^2; this unit is called the poise, after Poiseuille.

Since resistance (R) is the ratio of pressure difference ($P_1 - P_2$) to flow (Q), then

$$R = \frac{P_1 - P_2}{Q} = \frac{8n\,L}{\pi r^4}$$

The expression clearly shows that the resistance (R) is proportional to the length (L) of the tube and the viscosity (n) of the fluid within it. Note also that the resistance varies inversely with the fourth power of the radius, which means that a very small decrease in radius will increase the resistance considerably.

Poiseuille's law was developed to describe the flow of an ideal fluid with a constant viscosity. In addition, the law refers to laminar, that is, nonturbulent flow. In such a case, the velocity profile across the diameter is parabolic, with the peak velocity being twice the average velocity. Despite the fact that Poiseuille's law was developed with these constraints, the concepts that it embodies are generally applicable to cardiovascular physiology. Perhaps it is pertinent to note that flow in physiological systems may not be laminar; often the flow-velocity profile approximates a trapezoid across the vessel diameter. This flow pattern is called plug flow, because the profile approximates the shape of a plug. In addition, blood is not a simple fluid and its viscosity is not constant, being dependent on the packed-cell volume and the velocity of flow. Notwithstanding these features, the concept of Poiseuille's law is very useful in understanding physiological systems.

Poiseuille's law states that the flow in a given system is related to the driving pressure ($P_1 - P_2$) and the viscosity (n). The viscosity of blood is dependent on the packed-cell volume in a complex way. In fact, blood viscosity is difficult to measure accurately. Nonetheless, it is possible to illustrate the effect of changing viscosity on flow. Figure 4.21 illustrates this point. Note that for a given driving pressure, increasing viscosity decreases the volume flow.

Peripheral Resistance

In the cardiovascular system, the mean pressure decreases from the left ventricle to the capillaries. It must be recognized that the arterial system

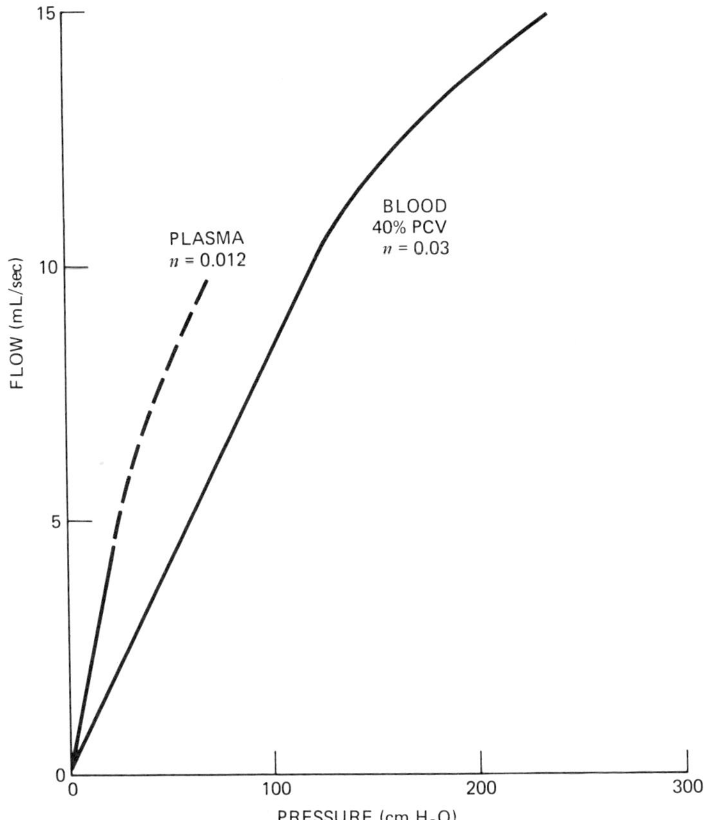

FIGURE 4.21. The relationship between flow and pressure for plasma and blood in a long slender tube. Note that with low pressure, flow is linearly proportional to the applied pressure, as predicted by Poiseuille's law. Note also that the flow for blood is less than that for plasma, which has a lower viscosity. With higher pressure, the velocity exceeds the limit for laminar flow, as predicted by the Reynolds number (980). Beyond this point, turbulence occurs and the flow is no longer linearly proportional to the applied pressure.

branches extensively along this route and, therefore, the total cross-sectional area facing the left ventricle increases. Figure 4.22 illustrates this point, which carries an important implication, namely, the velocity of blood flow through the capillaries is very slow. Because it is in the capillaries where metabolic exchange takes place, the low flow velocity along the many parallel capillary paths provides the time for this exchange to occur.

The total peripheral resistance is the opposition to blood flow presented to the left ventricle. To calculate peripheral resistance the mean pressure difference (mean aortic minus mean venous pressure) is divided

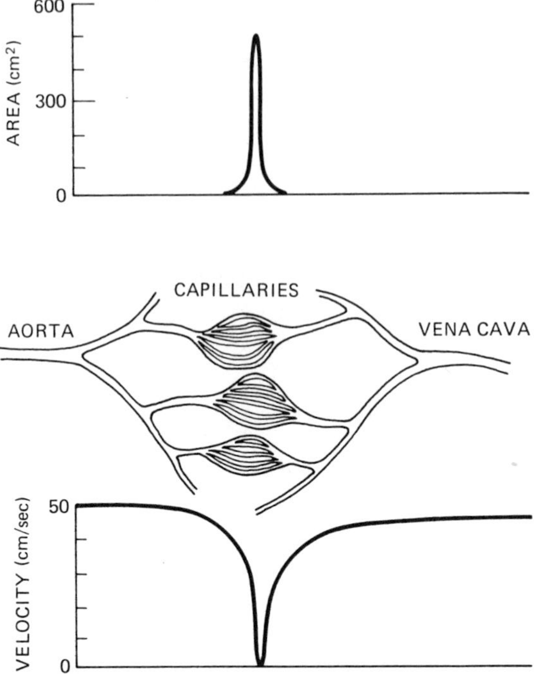

FIGURE 4.22. Total vascular cross-sectional area and blood flow velocity from the aorta to the vena cava.

by cardiac output. However, since mean venous pressure is usually negligible with respect to mean aortic pressure, it is often ignored. Hence, peripheral resistance is approximately mean aortic pressure divided by cardiac output. Pulmonary vascular resistance is calculated by dividing mean pulmonary artery pressure minus left atrial mean pressure by pulmonary blood flow. In a normal subject, pulmonary blood flow is essentially the same left ventricular (cardiac) output. In patients with cardiovascular shunts, this situation does not prevail.

Unfortunately in cardiovascular studies, several different systems of units are used to describe the resistance of blood flow. The most familiar units for pressure (mm Hg) and flow (L/min) are often converted into other units to perform the calculation of resistance. This situation has resulted in the appearance of three systems of units: peripheral resistance units (PRU), hybrid resistance units (HRU), and absolute resistance units (ARU). The quantities that underlie these units will now be discussed.

Peripheral Resistance Units (PRU). The earliest expressions for the resistance to blood flow employed two different methods to calculate resistance. One method expressed peripheral resistance as the mean pressure difference in mm Hg divided by the flow in mL/min. Another method expressed peripheral resistance in terms of mm Hg divided by mL/sec. This latter method provides a value for PRU near unity for the arterial system of a normal subject. With a mean aortic pressure of 93 mm Hg and a cardiac output of 5000 mL/min, the output per second is 5000/60 = 83.3; the peripheral resistance is then 93/83.3 = 1.12 PRU. In summary:

$$\text{PRU} = \frac{\text{mm Hg}}{\text{mL/sec}}$$

Hybrid Resistance Units (HRU). Ordinarily, pressure is in mm Hg and flow is in L/min; therefore, the number of hybrid resistance units (HRU) for these quantities is

$$\text{HRU} = \frac{\text{mm Hg}}{\text{L/min}}$$

For example, the pulmonary vascular resistance in HRU can be calculated from the pulmonary blood flow and the pressure drop across the pulmonary vascular circuit (i.e., mean pulmonary artery pressure minus mean left atrial pressure). Therefore, if the mean pulmonary artery pressure is 15 mm Hg and left atrial pressure is 8 mm Hg when the pulmonary blood flow is 5 L/min, the pulmonary vascular resistance R_p (in HRU) is

$$R_p = \frac{15 - 8}{5} = 1.4 \text{ HRU}$$

Absolute Resistance Units (ARU). In the absolute system, pressure is expressed in dyn/cm^2 and flow is expressed in mL/sec; mm Hg is converted to cm H_2O by multiplying by 13.6 and dividing by 10. In order to convert the resulting pressure to dyn/cm^2, it is necesary to multiply by the gravitation constant, 980. Cardiac output in L/min is multiplied by 1000 to obtain mL/min and divided by 60 to obtain mL/sec. Therefore,

$$\begin{aligned} \text{ARU} &= \frac{\text{mm Hg } (13.6/10)980}{\text{L/min } (1000/60)} \\ &= 79.95 \frac{\text{mmHg}}{\text{L/min}} = 79.95 \text{ HRU} \\ &\doteq 80 \text{ HRU} \end{aligned}$$

Therefore, it can be seen that by multiplying the resistance obtained in hybrid resistance units (HRU) by 80, the number of absolute resistance

TABLE 4.10. Vascular Resistance Values

	PRU[a]	ARU[b]	HRU[c]
Arterial system (normal)	0.71–0.98	950 – 1300	11.9–16.2
Pulmonary system (normal)	0.12–0.19	205 ± 50	1.94–3.19
Arterial system (moderate exercise)	0.47	626	7.82
Arterial system (essential hypertension)	1.50–4.35	2000 – 5800	25–72.5

[a]PRU = mm Hg/mL/sec.

[b]ARU = dyn/cm^2 per mL/sec.

[c]HRU = mm Hg/L/minute.

ARU = (HRU) 80.

ARU = (PRU) 1333.

units is obtained. It is interesting to note that the units contained in the HRU term are dyn-sec/cm^5.

Typical Values for Vascular Resistance. Table 4.10 presents the resistance to blood flow offered by two vascular beds. Note that all of the cardiac output flows through the lungs and the systemic circuit; but the pulmonary vascular resistance is much less than that of the arterial circuit.

An interesting sidelight on peripheral resistance is presented by subjects with hypertension (elevated arterial pressure). Interestingly, the cardiac output may be essentially normal but the peripheral resistance is elevated, being in the range of 2000–5800 dyn-sec/cm^5. The peripheral resistance in normal subjects is typically 950–1300 dyn-sec/cm^5.

In its early stages, hypertension may produce few symptoms. However, because the heart must develop more pressure and hence do more work per unit time, it hypertrophies and needs more oxygen to meet this need. Ultimately, it may not have an adequate coronary circulation for its oxygen requirements. If this happens, the heart will fail. In addition, because the blood vessels must sustain a higher pressure at all times, there is the danger of a vascular accident, that is, rupture of a blood vessel. Therefore, hypertension is a condition that must be treated as soon as detected.

TURBULENT FLOW AND THE REYNOLDS NUMBER

Poiseuille's law states that the volume flow per unit time (Q) is proportional to the driving pressure ($P_1 - P_2$). While this linear relationship is true, it applies only to a finite limit of flow velocity; beyond this point, turbulence occurs and the flow is no longer linearly proportional to the applied pressure. In practice, this transition point is not clearly defined as shown in Figure 4.21. The transition is identified by a dimensionless quantity known as the Reynolds number, named after the engineer who developed the concept of critical velocity for the appearance of turbulence, which is characterized by the presence of eddies. The resulting velocity profile is not parabolic, as is the case with laminar flow, to which Poiseuille's law applies.

In an experimental study, with long straight tubes of different diameters, Reynolds discovered that turbulence was associated with a dimensionless number N (later called the Reynolds number) that describes the ratio of inertial to viscous forces in a fluid. The inertial forces are identified by the density and the viscous forces by the viscosity. The Reynolds number (N) is given by the following

$$N = \frac{\bar{V}pr}{n}$$

In this expression $\bar{V}$ is the average velocity, p is the density, and n is the viscosity of the fluid flowing in a long tube of radius r. Reynolds found that when this dimensionless number exceeded 2000, laminar or streamline flow changed to turbulent flow in an hydraulic system.

The factors embodied in the Reynolds number are important because they identify that for any given fluid (i.e., density and viscosity are defined), there exists a critical relationship between diameter and flow velocity for the limit of laminar flow. In addition, it can be seen that the ratio of density to viscosity (p/n) plays an important role in identifying the point of turbulent flow. Figures 4.23 and 4.24 present approximate values for specific gravity and viscosity for blood.

By a simple rearrangement of the expression containing the Reynolds number, it is possible to illustrate the concept of a critical average velocity ($\bar{V}_c$) for the development of turbulence. Performing this rearrangement gives

$$\bar{V}_c = \frac{Nn}{rp}$$

The concept can be extended to identify a critical flow (Q_c) by recognizing that flow is equal to the mean velocity multiplied by the tube area (πr^2). Therefore, the idealized critical average flow for tubulence becomes

$$Q_c = \frac{\pi rnN}{p}$$

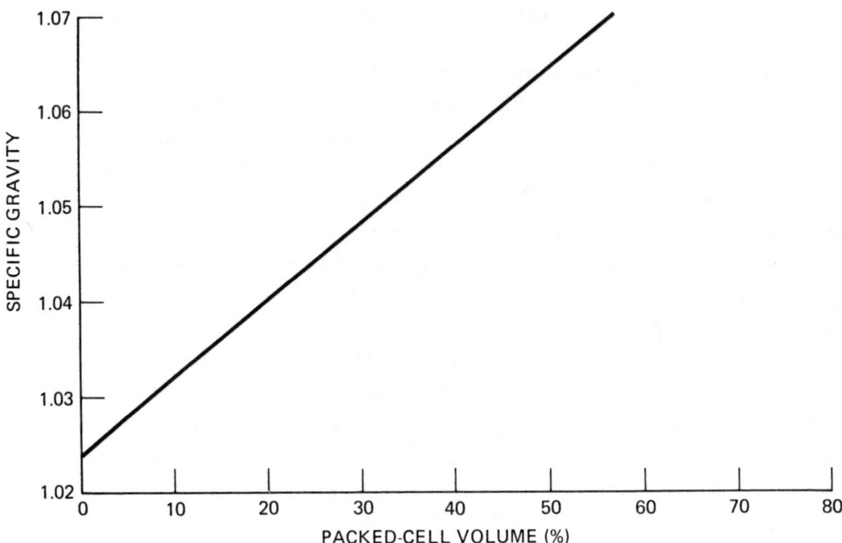

FIGURE 4.23. The relationship between specific gravity and packed-cell volume for blood.

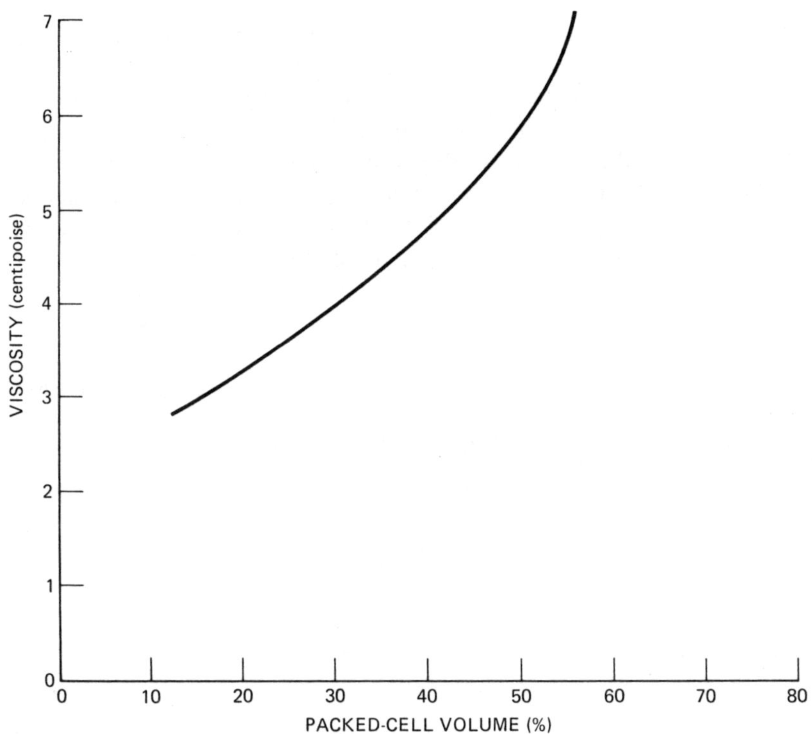

FIGURE 4.24. The relationship between blood viscosity and packed-cell volume.

In this expression, the symbols have the same meaning as before; r is the tube radius, n and p are the viscosity and density of the fluid, and N is the Reynolds number for the fluid.

The critical-flow equation merely serves to relate the factors that identify the flow for the development of turbulence. Although an acceptable value (2000) exists for the Reynolds number for water, it is possible to encounter much higher values in special circumstances. However, when this expression is applied to describe blood flow, difficulties are encountered. Although Coulter and Pappenheimer (1949) reported a Reynolds number of 980 ± 80 for bovine blood, the viscosity of blood is not only difficult to measure, but appears to be dependent on the size of the tube and flow velocity. Ideal, or Newtonian, fluids have a viscosity that is not dependent on velocity; blood is therefore a non-Newtonian fluid.

It should be emphasized that the change from laminar to turbulent flow is not an abrupt transition nor is it strictly associated with a given Reynolds number; length, smoothness, and tube geometry at the point where the fluid enters are also factors that affect the transition to turbulent flow. Nonetheless, the concept of turbulent flow occurring when a critical Reynolds number has been exceeded is an important one. Although turbulent flow dissipates some energy, and in some cases produces audible sound, it has the advantage of providing excellent mixing in the fluid.

BLOOD FLOWMETERS

Two types of flowmeter are used to measure blood flow in unopened vessels. One type is the electromagnetic blood flowmeter and the other is the Doppler flowmeter, which employs ultrasound. With the latter, blood flow can be measured transcutaneously in superficial vessels. Both types measure blood velocity and will now be described.

Electromagnetic Flowmeter

The principle underlying the electromagnetic blood flowmeter is elegantly simple, for it is a straightforward application of Faraday's law of induction which states that a voltage will appear across the ends of a conductor moving at right angles to a magnetic field. Since an electrolyte is a conductor, which can be caused to flow in a magnetic field, suitably placed electrodes can be used to detect the flow-dependent voltage. Figures 4.25*a* and 4.25*b* illustrate this principle. Note that the direction of the magnetic field, flow, and the electrode axis are mutually perpendicular (Figure 4.25*b*). The voltage developed is proportional to the strength of the magnetic field, the length of the moving conductor (i.e., the diameter

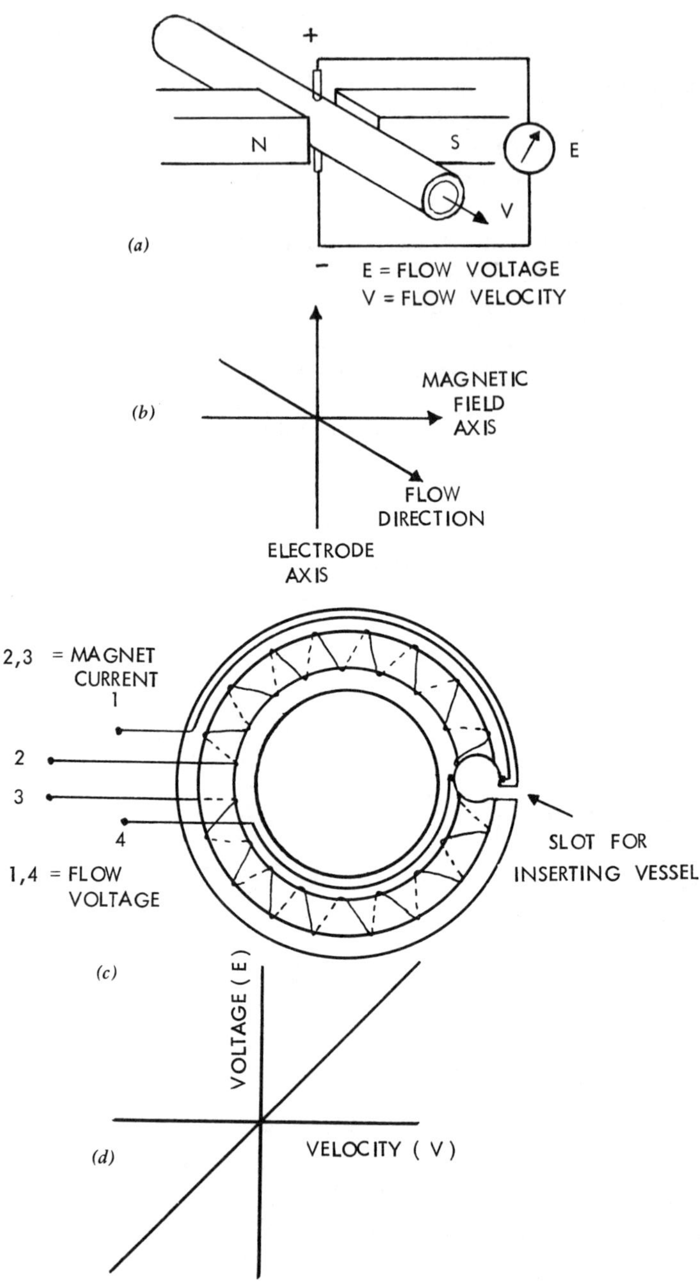

FIGURE 4.25. Basic principle underlying the operation of an electromagnetic flowmeter. (*a*) and (*b*) illustrate the direction of the electrodes and magnetic field with respect to the flow. (*c*) Shows the practical arrangement for a perivascular flow probe and (*d*) illustrates the fact that the flow voltage (*E*) is linearly related to flow velocity (*V*).

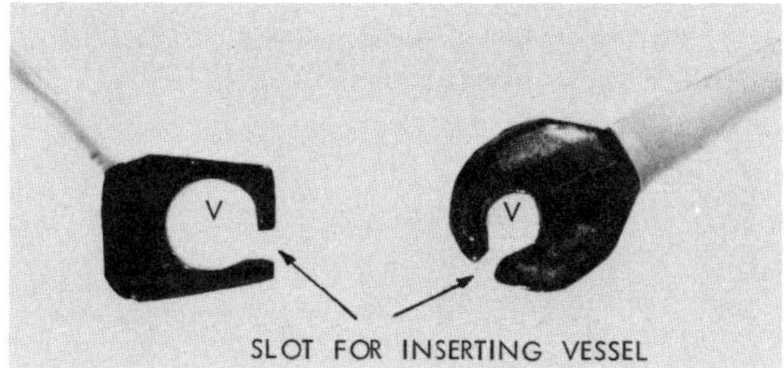

FIGURE 4.26. Perivascular electromagnetic blood flowmeter probes.

of the tube), and the velocity of flow. In a typical case, the first two are constant; therefore, the voltage appearing across the electrodes is proportional to the velocity. Since volume flow is equal to velocity multiplied by area, the voltage is proportional to volume flow.

The method of applying the principle to detect blood flow in an unopened vessel is shown in Figure 4.25*c*. The vessel is slipped into a slot and fills the opening in the magnet, which is a ring of magnetically permeable material surrounded by a coil (2,3 in Figure 4.25*c*). Current flowing in this coil produces the magnetic field in the gap through which the blood flows. In this probe assembly there are two electrodes that make firm contact with the vessel wall when it is in the gap. The electrodes are connected to wires (1,2) that deliver the flow-dependent voltage to the amplifying and display apparatus.

Figure 4.26 illustrates a typical flow probe, which is applied to an unopened vessel. Because the electrodes must embrace the vessel snugly, it is necessary to have a family of probes to fit the vessels of interest.

The concept illustrated in Figure 4.25*a* employs a constant magnetic field produced by a permanent magnet; in practice, an electromagnet is used (Figure 4.25*c*). In this case the polarity of the flow voltage depends on the direction of current in the electromagnet. Although the principle underlying the electromagnetic flowmeter is easy to understand, implementation of it to provide a practical and reliable flowmeter involves considerable technical difficulty. For example, the magnitude of the flow-dependent signal is small because blood vessels are small and the flow velocities are low. Moreover, it is desirable to make the flow probe as small as possible for widespread applicability. The end result is that stable amplification of the tiny flowmeter signals presents practical difficulties. To overcome these and to minimize electrode artifacts, recourse is taken to the use of an alternating rather than a static magnetic field. In this way the flow-dependent voltage becomes modulated by the type of signal used to generate the magnetic field. It is practically very easy to amplify this

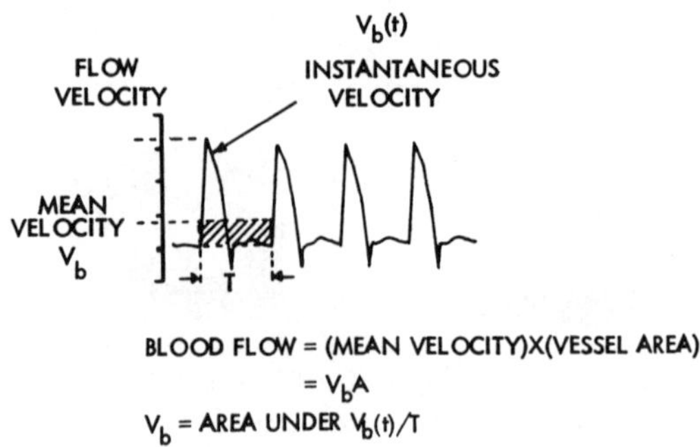

FIGURE 4.27. Instantaneous and mean flow velocity in the aorta detected by an electromagnetic flowmeter probe.

type of signal and recover the envelope, which contains the flow information. There are two types of electromagnetic blood flowmeter. In one, sinusoidal current is used to excite the magnet; in the other, a square wave is used. Usually, the frequency is in the neighborhood of 400 Hz. Thus the flow signal modulates a sine wave or a square wave. Within the flowmeter, electronic circuitry samples only the flow-dependent portion of the signal and provides an analog signal for recording.

Calibration of the output of an electromagnetic flowmeter is not easy. Some probes come with a calibration factor stamped on them and thus allow setting a control on the flowmeter so that its output can be specified. However, the accuracy of precalibrated probes is open to question, and, for high accuracy, it is desirable to hand calibrate the probe by placing a vessel in the probe and pumping blood through at a measured flow rate. For highest accuracy it is desirable to use blood with the same packed-cell volume as was used when the measurement was made. Since the output is linear with flow, a single flow rate calibration will suffice.

Many electromagnetic flowmeters provide an output that represents the instantaneous flow velocity, as shown in Figure 4.27, as well as an output which represents mean flow. Often a panel meter indicates continuously the mean flow.

The electromagnetic blood flowmeter is extremely popular, particularly among those who conduct animal-based research. Because electrodes are used to detect the flow signal, the instrument is susceptible to some types of interference, especially electromagnetic from diathermy or electrosurgical instruments. Often interference is encountered if two flowmeters are used on the same subject and the flow probes are not widely separated.

Ultrasonic Flowmeter

Blood flow velocity can be measured by directing a beam of ultrasound into flowing blood and detecting the echo that is produced by reflection from the moving blood cells. The frequency of the echo is different from that of the incident beam owing to the well-known Doppler frequency-shift phenomenon. If the blood is moving away from the source of ultrasound, the frequency of the reflected ultrasound is lower. Conversely, if the blood flows toward the incident beam, the frequency of the echo is higher. In both cases the frequency difference (shift) is proportional to the velocity of blood flow. Parenthetically, this Doppler frequency shift is familiar to all who have noted that the frequency of a sustained automobile horn appears to rise and fall as the automobile approaches, passes, and recedes.

The method of implementing the Doppler frequency-shift method to measure blood flow is illustrated in Figure 4.28. A generator (U) excites a piezoelectric element P_i to emit an incident beam of ultrasound of frequency f_i, which intercepts the blood flow with an angle θ. The moving blood cells reflect the ultrasound and the echo returning to piezoelectric element P_r has a different frequency f_r. The velocity V of blood flow is given by

$$V = \left(\frac{f_i - f_r}{f_i}\right)\frac{c}{2\cos\theta}$$

where f_i and f_r are the frequencies of the incident and reflected ultrasound and c is the velocity of ultrasound in blood ($\sim 1.5 \times 10^5$ cm/sec).

The incident and reflected signals are led to a processor P, which provides a signal proportional to $f_i - f_r$, thereby permitting analog recording of blood-flow velocity. Volume flow is velocity multiplied by the vessel cross-sectional area.

Because of the ultrasonic frequency used ($\sim$ 5 MHz) and the commonly encountered velocities in vessels (0–200 cm/sec), the difference frequency (0–1200 Hz) falls in the audible range. Therefore, many Doppler blood flowmeters include a loudspeaker for aural monitoring of blood flow. The pitch of the audible signal is proportional to blood-flow velocity.

Calibration of the difference-frequency signal in terms of volume flow is not easy, because it is necessary to know the vessel diameter and the angle θ that the ultrasonic beam makes with the direction of blood flow. According to Roberts (1973), when the velocity profile is uniform over the

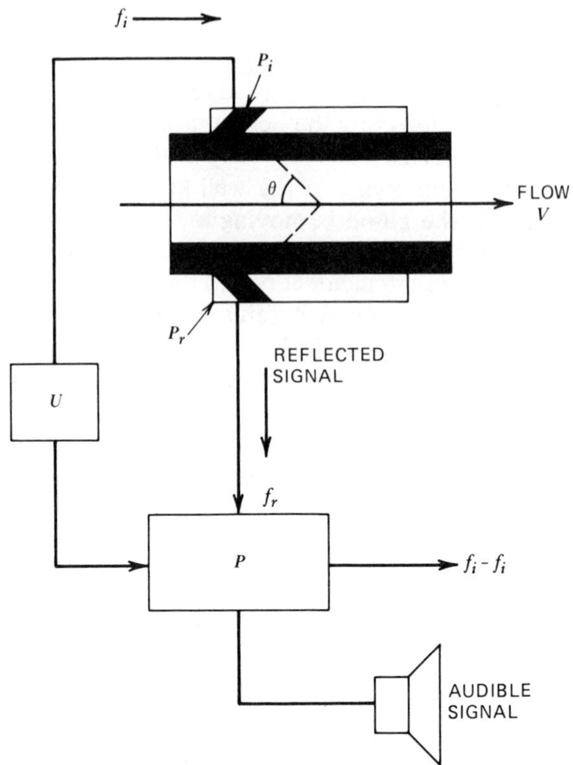

FIGURE 4.28. The Doppler frequency-shift blood flowmeter. An incident beam (P_i) of ultrasound intercepts the flowing blood with an angle θ to provide the reflected beam (P_r). The blood flow velocity (V) is given by $V = [(f_i - f_r)/f_i]\ (c/2 \cos \theta)$, where f_i and f_r are the frequencies of the incident and reflected ultrasound, respectively, and c is the velocity of ultrasound in blood ($\sim 1.5 \times 10^5$ cm/sec).

diameter of the vessel, flow can be calculated accurately. When the flow profile is parabolic, the flow is overestimated by about 16%.

In Figure 4.28, the piezoelectric elements are shown on opposite sides of the vessel. However, both can be placed on the same side of the vessel and mounted in a sleeve. In addition, blood flow in superficial vessels can be measured transcutaneously. In this application, the two piezoelectric elements are mounted side by side in a hand-held probe and a thick gel is used to couple the ultrasound into the tissues. By listening to the Doppler frequency-shift signal, it is relatively easy to adjust the probe to obtain a clear flow signal. It is also easy to distinguish between arterial and venous flow. Arterial flow produces a rhythmically fluctuating whistlelike increase and decrease in frequency. Venous flow is represented by a low pitched, rumbling sound with little variation in frequency.

The Doppler-shift blood flowmeter produces a velocity signal, identical to that produced by the electromagnetic blood flowmeter. The Doppler ultrasonic flowmeter can be applied to the unopened blood vessel as well as transcutaneously. Both types are very easy to use, and transcutaneous instruments have been made with the dimensions of a fountain pen, with the audible signal being monitored with stethoscope ear tubes. More-sophisticated units permit analog recording and aural monitoring. At present not all instruments indicate forward and backward flow; but this limitation is being removed in the newer instruments. The major difficulty with Doppler flowmeters relates to the need to determine θ, the interception angle with blood flow, and the diameter of the vessel, as well as the velocity profile. Considerable research is underway to electronically determine these quantities and thereby provide a signal calibrated in volume flow per second.

BALLOON-TIPPED (SWAN–GANZ) CATHETER

Although it is easy to advance a catheter into the right heart via the venous approach, it is difficult to place a catheter tip in the pulmonary artery—an important site for measuring pulmonary function and cardiac output, and for estimating left atrial pressure using the wedge technique. Development of flow-guided catheters for pulmonary-artery catheterization had been unsatisfactory until 1970 when Swan and Ganz described their balloon-tipped catheter. Illustrated in Figure 4.29, this catheter is available with diameters ranging from 4F to 7F and in 50 and 100 cm lengths. Single-, double-, and triple-lumen units are now available. Each catheter has a tiny lumen that communicates with the balloon and a

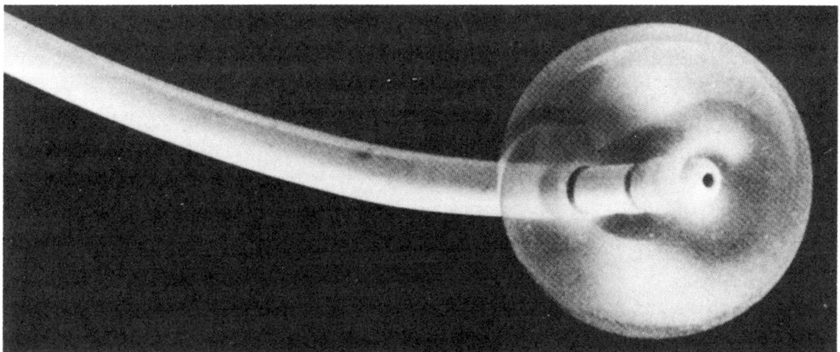

FIGURE 4.29. The Swan–Ganz balloon-tipped catheter with the balloon inflated.

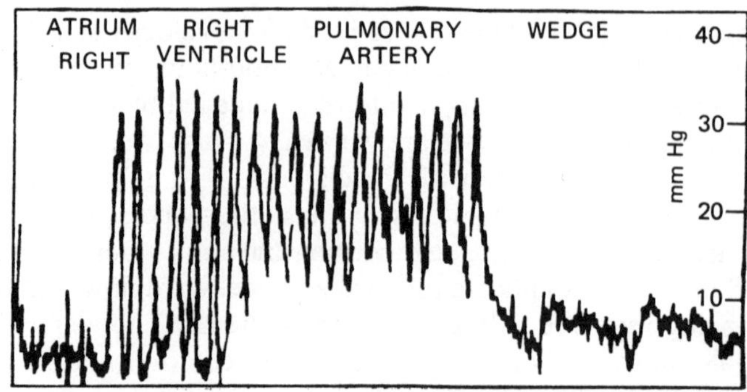

FIGURE 4.30. Continuous record of blood pressure as a balloon-tipped catheter is advanced through the right atrium and right ventricle, and into the pulmonary artery and finally into the wedge position. (Courtesy Electro-Catheter Corp., Rahway, NJ 07065.)

vented (volume-limited) syringe is used to inflate the balloon to the correct size.

The technique of catheterizing the pulmonary artery consists of inserting the catheter (with the balloon deflated) into a suitable vein. The catheter is usually filled with saline containing an anticoagulant and connected to a high-quality pressure-recording system. Continuous recording of pressure allows identification of the location of the catheter tip, as will be described subsequently. When the catheter tip is judged to be in the vena cava, the balloon is inflated and, as the catheter is advanced, blood flow guides the tip into the pulmonary artery. Usually the subject is directed to inhale deeply to facilitate passage of the tip through the right ventricle into the pulmonary artery. Figure 4.30 illustrates a sequence of pressure recording while the catheter is being advanced. When in the pulmonary artery, the balloon is deflated.

Because catheters are long and usually have a small lumen, it is necessary to use a high-quality pressure transducer to obtain an accurate reproduction of the pressure at the catheter tip. A typical high-quality pressure transducer has a volume displacement on the order of 0.01 mm^3/100 mm Hg. Transducers with a volume displacement on the order of 0.1 mm^3/100 mm Hg are unsuitable for recording with long, small-lumen catheters.

CARDIAC CATHETERIZATION

Cardiac catheterization is the name given to the technique in which a catheter is advanced into the heart chambers or associated great vessels in order to identify abnormal flow paths for blood or to evaluate the function of one or more of the four cardiac valves.

TABLE 4.11. Specifications of Balwedge Single-Pressure (Double-Lumen) Monitoring Catheter[a]

Catolog No. (Former No.)	Length (cm)	Size	Diameter Of Inflated Balloon (mm)	Lumen Area (mm^2)	Frequency Response (Hz)
31—1064 (08104)	110	4F	8	0.5	21
31—1065 (08105)	110	5F	9	0.8	25
31-1066 (08106)	110	6F	10	1.3	30
31—1067 (08107)	110	7F	11	1.6	35
31—1024 (08114)	50	4F	8	0.5	26

[a]Courtesy Electro-Catheter Corp., Rahway, New Jersey 07065.

In the following paragraphs, examples of the techniques for identifying abnormal flow will be presented. Elsewhere in this chapter are found examples of how the pressure across cardiac valves and the flow through them can be used to calculate valve area.

Cardiac catheterization is not a difficult procedure and is therefore performed routinely. Access to the right heart is gained by advancing a catheter up the median basilic vein in the arm or the saphenous vein in the thigh. The position of the catheter, which is radioopaque, is monitored with the aid of a fluoroscope. The left heart is reached by passing a catheter up the brachial or femoral artery. Electrocardiography is always used to monitor the procedure to identify the presence of arrhythmias. A defibrillator, "at the ready," is always on hand to arrest ventricular fibrillation if it occurs, which, although rare, is not unknown.

The method of specifying the fidelity of pressure recording is in terms of the sine wave frequency response of the recording channel. For a typical blood-pressure pulse, the sine wave frequency response of the recording system should extend from 0 Hz to at least six times the cardiac frequency (Geddes, 1970). Table 4.11 illustrates the sine wave frequency response capabilities of typical balloon-tipped catheters connected to a high-quality pressure-recording system.

The presence of the catheter tip in the pulmonary artery is easily confirmed by the pressure recording, which shows a systolic and diastolic pressure (well above zero) and a dicrotic notch on the pressure pulse.

Advancing the catheter farther will cause it to be wedged in a small branch of the pulmonary artery. In this situation the pressure seen by the catheter tip is pulmonary capillary wedge (PCW) pressure, which is close to left atrial pressure (Figure 4.30). An alternative method of obtaining wedge pressure employs partial inflation of the balloon while viewing the pressure recording. However, great care must be exercised to avoid over-stretching of the pulmonary-artery branch.

CARDIAC SHUNTS

Several types of abnormal or shunt paths for blood flow can occur between the left and right sides of the heart and its great vessels. For example, with a ventricular septal defect (VSD), blood that is rich in oxygen can flow from the left into the right ventricle, thereby increasing its oxygen content. With the same anatomical defect and in other circumstances, such as pulmonary stenosis, right ventricular pressure can exceed left ventricular pressure and right ventricular blood, which is low in oxygen content, can enter the left ventricle. Likewise, there can be an atrial septal defect (ASD) in which the blood of one atrium can enter the other. At birth, there is an opening (the foramen ovale) between the two atria which may not close in a few days as it does normally. In such a case, oxygen-rich left atrial blood can enter the right atrium. Likewise, a left-to-right shunt can occur if the ductus arteriosus, a communication between the pulmonary artery and aorta, does not close, as it usually does within a few days after birth. From the pressures and the oxygen contents of the blood in the various cardiac chambers and great vessels, it is possible to identify the presence of such shunts and calculate the amount of blood that flows through them.

Cardiac shunts can also be identified by injecting a detectable material into the cardiac chambers. For example, the indicator-dilution method, which is used to determine cardiac output, provides dilution curves that are characteristically altered by shunt flow. Cardiac shunts, diminished flow in vessels and incompetent valves can also be identified by injecting radioopaque material into a cardiac chamber (or great vessel) while the heart is viewed fluoroscopically; this technique is called angiography (*angio* meaning vessel).

Normal Heart

In the normal heart, Figure 4.31*a* presents the typical pressures in mm Hg. Table 4.12 lists the typical range of pressures encountered in normal subjects. Figure 4.31*b* identifies the oxygen content of the blood found in these chambers. Note that the oxygen content of the venous blood entering the right atrium is reduced slightly as it mixes with the low-oxygen-content blood entering from the coronary sinus, which is the venous outflow from most of the heart muscle. The heart muscle extracts more than one-half of the oxygen in the blood delivered to it. Therefore, the blood in the right ventricle and pulmonary artery have a slightly lower oxygen content than the blood entering the right atrium. Right-ventricular and pulmonary-artery blood contain typically 15 mL of oxygen per 100 mL of blood, that is, 15 V%.

After passing through the lungs, pulmonary artery blood has gained oxygen and contains, typically, 19.5 V% of oxygen. Recall that the majority of the oxygen is transported by the red cells, which contain hemoglobin; 1 g of hemoglobin combines with 1.34 mL of oxygen. In a typical normal subject, the blood contains 15 g of hemoglobin per 100 mL of blood. Therefore, the oxygen-carrying capacity of blood saturated with oxygen is $15 \times 1.34 = 20.1$ V%. However, pulmonary venous blood entering the left atrium is typically 95% saturated (owing to lung shunts) and, therefore, the red cells will transport $0.95 \times 20.1 = 19.1$ V% of oxygen. Since the plasma contains typically 0.4 V% of oxygen in simple solution, the total oxygen content of pulmonary venous, and left atrial blood, is $19.1 + 0.4 = 19.5$ V%, that is, each 100 mL of blood contains 19.5 mL of oxygen.

Pulmonary and Systemic Flows

Figure 4.32 illustrates the oxygen content of blood found in the four cardiac chambers. The direct Fick method can be used to calculate the blood flow in the pulmonary vascular circulations. An important requirement in using the Fick method is that steady-state conditions prevail. Recall that use of the Fick method requires a knowledge of the upstream and downstream concentrations of the indicator and the amount of indicator injected. With the direct Fick method the indicator is oxygen and its uptake is measured with a closed-circuit spirometer filled with oxygen and containing a CO_2 absorber. The O_2 uptake is identified by the reduction in volume in the spirometer during the period of breathing (Figure 4.4). The usual correction must be applied to bring the volume collected to BTPS (see Cardiac Output Measurement). The flow (Q) in mL/min, is equal to the mL of oxygen uptake per minute divided by the arteriovenous oxygen difference in volume percent. Mathematically,

$$Q = \frac{O_2 \text{ (mL/min)}}{\text{A-V difference}}$$

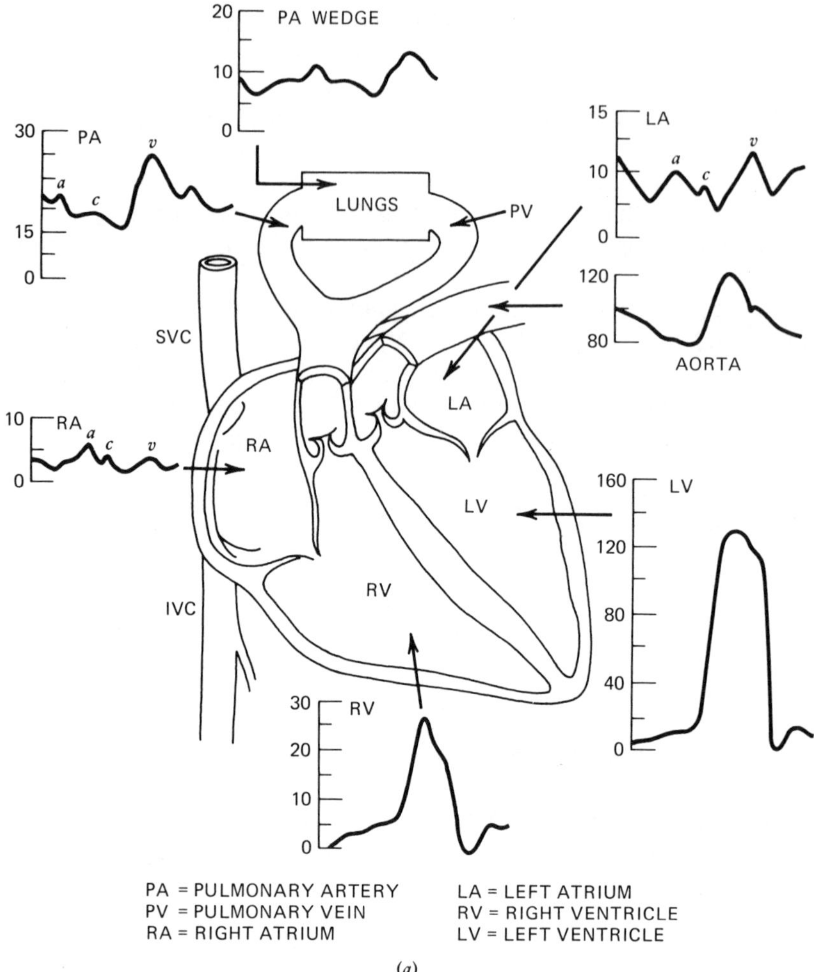

(*a*)

FIGURE 4.31a. (*a*) Pressures in the heart and great vessels.

The Fick expression will now be used to illustrate how it can be applied to calculate blood flow. For example, in Figure 4.32, the oxygen uptake (corrected to BTPS) is 244 mL/min. The blood in the pulmonary artery contains 15 V% and that in the pulmonary vein contains 19.5 V% of oxygen. Therefore, 19.5 − 15 = 4.5 V% was picked up by the blood flowing through the lungs. Consequently, the pulmonic blood flow (Q_p) is

$$Q_p = \frac{244}{(19.5 - 15)/100} = 5422 \text{ mL/min}$$

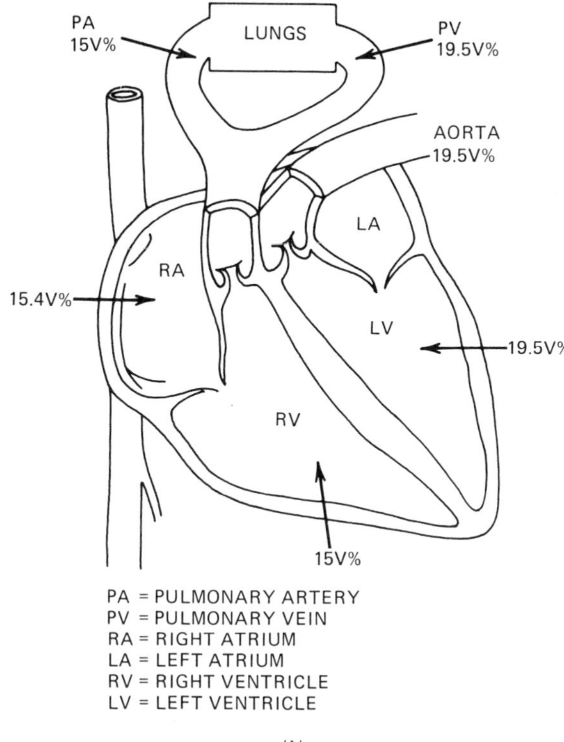

(*b*)

FIGURE 4.31b. (*b*) Normal values for oxygen saturation in volume percent.

TABLE 4.12. Caridovascular Pressures[a]

Site	Typical Pressure
PA	15–30/4–12 PA Wedge = 1–10
PV	Left Atrium (LA)
RA	0–8 mean; *a*, 2–10; *v* = 2–10
LA	1–10 mean
RV	15–30/0–8
LV	100–140/3–12; *a* = 3–15; *v* = 3–15
Aorta	100–140/60–90

[a]Data from *Cardiac Catheterization and Angiocardiography*. Grossman, Philadelphia 1974, p. 339.

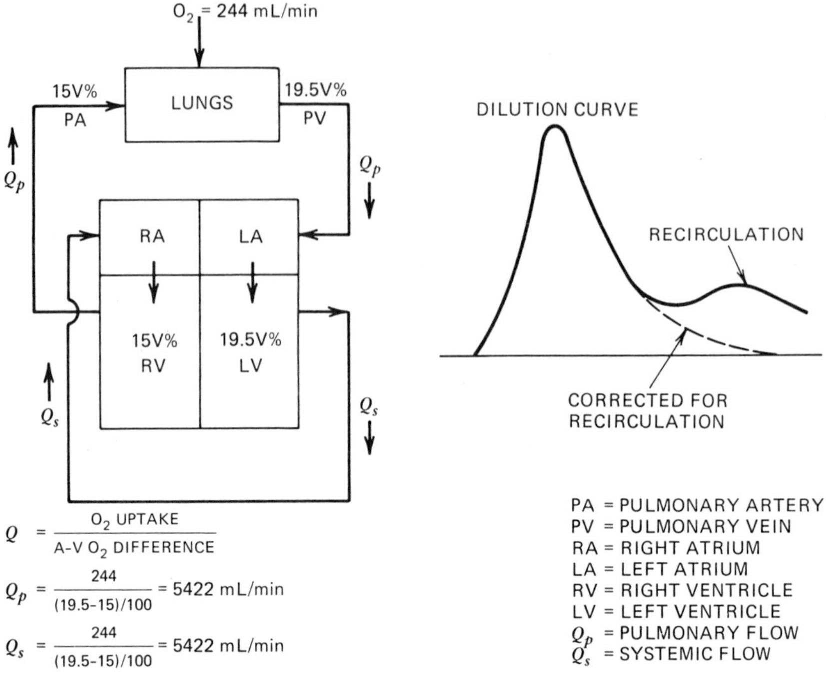

FIGURE 4.32. Cardiac output under normal conditions.

In the normal subject, there are no shunt paths within the heart and great vessels; therefore, the systemic flow (Q_s) is equal to the pulmonary flow (Q_p). Figure 4.32 also shows the typical dilution curve obtained from a normal subject in whom the indicator was injected into the right atrium ventricle or pulmonary artery and detected in the aorta. The dilution curve exhibits a typical recirculation, which was corrected for by semilogarithmic plotting and extrapolation as discussed earlier in this chapter.

Left-to-Right Shunts

A left-to-right shunt can occur between the aorta and pulmonary artery (patent ductus arteriosus), the left and right atria (patent foramen ovale or atrial septal defect), and the left and right ventricles (ventricular septal defect). As a result of any of these defects, oxygen-rich blood can flow from the left side of the circulation into the right through the particular defect. This fact forms the basis for identifying the presence of the shunt. In practice, the oxygen content of blood in the pulmonary artery, right ventricle, right atrium, and vena cava are determined by withdrawing samples for chemical analysis or by withdrawing the blood from a catheter located at a chosen site into a cuvette oximeter. Alternatively, a fiberoptic catheter oximeter can be used to measure the oxygen saturation at the tip of the catheter.

With a knowledge of the range of normal values for oxygen content in the right side of the heart and pulmonary artery, it is possible to identify the presence of left-to-right shunts. For example if there is a stepup in oxygen concentration as the catheter moves from the vena cava to the right atrium, then there is an atrial septal defect. If an increase in oxygen concentration occurs as the catheter moves from the right atrium to the right ventricle, then there is a ventricular septal defect. If the stepup in concentration occurs when the catheter leaves the right ventricle and is advanced along the pulmonary artery, then there is a shunt between the aorta and pulmonary artery.

Ventricular Septal Defect (VSD)

The information just presented can be used to demonstrate the presence of a ventricular septal defect. Figure 4.33 illustrates the situation in which there is an opening in the septum between the left and right ventricles. In a typical situation, the left ventricular pressure exceeds right ventricular pressure and, therefore, oxygen-rich blood will enter the right ventricle. In addition, the septal defect will also cause an increase the pressure in the right ventricle by an amount which is dependent on the size of the septal defect and left ventricular pressure. Thus, with a left-to-right ventricular shunt, the oxygen content and pressure in the right ventricle are above the values found in normal subjects.

Figure 4.33 illustrates the blood-oxygen values when blood flows through the defect from the left to right ventricle. Using these values it is easy to calculate the shunt flow (*SF*). To do so requires that the pulmonary blood flow (Q_p) is known. The blood flowing into the pulmonary vascular circuit contains 16.6 V% and on emerging from the lungs it contains 19.5 V% of oxygen, providing an A-V O_2 difference of 2.9 V%. The O_2 uptake is 244 mL/min; therefore, the pulmonary blood flow Q_p is calculated as follows:

$$Q_p = \frac{244}{(19.5 - 16.6)/100} = 8414 \text{ mL/min}$$

The systemic blood flow (Q_s) can be calculated in a similar manner. To calculate this flow, a mixed venous sample is obtained from the chamber

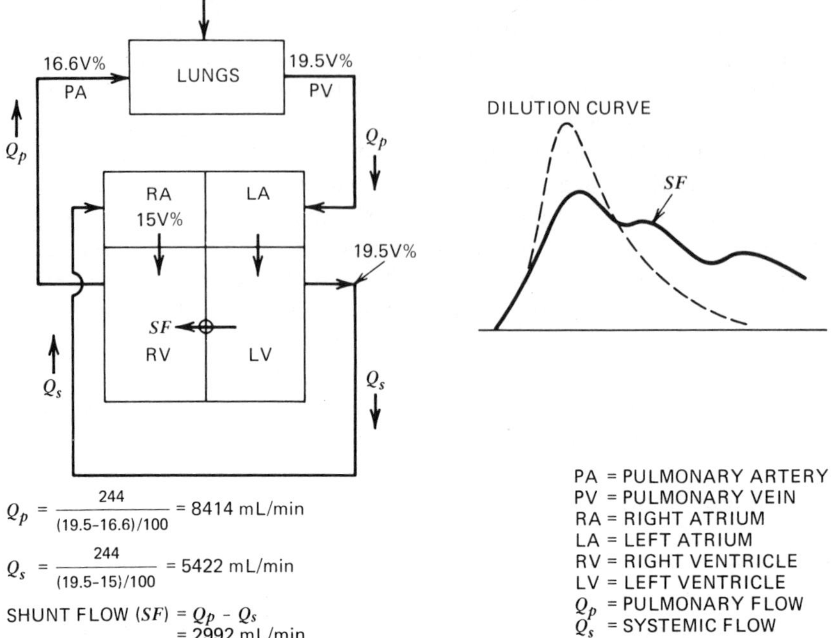

FIGURE 4.33. Conditions with a ventricular septal defect with a left-to-right shunt.

ahead of the site of the shunt. The O_2 content of the blood entering the right ventricle is 15 V% and the arterial blood oxygen content is 19.5 V%; therefore, the systemic flow Q_s is calculated as follows:

$$Q_s = \frac{244}{(19.5 - 15)/100} = 5422 \text{ mL/min}$$

Consequently, the shunt flow (Q_{SF}) is merely the difference in these two flows, that is,

$$Q_{SF} = 8414 - 5422 = 2992 \text{ mL/min}$$

Note that in this case of left-to-right ventricular shunt, the pulmonary flow is 1.55 times that of the systemic flow. The pressure in the right ventricle is also elevated.

If the indicator-dilution method had been employed in this subject, the shunt flow would reveal itself by an early appearance of a "recirculation wave" (SF) on the downslope of the dilution curve, as shown in Figure

4.33. In a typical case the dilution curve may not show a prominent recirculation, but instead would be considerably prolonged and difficult to use to calculate flow. The dashed curve represents the corrected dilution curve with no shunt flow.

Right-to-Left Shunts

In normal circumstances, the oxygen content of the blood in the left-heart chambers (left atrium and ventricle) is much higher than that of the right-heart chambers. A defect in the atrial or ventricular septum can, in circumstances when the pressure in the right side of the heart exceeds that in the left, cause venous blood to pass through the defect and reduce the oxygen content of the chamber into which it flows. Likewise, a communication between the aorta and pulmonary artery can, in the presence of a much elevated pulmonary artery pressure, cause venous blood to appear in the systemic circulation. When this occurs, a subject demonstrates it by the blush color called cyanosis. The situation is called hypoxemia, or blood with less oxygen than it can transport. It should be immediately apparent that the condition could be due to an impairment in respiratory function as well as a cardiac defect.

Right-to-left shunts are slightly more difficult to quantify than left-to-right shunts. Angiography can be used to follow the injection of a radioopaque indicator as it flows through the shunt. However, this technique is not without its difficulties and is only qualitative.

The two techniques described previously, namely, the measurement of oxygen content in the heart and great vessels and the indicator-dilution method, are used to identify the presence of right-to-left shunts and, in some cases, to quantify the flow.

With the concept just presented it is clear that if the oxygen content in the left atrial blood is less than that in the pulmonary vein, venous blood is flowing through an atrial septal defect. If the pulmonary vein and left atrial blood contain the same amount of oxygen, but left ventricular blood contains less oxygen, venous blood from the right ventricle is entering the left ventricle. Likewise if the oxygen content of the pulmonary vein, left atrium, and left ventricle is higher than that in the aorta, then pulmonary artery venous blood is flowing into the aorta. Although it is straightforward to state the basic procedures used to make these determinations, carrying them out is far from easy, because the pulmonary vein and left atrium are relatively inaccessible to catheterization; therefore, the indicator-dilution method is often employed to identify right-to-left shunts.

Before describing use of the indicator-dilution method, it is of value to illustrate use of the oxygen-content method to quantify the flow through a

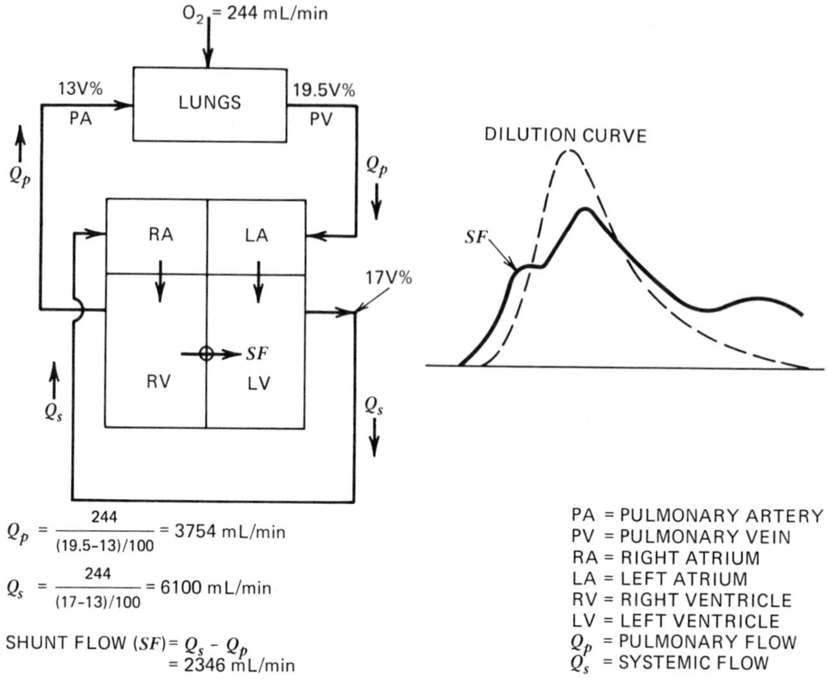

FIGURE 4.34. Conditions with a ventricular septal defect with a right-to-left shunt.

ventricular septal defect in which right ventricular pressure exceeds left ventricular pressure, thereby causing a net flow of venous blood into the left ventricle and systemic circulation. Figure 4.34 illustrates this example in which blood emerging from the lungs contains 19.5 V% of oxygen. When the blood appears in the aorta, the oxygen content is only 17 V% owing to the right-to-left shunt. As before, the Fick method can be used to calculate the pulmonary (Q_p) and systemic (Q_s) blood flow. The pulmonary blood flow (Q_p) is as follows:

$$Q_p = \frac{244}{(19.5 - 13)/100} = 3754 \text{ mL/min}$$

The systemic blood flow (Q_s) is calculated in a similar manner:

$$Q_s = \frac{244}{(17 - 13)/100} = 6100 \text{ mL/min}$$

Therefore, the shunt flow (Q_{SF}) from the right to left ventricle is as follows:

$$Q_{SF} = Q_s - Q_p$$
$$= 6100 - 3754 = 2346 \text{ mL/min}$$

The indicator-dilution method is used in an ingenious way to identify the presence of a right-to-left shunt. If the shunt occurs downstream to the site of injection of the indicator, the shunt flow will cause an early appearance wave on the rising phase of the dilution curve. If the shunt is upstream, that is, the indicator is injected beyond the site of the shunt, no early appearance wave will appear on the rising phase of the dilution curve.

To illustrate the principle just presented, consider the situation when blood flows from the right ventricle to the left. If the indicator is injected in the superior or inferior vena cava, or right ventricle, the blood carrying the indicator will appear in the aorta almost immediately and blood carrying the indicator will flow through the pulmonary circuit and appear much later in the aorta. Thus a dilution curve recorded from the aorta will show an early shunt flow (*SF*) wave on the ascending limb of the dilution curve, as shown in Figure 4.34.

By using the simple technique of injecting the indicator ahead of and beyond the point of a suspected shunt, the indicator-dilution curve will reveal the site of the shunt. An early arrival wave will be seen only on the ascending limb of the curve when the injection site is upstream from the shunt. Successive injection into the vena cava, right atrium, right ventricle, and pulmonary artery can identify atrial and ventricular shunts and flow from the pulmonary artery to the aorta.

Origin and Significance of Cardiovascular Shunts

The functional significance of a cardiovascular shunt depends on its location and the amount of blood that flows through it. It is interesting to note that we, and a large number of animals, start left with cardiovascular shunts. This point can be verified by examining Figure 4.35, which illustrates the fetal circulation schematically. During fetal life, the lungs are not functional and the O_2–CO_2 transport role that they serve postnatally is carried out by the placenta, which provides a chemical communication between the mother and fetus. In addition, across the placental membrane pass nutrients and many other substances that are necessary for fetal development.

Examination of Figure 4.35 will reveal the origin of a few cardiovascu-

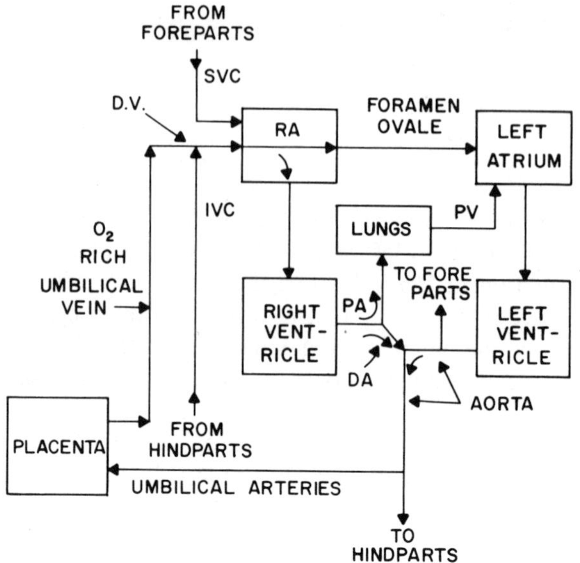

FIGURE 4.35. The fetal circulation.

lar shunts. *In utero,* blood which is low in oxygen content is pumped from the fetal aorta to the placenta via the two umbilical arteries. Oxygen-rich blood leaves the placenta via the umbilical vein, which joins the inferior vena cava (IVC) at the ductus venosus (DV), which is near the right heart. About three-quarters of the venous blood from the inferior vena cava and the oxygen-rich blood from the umbilical vein pass through the right atrium into the left atrium via the foramen ovale (FO). Thus, a considerable amount of oxygen-rich blood is delivered directly to the left heart. A small amount of venous blood from the superior vena cava, which drains the foreparts, joins this flow. A portion of the blood from the right atrium passes into the right ventricle, from where it is pumped through the vascular circuit of the lungs. Since the lungs are not functional *in utero,* the blood emerging from the pulmonary circuit and entering the left atrium has the same oxygen content as it had in the right ventricle. Blood from the left atrium is pumped from the left ventricle into the aorta. Interestingly enough, the pressure in the pulmonary artery is slightly higher than that in the aorta and blood flows through the ductus arteriosus (DA), which is a communication between the pulmonary artery and aorta. Thus the aorta receives blood from the right and left ventricles and distributes about one-half of it to the fetus and the other half to the placenta.

It is interesting to observe that there are three cardiovascular communications that normally close following birth. The ductus venosus

(DV) is a sphincterlike structure that closes and prevents loss of venous blood. The foramen ovale (FO) between the atria closes, as does the ductus arteriosus (DA) between the pulmonary artery and aorta. In a very small percentage of births, the foramen ovale and ductus arteriosus do not close, and surgical closure is required.

In uterine life, the pulmonary artery and aortic pressures are nearly equal. The pulmonary vascular resistance is high and the systemic vascular resistance is low, owing mainly to the placental bed. At birth, the placental circulation is shut off because flow ceases in the umbilical arteries. This causes an increase in arterial pressure. The pulmonary vascular resistance falls when the lungs are inflated with the first breath. Consequently, the pulmonary vascular resistance falls and, therefore, pulmonary artery pressure falls. The left atrial pressure exceeds the right atrial pressure and blood will flow through the foramen ovale creating a left-to-right shunt. Fortunately, a flap of tissue over the foramen acts like a valve and soon closes the opening. This tissue flap later becomes permanently adhered to the atrial septum.

After birth, blood flows from the aorta into the pulmonary artery via the ductus arterosus. Within a few days, this communication closes, thereby eliminating the second left-to-right shunt.

In some subjects these shunts persist and, as stated previously, the significance of a cardiovascular shunt depends on its location and the amount of blood that flows through it. Shunts can be so small that no serious impairment results, and surgical correction is unnecessary. However, a shunt can be so large that the subject is incapacitated, and surgical repair is required. With a left-to-right shunt, arterial blood is well oxygenated and the subject appears normal at rest. The pulmonary blood flow exceeds the systemic flow by an amount that depends on the shunt flow. The impairment encountered by a person with a left-to-right shunt relates to an inability to tolerate exercise, which requires an increase in systemic cardiac output. In addition, the added load placed on the right ventricle leads to increased pulmonary pressure and congestion. Ultimately, right ventricular failure occurs if the shunt is large and persists.

A right-to-left shunt causes venous blood to enter the arterial system, producing arterial hypoxemia. Such a situation is serious, and if present at birth, results in a falure to develop if not corrected. In adults, the impaired oxygen transport can result in an intolerance to exercise if the shunt is small, or in unconsciousness and death if the shunt is large.

Vessel Dilation

Major arteries often develop localized narrowing due to atheromatous deposits, which can dramatically reduce blood flow. About three decades

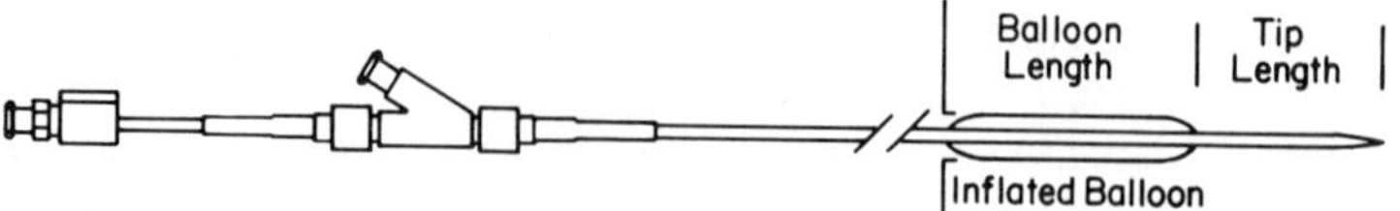

FIGURE 4.36. The Gruntzig vessel-dilating balloon catheter. (Courtesy Cook Catheter Co., Bloomington, IN.)

ago it was discovered that an implanted bypass could be used to carry blood beyond the stenosis. Shortly thereafter, it became customary to replace the stenosed region with any one of a number of different types of flexible tubing, often made from woven plastic fibers. The success of such vascular grafts is well known. However, more recently a new technique for widening the stenotic region has been introduced and is now in widespread use.

Dotter and Judkins (1964) introduced the technique of using a catheter with an expandable device to dilate arteries that had become narrowed by atherosclerotic plaques. The dilator consists of a sturdy balloon on a tapered catheter that can be inserted percutaneously and the balloon maneuvered into the region of the stenosis. The technique (called angioplasty) has been applied to widen stenosed regions of the femoral, iliac, popliteal, renal, and coronary arteries.

Figure 4.36 is a sketch of the vessel-dilating balloon-tipped catheter. The outside diameter is typically 8F (2.8 mm). The balloon is about 2–4 cm long and when inflated fully is 4–6 mm in diameter. A 2-mL syringe is used to inflate the balloon. Alternately air at 3–5 atmospheres pressure can be used. During balloon inflation, the pressure is measured with a dial guage.

The modern version of the dilator catheter was described by Gruntzig and Kumpe (1979); they also provided a detailed account of the technique of insertion and use. They recommended dilating stenotic regions that were less than 10 mm in length. The stenotic region is identified by fluoroscopy, using a catheter to inject the contrast medium. The ends of the stenotic region are marked on the skin. A slender catheter with a guidewire inside is advanced through the stenotic region and the catheter is then removed. Then the dilator catheter is advanced into the vessel over the guidewire. The skin markings and those on the catheter allow determination of the position of the (deflated) balloon. When in the desired location, the balloon is inflated partially for about 30 sec. The balloon is then deflated; the catheter is advanced and the procedure is repeated if necessary. Fluoroscopy, with contrast material, is used periodically to evaluate the degree of widening of the stenosis.

According to Gruntzig and Kumpe (1979), who used the method for dilating arteries in the thigh region, there are few complications and a high success rate. The method is applied using local anesthesia, and the patients are ambulatory on the following day.

CARDIAC FUNCTION

Although it is very useful to measure cardiac output, it is more desirable to evaluate the ability of the heart to eject blood against the outflow pressure (afterload). Unfortunately, it is difficult to measure the pumping capability of the heart directly. For this reason, indirect measurements are made or stresses are imposed on the heart to evaluate its ability to perform an increasing workload. To understand the bases of these tests, it is useful to first examine the function of the heart as a pump and discuss the very important terms: work and power.

Heart Work and Power

The heart is a double stroke pump, ejecting blood against an outflow pressure which identifies the vascular resistance. The outflow resistance is often termed the afterload. The right ventricle ejects its stroke volume against the prevailing pulmonary-artery diastolic pressure, and the left ventricle ejects its stroke volume against the prevailing aortic diastolic pressure. Normally, little opposition to flow is offered by the pulmonic and aortic valves. In addition, the two atria pump blood into the ventricles against the normally insignificant resistance of the large-area atrioventricular valves. The whole heart is therefore a mechanical pump that consumes chemical energy and produces mechanical energy.

It is becoming diagnostically important to study the energetics of the heart in order to evaluate its pumping capabilities. Terms such as heart work, stroke work, heart work per minute, and heart power are used with increasing frequency, sometimes without a clear recognition of their significance. In order to remove this ambiguity, it is of value to provide a simplified physical picture to illustrate how the heart functions as a pump and to identify the input and output parameters of this remarkable tireless organ.

Energy is the ability to perform work; the units most frequently used are the g-cm, dyn-cm, erg, and joule. Work is performed when a force moves an object through a distance. The work performed is the product of force and distance. Stated in another way, work is performed when a weight is raised to a height; the work is the weight multiplied by the height. The practical unit of work is the g-cm. When converted to absolute units (by multiplication by the gravitational constant, 980), the unit becomes the dyn-cm or erg. One joule is 10^7 ergs.

These concepts can be applied to the heart very easily. The output work performed by the left ventricle can be described as the work expended by ejecting the stroke volume against the aortic pressure. Neglecting the small amount of work (kinetic energy) done in imparting velocity to the stroke volume, the average output work performed by the left ventricle can be visualized as raising the weight of the stroke volume to a height that is equivalent to the mean aortic pressure. For example, the weight of the stroke volume (SV) is equal to its volume multiplied by the density (d) of the blood. The equivalent height for the mean aortic pressure ($\bar{P}_a$ in mm Hg) is obtained by multiplication by 13.6, which is the density of mercury; this product must then be divided by 10 to obtain the height in centimeters. Therefore, the output work (W_l) of the left ventricle (neglecting kinetic energy) in g-cm is

$$W_l = \bar{P}_a\,(13.6/10)\,(SV)d$$

The average output power developed by the left ventricle is the work per second. The work must first be converted to absolute units (by multiplying by 980) and then multiplied by the number of beats per second, that is, heart rate (HR) in beats per minute divided by 60. Therefore, the average output power (P_l) of the left ventricle (neglecting the kinetic energy) in dyn-cm/sec or erg/sec is

$$P_l = \frac{\bar{P}_a\,(13.6/10)\,(SV)\,(d)\,(HR) \times 980}{60}$$

In cardiovascular studies the terms heart power and ventricular power are rarely used. However, the unit of power that is frequently used is minute work, that is, the work performed in 1 min.

The information just presented can be put to use to calculate the approximate average power output of the left ventricle. For example, in a resting 70-kg adult with a heart rate of 72 beats per minute, the cardiac output is typically 5 L/min and the aortic pressure is about 120/80 mm Hg. Therefore, the stroke volume (SV) is $5000/72 \times 69.4$ mL. The density (d) of blood is typically 1.06 g/mL and the weight of the stroke volume is $69.4 \times 1.06 = 73.6$ g. The mean aortic pressure ($\bar{P}_a$) is approximately equal to diastolic pressure plus one-third of pulse pressure, that is, $\bar{P}_a \times 80 + (120 - 80)/3 = 93.3$ mm Hg. The equivalent height for this pressure is therefore 93.3 × 13.6/10 = 126.9 cm. Therefore, the work performed by the left ventricle each time it beats is the product of weight and height, that is,

$$W_l = \left(\frac{5000}{72} \times 1.06\right)\left(\frac{93.3 \times 13.6}{10}\right) = 9340 \text{ g-cm}$$

The work performed in dyn-cm or ergs is therefore:

$$9340 \times 980 = 9.15 \times 10^6$$

Since power is the time rate of performing work, the output power of the left ventricle is calculated by determining the number of times that this work is performed in each second. The heart rate is 72 beats per minute or 72/60 = 1.2 beats/sec; therefore, the average power (P_l) of the left ventricle in dyn-cm/sec or ergs/sec is

$$P_l = 9.15 \times 10^6 \times 72/60 = 10.98 \times 10^6 \text{ ergs/sec}$$

Since 10^7 ergs = 1 J (joule) and 1 J/sec = 1 W (watt), the average output power of the left ventricle in watts is

$$P_l = \frac{10.98 \times 10^6 \text{ ergs/sec}}{10^7 \text{ ergs/J}} = 1.098 \text{ W}$$

By a similar calculation, it is possible to determine the approximate average output power of the right ventricle which ejects the stroke volume against an afterload of 25/10 mm Hg of pressure (mean pressure approximately diastolic plus one-third pulse). Performing this calculation gives a power output (P_r) for the right ventricle as follows:

$$\begin{aligned} P_r &= \frac{(10 + 15/3)\,(13.6)\,(69.4)\,(1.06)\;72 \times 980}{10 \times 60} \\ &= 1.76 \times 10^6 \text{ dyn-cm/sec} \\ &= 0.176 \text{ W} \end{aligned}$$

Therefore, the total average power (P_t) of the right and left ventricles is (neglecting the kinetic energy required to accelerate the blood)

$$P_t = P_r + P_l = 0.176 + 1.098 = 1.27 \text{ W}$$

The left ventricle performs the major work of the heart. Therefore, it is useful to rearrange the left-ventricular power expression by recognizing that cardiac ouput (CO) is equal to heart rate multiplied by stroke volume. Therefore, by substituting for stroke volume in mL/min (CO/HR), the average left-ventricular power output in watts is

$$P_l = \frac{\bar{P}_a\,(13.6/10)\,d(CO)\,980}{60} = \bar{P}_a\,(CO)\,(0.002355)$$

where P_l is in W, $\bar{P}_a$ is in mm Hg, and CO is in L/min.

Since the myocardial oxygen uptake (in mL/min) is directly related to the power developed by the heart, the foregoing expression indicates that the oxygen used per minute by the left ventricle depends on mean aortic pressure ($\bar{P}_a$) and cardiac output (CO). A similar statement can be made for the right ventricle by substituting mean pulmonary artery pressure ($\bar{P}_p$) for mean aortic pressure. Thus, the oxygen uptake of the heart is increased if cardic output (CO), mean aortic ($\bar{P}_a$) and mean pulmonary ($\bar{P}_p$) artery pressures are increased. State mathematically,

$$\frac{\text{O}_2 \text{ uptake}}{\text{min}} = K\,(\bar{P}_a + \bar{P}_p)\,CO$$

where K is a constant.

At this point it is important to digress on the difference between the energy cost of work in physical systems and the cost in physiological systems. As stated previously, energy is expended when a weight is raised through a height. In physical systems, no energy is expended in maintaining the weight at the new height. However, in physiological systems, if the weight is lifted by muscle force, energy is expended in raising the weight. If the weight is held at the new height, muscular energy is used for the duration of time that it is held at the new elevation. Thus, oxygen will be consumed in raising the weight and in maintaining it at its new elevation. In maintaining the elevated weight, tension (i.e., force) is developed in the muscle, and the oxygen consumed is dependent on the duration of the tension. This concept has become known as the tension–time relationship. Stated simply, it means that if forces are developed in physiological systems without the production of physical work, oxygen is consumed. An interesting example in the heart is the rise in ventricular pressure during the period of isovolumic (isometric) contraction when ventricular pressure is raised prior to ejection. The consequence of this fact is that the oxygen consumption of the heart is in excess of that required to produce output work.

Efficiency of the Heart

The output power of the heart is developed from the energy of metabolism. The amount of oxygen consumed per minute is directly related to the output power, which, of course is dependent on heart rate, cardiac output, and blood pressure. The oxygen consumed by the heart is identifiable by the difference in coronary arterial and venous oxygen concentrations. The number of calories liberated by oxygen consumption is dependent on the calorific equivalent of oxygen when a particular type of substrate (carbohydrate, protein, or fat) is metabolized. The calorie is a unit of energy and there are 4.18 J liberated for each physical (standard) calorie produced.

These facts can be used to estimate the power input to the heart that produced the average output power just calculated, that is, 1.27 W. The starting point is a knowledge of the coronary blood flow and the arterial and venous oxygen content of the blood entering and leaving the coronary circulation. In a typical 70-kg subject, the coronary artery blood flow is 5% of the cardiac output. Therefore, the coronary flow is $5000 \times 5/100 =$ 250 mL/min or $250/60 = 4.17$ mL/sec. Typically, arterial blood contains 19.5 mL of oxygen per 100 mL of blood. The coronary sinus blood draining most of the heart muscle contains only about 40% of this amount of oxygen, that is, $19.5 \times 0.4 = 7.8$ mL O_2/100 mL blood. Therefore, the heart consumed $19.5 - 7.8 = 11.7$ mL O_2 per 100 mL of blood flowing through it, meaning the amount of oxygen consumed in each second is $4.17 \times 11.7/100 = 0.488$ mL. For a typical substrate, 1L of oxygen consumed liberates 4.8 large (kilo) calories, or 4.8 standard calories per mL oxygen. Consequently, the number of standard calories liberated per second by the myocardial oxygen consumption is $4.8 \times 0.488 = 2.34$ calories/sec. The mechanical equivalent of heat is 4.18 J/calorie; therefore, the number of joules per second (i.e., watts) of input power (P_i) is $4.18 \times 2.34 = 9.78$ W.

The percent efficiency of a device is defined as the ratio of output (P_o) to total input (P_t) power multiplied by 100. Therefore, the percent efficiency (N) is

$$N = \frac{P_o}{P_t} = \frac{1.27}{9.78} = 0.129 \text{ or } 12.9\%$$

This value for efficiency (at rest) is slightly low because the small amount of output produced in imparting velocity to the blood has been neglected; the power developed by the atria was also neglected. Nonethe-

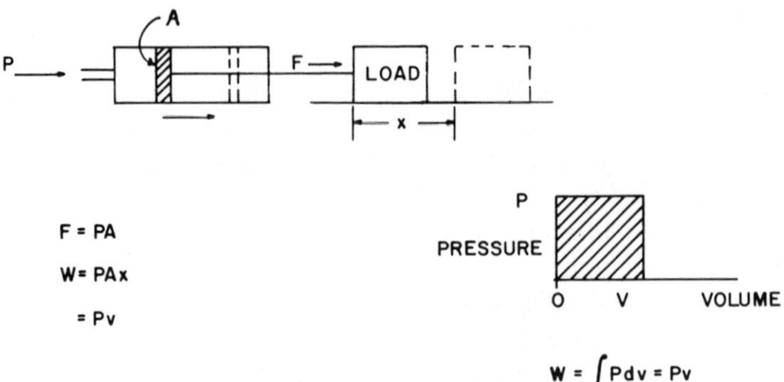

FIGURE 4.37. Work and pressure–volume diagram.

less, the value obtained is consistent with efficiency figures obtained for other chemical engines.

In the preceding discussion the kinetic energy was neglected. Because the stroke volume is ejected into the aorta with a velocity v, the kinetic energy is equal to the mass of the stroke volume (m) and the velocity squared, divided by two. The kinetic energy is therefore $mv^2/2$. At rest, this component represents only a small percentage of the energy required to eject blood against aortic pressure. However, during vigorous exercise, the kinetic energy can amount up to 20% or more of the energy required to eject blood against aortic pressure.

The Pressure–Volume Diagram

The behavior of the heart as a pump can be understood better if it is likened to a mechanical engine. In order to do so, it is necessary to recall that work is performed when a force acts through a distance. Therefore, consider a loaded piston in which a gas under a constant pressure (P) is admitted as shown in Figure 4.37. The force (F) on the piston is the pressure multiplied by the area (A) of the piston, that is, $F = PA$. Now if the piston moves the load through a distance X, the work performed is PAX. Note that AX is the volume of gas admitted; therefore, the work performed (W) is the product of the pressure and volume,

$$W = PV$$

In the heart and in other engines, both the pressure and volume vary throughout the cycle. For this reason it is necessary to integrate the pressure–volume relationship; therefore, the work (W) is

$$W = \int_{t_1}^{t_2} PdV$$

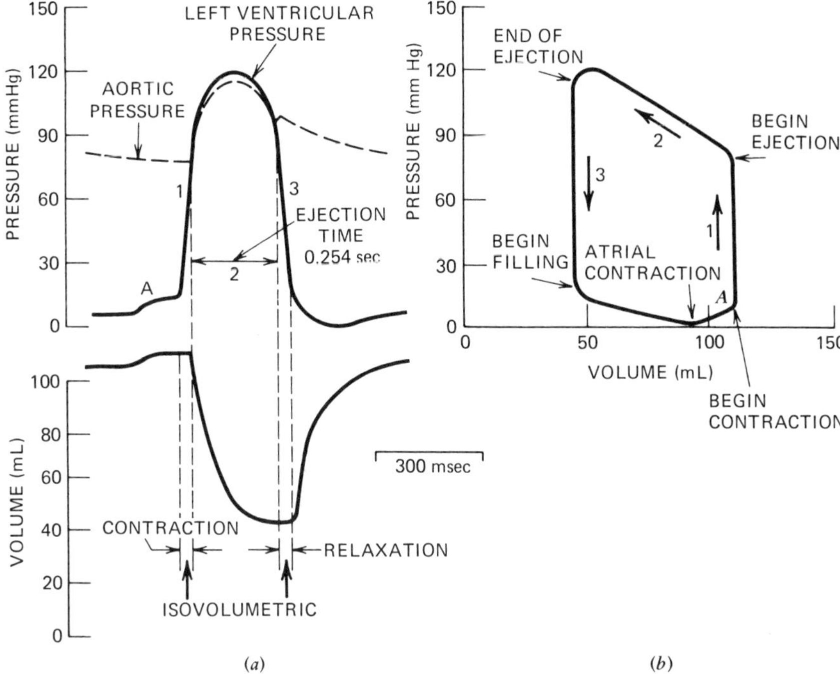

FIGURE 4.38. (*a*) Left ventricular pressure and volume curves and (*b*) pressure–volume diagram.

where P is the pressure that exists for the incremental volume change dV. The integration time $(t_1–t_2)$ is the ejection period of the heart. It is interesting to note that $\int PdV$ is the area under a pressure–volume curve, when pressure is plotted versus volume.

The simple concept just developed can be applied to the analysis of the heart as a pump. Figure 4.38 illustrates the left-ventricular and aortic pressure and the left-ventricular volume during systole and diastole. Referring to Figure 4.38*a*, the cardiac cycle starts with atrial contraction, which propels a small amount of blood into the left ventricle causing a slight rise in pressure (A) and a slight increase in ventricular volume. Ventricular contraction starts and ventricular pressure rises (1) with no change in ventricular volume; this portion of the cycle is called the isometric or isovolumetric phase of contraction. When ventricular pressure rises to aortic diastolic pressure, the aortic valve opens, blood is ejected (2), and output work is performed on the blood. As ejection continues, pressure rises then falls late in systole. When the ventricular pressure falls below aortic pressure, the aortic valve closes and ventricular pressure falls with little change in ventricular volume (3). When ventricular pressure falls below left atrial pressure, the mitral valve opens and the left ventricle starts to fill passively, that is, the volume starts to increase as shown. Ventricular filling is rapid at first, owing to the accumulation of blood in the left atrium while the left ventricle was contracting.

When the left ventricular cycle is expressed as a pressure–volume diagram, as shown in Figure 4.38*b*, the various phases can be identified clearly. The interesting feature of such a pressure–volume diagram is that its area represents the work performed by the left ventricle. In the example shown the area is 6090 mm Hg-mL, which when converted to ergs (by multiplying by 1413)* is 8.6×10^6. The power developed is this work divided by the time taken to complete the *PV* loop (the ejection time), that is, 0.245 sec; therefore, the power is $8.6 \times 10^6/0.254 \times 10^7 = 3.38$ W. (The time required to complete the loop is, however, slightly in excess of the ejection time.) Note that it is during the ejection phase that the ventricles are working maximally, and that the peak power developed during this time is about three times the average power.

Approximation of Cardiac Work and Power

Unfortunately, there is no accurate method for recording volume throughout the ventricular cycle. However, it is easy to record ventricular and aortic pressure; from the latter, ejection time can be measured. Cardiac output can be determined easily and various indices that use these quantities have been developed to express the performance of the left ventricle as a pump. A few of these will now be presented.

VENTRICULAR DYNAMICS TESTS

It is of considerable importance to be able to assess the pumping capability of the heart in humans. Perhaps the best test is embodied in Starling's law, which will be described subsequently. There are, however, other direct and indirect tests that have been designed to measure ventricular function. A remarkable number of terms, such as index of cardiac effort, pressure–time per beat, force–time per beat, tension–time index, contractile element work, contractile element work index per minute, have been created to describe some aspect of ventricular function; Yang *et al.* (1972) defined and discussed all of them. Only the most frequently used tests will be described in the following paragraphs.

*Assuming $g = 980$; 1.06 and 13.6 for the density of blood and mercury, respectively; and dividing by 10 for mm Hg units.

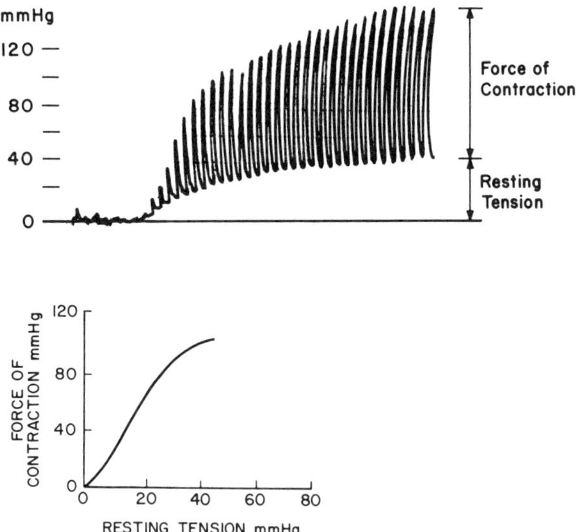

FIGURE 4.39. Starling's law of the heart, which states that an increase in resting (diastolic) tension results in an increased force of contraction. (Illustrated courtesy of M. Niebauer.)

Starling's Law

In the latter part of the 19th century, Ernest Starling, the eminent British physician–physiologist, enunciated the law that describes the response of cardiac (and skeletal) muscle to loading. Stated simply, Starling's law states that an increase in resting (diastolic) fiber length results in an increased force of contraction. This law can be demonstrated by applying mechanical stretch directly to myocardial fibers or by increasing the diastolic filling, which accomplishes the same end. Stated functionally, the law predicts that increased diastolic filling results in an increase in stroke volume. There is, of course, a limit to this response, as Starling clearly demonstrated.

Figure 4.39 illustrates Starling's law demonstrated on the isolated canine heart in which the left ventricle was beating isovolumically. A catheter in the left ventricle permitted recording pressure and gradually increasing filling as shown. With a continued increase in diastolic loading, the force of contraction increased. Beyond a point, a further increase in loading no longer produced an increase in the force of contraction. In the normal heart, unloading usually restores the contractile force. In the diseased heart temporary unloading is frequently employed to permit recovery to occur.

Tension–Time Index

It was stated earlier that oxygen is consumed by a muscle if it exerts a force through a distance and if it sustains a force without a change in length. Thus the physiological cost of work is in excess of the mechanical work performed, because in most situations of muscular contraction, at least for a portion of the contraction phase, metabolic energy is consumed without accomplishing mechanical work. The sustained muscle force that does not move a load is described as muscle tension, and the amount of oxygen consumed is related to the amount of tension and the time it is present. This is the idea behind the tension–time index.

Perhaps nowhere is the tension–time concept more important than in the heart muscle, which is extremely oxygen hungry. Cardiac muscle is totally dependent on its coronary circulation, from which it removes about 60% of the oxygen it contains. Therefore, it is of considerable value to develop techniques, preferably indirect, that can identify changes in myocardial oxygen consumption.

Recall that the power output of the heart dictates the oxygen need per unit of time and that heart rate, stroke volume, and outflow pressure (afterload) are the important determinants of oxygen need. Also recall that the work done per beat by the left ventricle is the area of the pressure–volume loop (Figure 4.38). The power output is the area of the loop divided by the time required to complete it, which is very close to the ejection time. These important theoretical concepts underlie the tension–time index developed by Sarnoff et al. (1958). Figure 4.40 provides graphic representation of the definition of the tension–time index, which is the mean left ventricular pressure (detertmined during the ejection period) multiplied by the ejection period; this product is then multiplied by the heart rate in beats per minute. Conceptually, therefore, the tension–time index identifies mean left ventricular pressure which is sustained for a time (the number of seconds for each minute) that ejection occurs. Note that the stroke volume is not included in the tension–time index. Nonetheless, it has been found that the tension–time index is a reasonably good descriptor of myocardial oxygen consumption. In a series of isolated-heart experiments Sarnoff and his associates proved this point by varying heart rate, stroke volume, and outflow resistance.

Systolic-Time Intervals

The time between the onset of ventricular excitation and the ejection of blood from the left ventricle into the aorta is called the pre-ejection period (PEP). The time when the left ventricle ejects blood is called the left

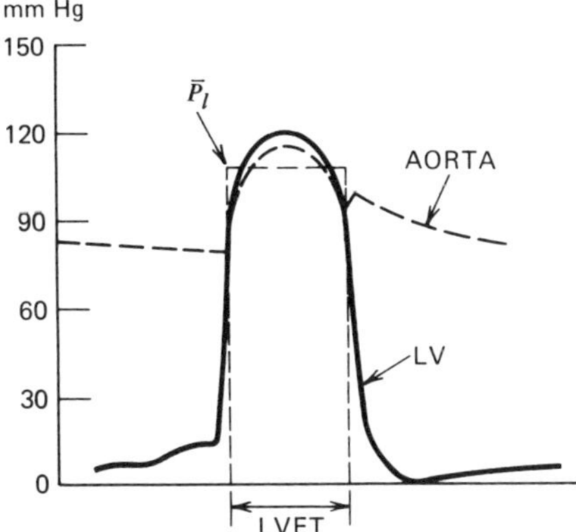

FIGURE 4.40. The tension–time index is a measure of the duration in 1 min that the left ventricle develops pressure. The tension–time index (TTI) is the product of the mean left ventricular pressure (P_l) in mm Hg during the ejection time, the duration of the left ventricular ejection time (LVET) in seconds, and the heart rate in beats per minute; TTI = $\bar{P}_l$ × LVET × *HR*.

ventricular ejection time (LVET). These two times, which are illustrated in Figure 4.41, are indicative of the status of the heart. The ratio of PEP to LVET has been found to be a good indicator of the condition of the heart, and as will be shown, there is a normal and abnormal range for this cardiac parameter.

In practice the preejection period is calculated in the following manner. The time between the onset of the Q wave of the ECG identifies the onset of ventricular excitation in a very precise way. The onset of the second heart sound (S_2) signals the end of ventricular ejection accurately. The left ventricular ejection time is found by recording the output of a pulse pickup placed over an artery close to the heart (e.g., carotid). Although there is a pulse transit time between the ECG and the arterial site, this time contributes no error because the arterial pulse is used only to measure the left ventricular ejection time (LVET): Thus the preejection period is calculated by subtracting the LVET from the QS_2 interval as shown in Figure 4.41.

It has been found that the systolic time intervals are quite sensitive to the pumping ability of the left ventricle. For example, if left ventricular performance is diminished by cardiac disease, the preejection period lengthens and the left-ventricular ejection time decreases, while the QS_2 time remains relatively unchanged. It has been found that the ratio PEP/LVET is 0.35 ± 0.04 in normal subjects with heart rates of 50–110 beats per minute. With cardiac disease, the ratio increases. Mild, moderate, and

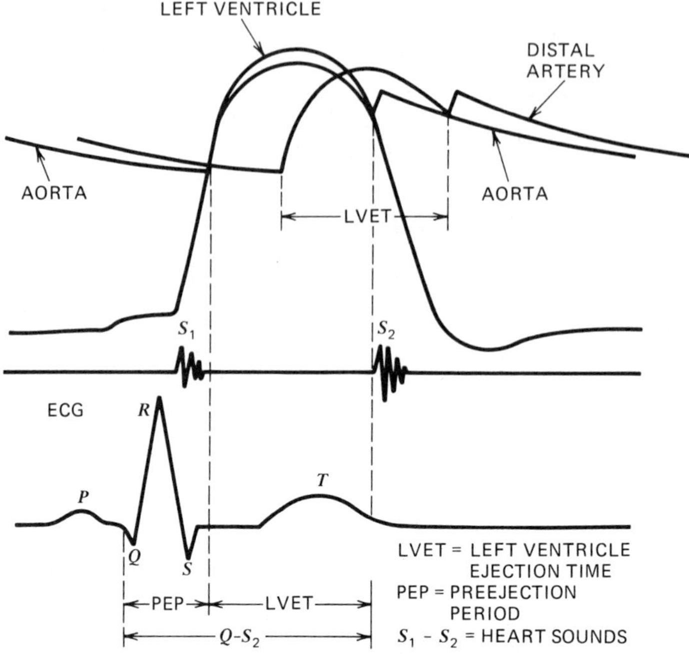

FIGURE 4.41. Left ventricle aortic and distal artery pressure, along with heart sounds and the ECG. These data are used to calculate the preejection period (PEP) as shown.

severe myocardial impairment are associated with ratios of 0.44–0.52, 0.53–0.60, and greater than 0.60, respectively (Weissler, 1977).

The systolic time intervals are good indicators of myocardial function. They can be recorded noninvasively and will undoubtedly see widespread use. However, there are situations in which the ratio of PEP/LVET must be viewed critically to avoid misinterpretation of the extent of cardiac disease.

Stroke-Work Index

The fact that it is now relatively easy to measure cardiac output at the bedside (with the thermal-dilution technique) makes it possible to obtain quantitative information on the ability of the heart to pump blood. Dividing cardiac output by heart rate yields stroke volume. By knowing stroke volume, arterial blood pressure and left-ventricular end-diastolic pressure, the work per beat (stroke work) can be calculated for the left ventricle. By knowing body weight and height, body surface area can be calculated. Therefore, the stroke work per square meter of body surface area

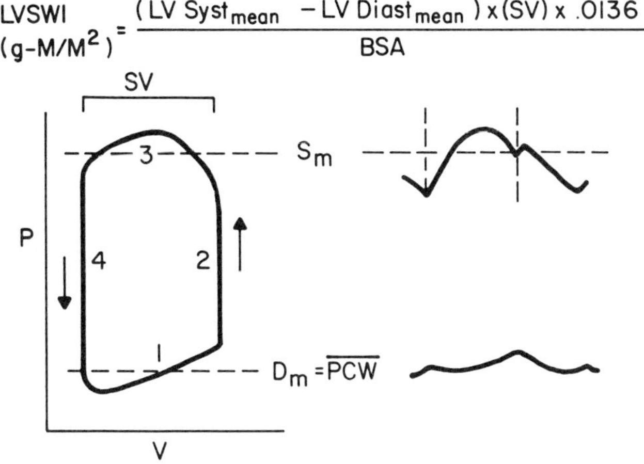

Sm ~ SYSTOLIC BP − 1/3 (SYSTOLIC−DIASTOLIC BP)
SV = CO/HR

FIGURE 4.42. Method of calculating left-ventricular stroke-work index. [Redrawn from Parmley (1978).]

can be calculated. Parmley (1978) designated this quantity "stroke-work index" and has found that it, along with left-ventricular end-diastolic pressure, is a useful descriptor of a failing heart.

Calculation of the stroke-work index is based on the fact that the work performed by the left ventricle is represented by the area of the pressure–volume loop (Figure 4.38), which is a plot of pressure versus volume. The method used by Parmley to estimate stroke work, without recording the pressure–volume loop, is illustrated in Figure 4.42. To determine the area of the loop, simplifying assumptions are made in reference to the pressure. The aortic pressure is shown on the upper right of Figure 4.42. Mean ejection pressure (S_m) for the loop is taken by Parmley as aortic systolic pressure minus one-third of pulse pressure (systolic minus diastolic pressure). End-diastolic mean pressure (D_m) is taken as pulmonary capillary wedge (PCW) pressure. Thus the mean pressure difference during one cardiac cycle is (S_m − PCW). The volume ejected is stroke volume (SV), which is calculated by dividing cardiac output by heart rate. Stroke-work index is this product divided by body surface area (BSA) calculated from body weight and height according to the standard expression

$$\text{BSA} = 3.81\ W^{0.425} H^{0.725}$$

where W is weight in g and H is the height in cm; the area is in cm^2.

The stroke-work index (SWI) is therefore

$$\text{SWI} = \frac{(S_m - \text{PCW})(SV)\,0.0136}{\text{BSA}}$$

where 0.0136 is a constant employed to allow use of the conventional units (mm Hg and mL) and obtain SWI in g-m/m^2 of body surface area.

An example will illustrate a typical calculation. Suppose that aortic pressure is 120/80 mm Hg, pulmonary capillary wedge pressure is 10 mm Hg, cardiac output is 5 L/min with a heart rate of 70 beats per minute; the subject is 165 cm tall and weighs 70 kg. Therefore,

$$S_m = 120 - \tfrac{1}{3}(120 - 80) = 106.7 \text{ mm Hg}$$

$$\text{PCW} = 10 \text{ mm Hg}$$

$$SV = 5000/70 = 71.4 \text{ mL}$$

$$\text{BSA} = 3.81 \times 70{,}000^{0.425} \times 165^{0.725} = 17{,}700 \text{ cm}^2$$

$$\text{SWI} = \frac{(106.7 - 10) \times 71.4 \times 0.0136}{1.77} = 53.05 \text{ g-m/m}^2$$

Parmley (1978) found that SWI is a good descriptor of the ability of the left ventricle to pump blood when presented with a load, expressed as left-ventricular filling pressure. This relationship is shown in Figure 4.43 for subjects who have hyperreactive, normal, adequate, and depressed cardiac function and subjects in shock. The SWI is particularly useful in evaluating the ability of the left ventricle to pump following myocardial infarction. Table 4.13 presents data reported by Parmley (1978).

Exercise-Stress Testing

The exercise-stress test is designed to identify the ability of the coronary arteries to deliver an adequate amount of oxygenated blood to the heart muscle. The test consists of imposing a work load of sufficient intensity and duration to produce electrocardiographic changes in patients suspected of having coronary heart disease.

In the normal subject, the ability to tolerate exercise decreases with increasing age. Many studies have been carried out in which it has been found that for a given age, the maximum heart rate is a good descriptor of exercise tolerance. Figure 4.44 illustrates the type of relationship. There are tables to be used in stress testing that contain the same information. In a patient with suspected coronary heart disease, the exercise load may be

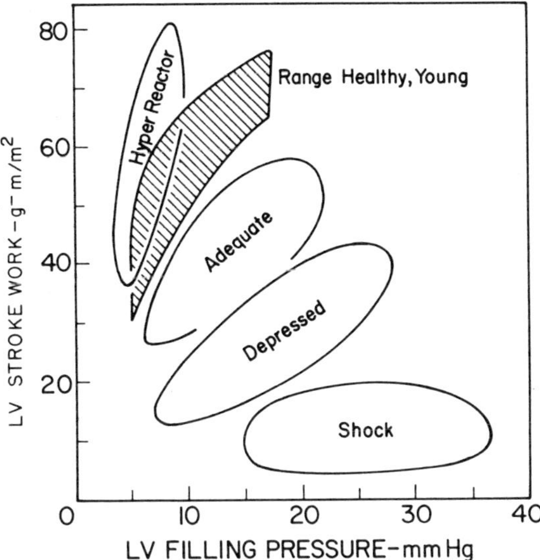

FIGURE 4.43. Relationship between left-ventricular stroke-work index and left-ventricular filling pressure. [Redrawn from Parmley (1978).]

adjusted to 80–100% of the predicted heart rate for the subject's age. However, if severe dyspnea, angina, or arrhythmias occur, the test is terminated.

The indicator of inadequate coronary circulation is a change in the ECG. Although the *QRS*, *T*, and *U* (if present) waves have been proposed as indicators of ischemia, it is a change in the *S-T* segment that is the most sensitive and consistent indicator. Figure 4.45 identifies the *S-T* segment and the *J* point (the end of the ventricular excitation and the beginning of the *S-T* segment) which feature prominently in describing the ECG in myocardial ischemia.

There are three important factors that underlie identification of a posi-

TABLE 4.13. Stroke Work Index (SWI) in Subjects with Impaired Left-Ventricular Function in Myocardial Infarction[a]

LV Filling Pressure (mm Hg)	SWI (g-m/m^2)	Description
<15	20	Without therapy, morality near zero
>15	<20	With conventional therapy, mortality about 85%
>15	>20	About 10–20% mortality

[a] Data from Parmley (1978).

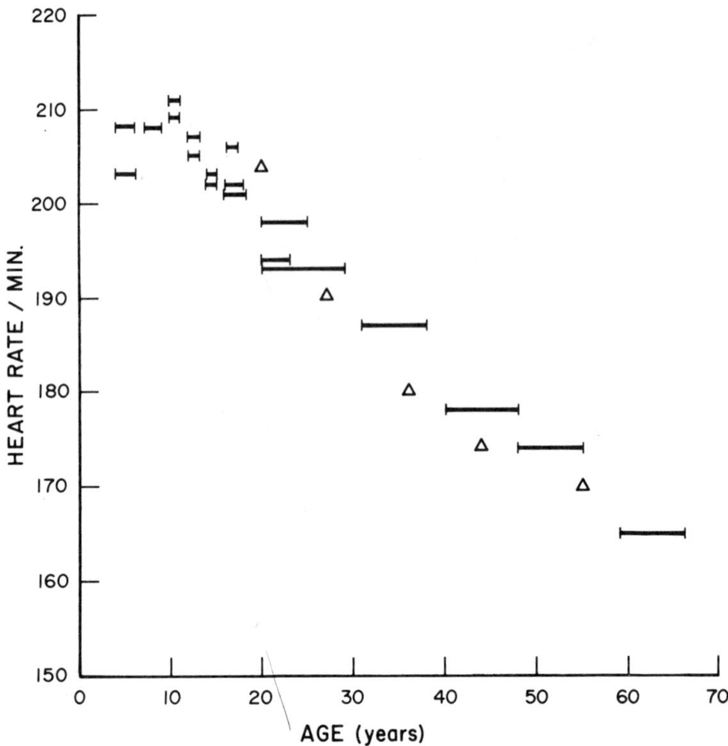

FIGURE 4.44. The relationship between maximum heart rate and age for males. [x from Bruce et al. (1965); other data from *Handbooks of Circulation* (1959) and *Respiration* (1959). Ditmer, D. S. (Ed.). WADC Tech. Rep. Oct 1957 and August 1958. ASTIC, Arlington, VA.]

tive exercise-stress test for coronary heart disease: (1) nature and severity of the imposed exercise, (2) the leads used for recording the ECG, and (3) the criteria used to evaluate the ECG. These points will be discussed subsequently.

Most exercise tests consist of running on a treadmill or pedaling a bicycle ergometer. The exercise load is increased (or prolonged) to attain a desired percentage of the predicted heart rate for the subject's age. The test may be discontinued before the desired heart rate is reached if ominous clinical signs supervene. Conversely, the test may be prolonged to bring out the sought-for changes in patients with suspected coronary heart disease.

There are many conditions which exclude application of the exercise test, such as valvular disease, cardiomyopathy, severe anemia, hypokalemia, corpulmonale, and vasoregulatory abnormalities. Digitalis therapy, if used, must be discontinued for several weeks before the test.

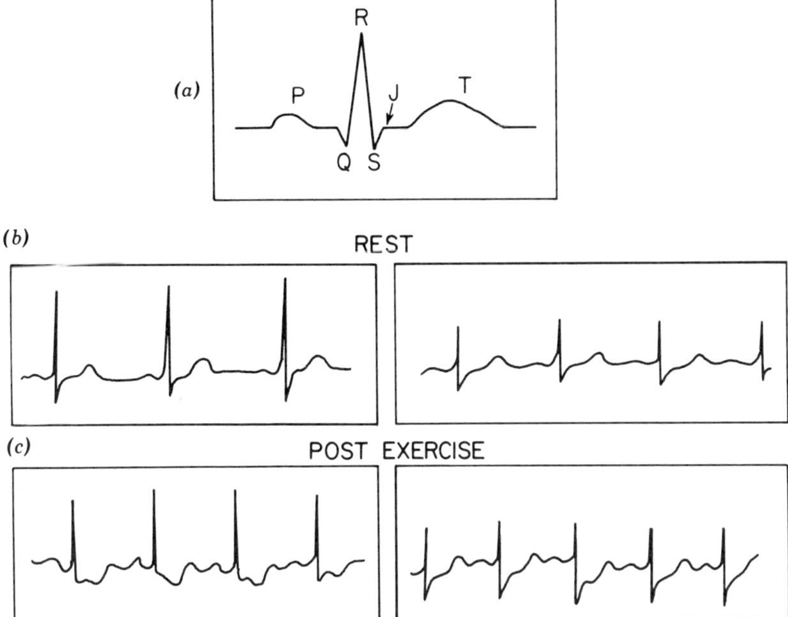

FIGURE 4.45. (*a*) The normal ECG showing the *J* point, which identifies the beginning of the *S-T* segment in a normal subject. (*b*) and (*c*) show control and postexercise lead V4-ECGs from patients with coronary heart disease; (*b*) illustrates and *S-T* segment shift of 0.2 mV with a downward slope in the *S-T* segment and (*c*) illustrates an 0.26 mV horizontal shift in the *S-T* segment.

Because the exercise test is designed to stress the ventricular myocardium, there is risk of arrhythmias. The test should not be performed without emergency medical aid available. A defibrillator should always be on hand.

The leads selected for recording the exercise ECG are important; those that are closest to the ventricles are the best. In practice, V2 and V5, which see the right and left ventricles, are most frequently used. Less often, the limb leads 2,3 and aVF are used. It is essential that a preexercise ECG be taken and it is highly desirable to monitor the ECG during, as well as after, the test.

The most controversial item in the exercise test is the criterion used to evaluate the ECG. As stated previously, the ischemia information is contained in the *S-T* segment. Many clinicians consider a shift of 0.1 mV or more in the *S-T* segment as an indicator of myocardial ischemia; some require slightly more displacement. The nature of the *S-T* segment shift is also believed to be important; a segment shift that is horizontal (for more than 0.08 sec) or slopes downward are indicative of myocardial ischemia. Figure 4.45 illustrates both types of *S-T* segment shift.

At this time, it is difficult to evaluate the exercise-stress test as an indicator of coronary heart disease. This is because many different criteria are used to identify a positive test. Although chest pain (angina pectoris) is a classic sign of coronary heart disease, many patients with effort-induced angina do not exhibit *S-T* segment shifts. But this does not mean that they are free from coronary heart disease; it may mean that the electrocardiographic leads used did not see the ischemic myocardium.

HISTORICAL POSTSCRIPT

Cardiac Output

In 1870 A. Fick proposed his now-famous method of measuring cardiac output, although he did not use the method himself. Nonetheless, its value was soon established. The original account of Fick's paper (translated by Hoff, 1965) provides the essential facts.

> Herr Fick gave a lecture on the measurement of the quantity of blood ejected by the ventricle of the heart in each systole, a figure which is without doubt of the greatest importance to determine. Nevertheless the most different opinions have been given of it. While Th. Young placed the value in question at 45 cc., the newer textbooks of physiology give much higher values, which, based on the estimations of Volkmann and Vierordt, run as high as 180. In such circumstances it is unusual that no one has yet hit upon the following obvious method by which this important value may be determined directly, at least in animals. One determines how much oxygen an animal takes out of the air in a given time and how much carbon dioxide it gives off. During the experiment one obtains a sample of arterial and a sample of venous blood. In both, the content of oxygen and the content of carbon dioxide are to be determined. The difference in oxygen contents tells how much oxygen each cubic centimeter of blood takes up in its course through the lungs, and since one knows the total quantity of oxygen absorbed in a given time, one can calculate how many cubic centimeters of blood passed through the lungs in this time, or, if one divides by the number of heart beats in this time, how many cubic centimeters of blood are ejected with each beat of the heart. The corresponding calculation with the quantities of carbon dioxide gives a determination of the same value, which serves as a control for the first.
>
> Since two gas pumps are required to carry out this method, the lecturer is unfortunately not able to report experimental findings. He will therefore give only a calculation of the extent of the circulation in man according to

> the schema of the method here described, based on more or less arbitrary data. According to experiments carried out by Schaeffer in Ludwig's laboratory, one cc. of arterial blood of the dog contains 0.146 cc. of oxygen (measured at 0° temperature and 1 meter Hg pressure); 1 cc. of venous dog's blood contains 0.0905 cc. of oxygen. Each cubic centimeter of blood takes up in its passage through the lungs 0.0555 cc. Assume that this were also true in man. Assume further that a man absorbs 833 g. of oxygen out of the air in 24 hours. At 0° and 1 m. pressure this would occupy a space of 433,200 cc. Accordingly 5 cc of oxygen would be absorbed by the lungs every second. In order to make possible this absorption, there must be, according to the above assumption, a blood flow through the lungs of 5 ÷ 0.0555 cc., or 90 cc. per second. assuming finally that 7 systoles take place in 6 seconds, 77 cc. of blood would be ejected with each systole of the ventricle.

Evidently the needed "pumps" for obtaining O_2 concentrations were not available. Nonetheless, the method was put to use in animals sometime before 1900, and it was quickly learned that right-ventricular or, even better, pulmonary artery blood was required for the mixed venous sample. It was, however, the development of cardiac catheterization in humans that permitted use of the Fick method to calculate cardiac output accurately.

The indicator-dilution method was first used by G. N. Stewart in England in 1898. The indicator was a saline solution infused continuously. Later, in 1921, he reported the single-injection method of using the same indicator. In both studies, the detector was a conductivity cell placed in a major artery.

The use of dyes as indicators for the measurement of cardiac output was developed by Hamilton and his colleagues in the late 1920s and early 1930s. Because there were no densitometers to permit inscription of the dilution curve, Hamilton and his colleagues developed an ingenious method for overcoming this limitation. The sampling method consisted of allowing arterial blood to flow via a small-bore tube into a series of test tubes affixed to the periphery of a slowly rotating drum (kymograph). A typical blood "withdrawal" sequence consisted of starting the kymograph about 5–15 sec after dye injection. The test tubes passed the blood-delivery tube at about 1 sec intervals. Although a little blood was lost between passage of the test tubes, this was unimportant, since it is only the concentration of dye in each tube that is important. The concentration of dye in the plasma of each sample was measured in a spectrophotometer. A plot of the magnitude of these individual concentrations versus time constituted the dilution curve. This technique was applied to animals and even to humans (Hamilton et al., 1932) using the femoral artery as the sampling site.

Recirculation of indicator obscured the downslope of the dilution curve, and there was much uncertainty about the end of the first pass. In a series of elegant studies with a water-filled, branching-tube model of the vascular system, Kinsman et al. (1929) used dyes as indicators and showed that the downslope of the dilution curve was essentially exponential. By plotting these concentration values on semilogarithmic paper, the descending limb of the first pass became a straight line. Extrapolation of this line to a negligible concentration provided the necessary data points that allowed reconstruction of the tail of dilution curve to eliminate recirculation, thereby allowing an accurate measurement of the area under the dilution curve.

Cardiac Catheterization

The first cardiac catheterizations were performed in France by Magendie and Bernard, who passed thermometers into the left and right ventricles to determine the temperature of the blood therein (Geddes et al., 1965). These studies were conducted to demonstrate that venous blood was hotter than artertial blood. Soon thereafter, Chauveau and Marey, also in France, passed catheters into the right atrium and right and left ventricle of the unanesthetized horse and recorded the pressures in these cardiac chambers in the 1870s. Figures 2.46 and 2.47 illustrate their catheters and pneumatic recording system, along with chamber-pressure records.

Cardiac catheterization in humans was accomplished by Forsmann in 1929. He passed a catheter into his own right atrium via a vein opened at the left elbow. He then walked the considerable distance from his laboratory to the X-ray room to verify the catheter position radiographically. Forsmann carried out this procedure because he wanted to develop a method of introducing drugs directly into the heart. It was Cournand and his associates who exploited cardiac catheterization in 1945 to obtain right ventricular blood for Fick cardiac output studies.

Fluid Flow

Jean Louis Marie Poiseuille (1799–1869) was the first to identify and quantify the factors that control the flow of fluids. It is somewhat surprising to note that despite the widespread use of aqueducts by the Romans, they had only superficial knowledge of fluid dynamics.

Poiseuille was the first to use the mercury-filled U-tube to measure blood pressure. The results of this study are contained in his doctoral thesis for the medical degree. Poiseuille's work gave us mm Hg as the units for measuring blood pressure. However, Poiseuille did not continue in medical practice and research; he transferred his attention to the flow of fluids in physical systems and his law, derived from this research, led him to an investigation of the flow of all materials. These studies founded the field of rheology. The unit of viscosity, the poise, was named after him.

Although Poiseuille recognized that the volume flow per unit time did not increase linearly with an increase in driving pressure, it remained for Osborne Reynolds (1842–1912) to point out that the flow changed from laminar to turbulent as flow velocity is increased in a given tube. He studied the relationship between the point where flow became turbulent in tubes of different diameters using a colored dye injected into the flowing stream. There are perhaps no better words than his own, written in 1883, which are

> When the velocities were sufficiently low, the streak of colour (sic) extended in a beautiful straight line through the tube. . . . As the velocity was increased by small stages, at some point in the tube, always at a considerable distance from the trumpet or intake, the colour band would all at once mix up with the surrounding water, and fill the rest of the tube with a mass of coloured water, ...

From this simple experiment, which is seldom repeated today, came the Reynolds number which identifies the flow velocity for the development of turbulence. Reynolds later developed the mathematical framework which underlies the number named after him.

Starling's Law of the Heart

Ernest H. Starling, the English physiologist, was a prolific researcher and made many important discoveries relative to the heart, circulation, and fluid transport. His law of the heart is elegantly described in the Linacre Lecture (1928). He used his isolated canine heart–lung preparation connected to an artificial resistance and venous reservoir to make his discovery. Ventricular volume was measured by a glass globe (oncometer), surrounding the heart and connected to piston recorder. Arterial and venous pressure and ventricular volume were recorded on a smoked-drum kymograph and cardiac output was measured by collecting the outflow from the heart in a graduate. By using several manipulations, Starling showed that the pressure developed was related to ventricular filling. He clearly showed that it was not filling pressure but diastolic ventricular volume that determined the force of contraction. He stated his law as follows: "the energy of contraction, however measured, is a function of the length of the muscle fiber." In another place in the Lecture, he stated that "within physiological limits the larger the volume of the heart, the greater are the energy of its contractions and the amount of chemical change at each contraction." He was, of course, referring to the increased oxygen uptake and carbon dioxide liberation.

REFERENCES

Allison, R. D. (1966). Stroke volume, cardiac output and impedance measurements. *Proc. Ann. Conf. Eng. Med. Biol.*, paper 8.5.

Andrews, F. A. and Wheeler, H. B. (1979). Venous occlusion plethysmography for detection of venous thrombosis. *Med. Instr.* **13,** 350–354.

Bache, R. J. (1969). Evaluation of thoracic impedance plethysmography as an indicator of stroke volume in man. *Amer. J. Med. Sci.* **258,** 100–113.

Baker, L. E., Judy, W. V., Geddes, L. E., Langley, F. M., and Hill, D. W. (1971). The measurement of cardiac output by electrical impedance. *Cardiovasc. Res. Ctr. Bull.* **9,** 135–145.

Bruce, R. A., Rowell, L. B., Blackmon, J. R. and Doan, A. (1954). Cardiovascular function tests. *Heart Bull.* **14,** 8.

Chauveau, J. B. A. and Marey, E. J. (1861). Determination graphique des rapports de la pulsations cardiaque avec les monvements de l'artericlle et du ventricule obtenu au moyen d'un appareil enregistreur. *C. R. Mem. Soc. de Biol.* **353,** Mem 3–11.

Chinard, F. P., Enns, T., and Nolan, M. F. (1962). Indicator-dilution studies with diffusible indicators. *Circ. Res.* **10,** 473–490.

Coulter, N. A. and Pappenheimer, J. R. (1949). Development of turbulence in flowing blood. *Amer. J. Physiol.* **159,** 401–408.

Cournand, A., Riley, R. L., Breed, E. S., Baldwin, E. de F., and Richards, R. W. (1945). Measurement of cardiac output in man using technique of catheterization of right airicle and ventricle. *J. Clin. Invest.* **24,** 106–116.

Denniston, J., Maher, J. T., Reeves, F. T., Cruz, J. C., Gymerman, A., and Grover, R. F. (1976). Measurement of cardiac output by electrical impedance at rest and during exercise. *J. Appl. Physiol.* **40,** 91–95.

Dotter, C. T., and Judkins, M. P. (1964). Transluminal treatment of arteriosclerotic obstruction. *Circulation* **30,** 654–670.

Fegler, G. (1954). Measurement of cardiac output in anesthetized animals by a thermodilution method. *Q. Journ. Exp. Physiol.* **39,** 153–164.

Fick, A. (1870). Uber die Messung des Blutstroms in den Hertzventrikle. Verhandl. d. phys. Med. Ges zu Wurzburg **2,** XVI. (See Hoff, 1965.)

Forrester, J. S., Ganz, W., Diamond, G., McHugh, T. Chanette, D. W., and Swan, H. J. C. (1972). Thermodilution cardiac output determination with a single flow-directed catheter. *Am. Heart J.* **83,** 306–311.

Forsmann, W. (1929). Die Sondierung des rechten Herzen. *Klin Wochnschr.* **8,** 2085–2087.

Ganz, W., Donoso, R., Marcus, H., Forester, J. S., and Swan, H. J. C. (1971). A new technique for measurement of cardiac output by thermodilution in man. *Am. J. Cardiol.* **27,** 392–396.

Geddes, L. A. (1970). *The Direct and Indirect Measurement of Blood Pressure*. Year Book Publishers, Chicago.

Geddes, L. A., and Baker, L. E. (1975). *Principles of Applied Biomedical Instrumentation*, Wiley, New York.

Geddes, L. A., McCrady, J. D., and Hoff, H. E. (1965). Contributions of the horse to knowledge of the heart and circulation. II. Cardiac catheterization and ventricular dynamics. *Connecticut Med.* **29**, 864–873.

Goodyer, A. V. N., *et al.* (1959). Thermal dilution curves in the intact animal. *Circ. Res.* **7**, 432–441.

Gruntzig, A., and Kumpe, D. A. (1979). Technique of percutaneous transluminal angioplasty with the Gruntzig balloon catheter. *Amer. J. Radiol.* **132**, 547–552.

Geddes, L. A. and Bobbs, C. F. (1980). A new technique for repeated measurements of cardiac output during cardiopulmonary resuscitation. *Crit. Care Med.*, **8**, 131–133.

Grubbs, D. S., Geddes, L. A., and Kusmic, J. (1983). Loss of indication in the pulmonary circuit when measuring cardiac output. *Jpn. Heart J.* (in press).

Grubbs, D. S., Geddes, L. A., and Voorhees, W. (1983). Right heart output using saline without indicator loss and with a new type of electrically calibrated catheter-tip conductivity cell. *Jpn. Heart J.* (in press).

Hamilton, W. F., Moore, J. W., Kinsman, J. M., and Spurling, R. G. (1932). Studies on the circulation. *Am. J. Physiol.* **99**, 534–555.

Handbook of Circulation (1949). Analysis and Compilation by P. L. Altman. Div. Biol. & Agr. Natl. Acad. Sci. Natl. Res. Council. ASTIA Document Proj. 7158, Task 71801.

Handbook of Respiration (1958). Compiled by Altman, J., Gilson, J. F., and Wang, C. C. Div. Biol. & Agr. Natl. Acad. Sci. Natl. Res. Council. Arlington, VA. ASTIA Document AD-15823.

Harley, A. and Greenfield, J. C. (1968). Determination of cardiac output in man by means of impedance plethysmography. *Aerosp. Med.* **39**, 248–252.

Hoff, H. E. in Geddes et al. (1965). Fick A. (1870). Uber die Messung des Blutstroms in den Herzventrikle. *Verhandl. phys. Med. Ges.* Wurzburg. **2**, XVI.

Judy, W. V., Langley, F. M., McGowen, K. D., Sternett, D. M., Baker, L. E., and Johnson, P. C. (1969). Comparative evaluation of the thoracic impedance and isotope dilution methods for measuring cardiac output. *Aerosp. Med.* **40**, 532–536.

Kinnen, E. and Duff, C. (1970). Cardiac ouput from transthoracic impedance records using discriminant analysis. *JAAMI (Med. Instr.)* **4**, 73–78.

Kinsman, M., Moore, J. W., and Hamilton, W. F. (1929). Studies on the circulation. *Am. J. Physiol.* **89**, 322–330.

Kubicek, W. G., Kanegris, J. N., Patterson, R. P., Witsoe, D. A., and Mattson, R. H. (1966). Development and evaluation of an impedance cardiac output system. *Aerosp. Med.* **37**, 1208–1212.

Kubicek, W. G., From, A. H. I., Patterson, R. P., Witsoe, D. A., Castenda, A., Lillehi, R. C. and Ersek, R. (1970). Impedance cardiography as a noninvasive means to monitor cardiac function. *J.A.A.M.I. (Med. Instr.)* **4**, 79–84.

Lababidi, Z. Ehmke, D. A., Durnin, R. E., Leaverton, P. D., and Lauer, R. M. (1971). Evaluation of impedance cardiac output in children. *Pediatrics* **47**, 870–879.

Mohapatra, S. N., Costeloe, K. L., and Hill, D. W. (1977). Blood resistivity and its implications for calculation of cardiac output by the thoracic electrical impedance technique. *Intensive Care Med.* **3**, 1–5.

Parmley, W. W. (1978). Hemodynamic monitoring in acute ischemic disease. In *Heart Failure,* A. P. Fishman (ed.), Hemisphere Publications, Washington, D. C.

Poiseuille, J. L. M. (1828). Recherches sur la force due coeur aortique. (These No. 166). Paris, 1828, v. 218, pp. 7–45.

Poiseuille, J. L. M. (1840–1841). Recherches experimentales sur le mouvement des liquids dans les tubes de tres petits diametres. *Comptes Rendus.* **11,** 961–967; *Comptes Rendus.* **11,** 1041–1048; *Comptes Rendus.* **12,** 112–115.

Reynolds O. (1883). An experimental investigation of the circumstances which determine whether the motion of water shall be direct or sinuous. *Proc. Roy. Soc. London* **30,** 84–99; *Nature* **28,** 627–632; *Phil. Trans. Roy. Soc.* **174,** 935–982.

Roberts, V. C. (1973). The measurement of flow in intact blood vessels. *Crit. Rev. Bioeng.* **1,** 419–447.

Sarnoff, S. J., Braunwald, E., Welch, G. H., Case, R. B., and Stairsby, W. N. and Macruz, R. Hemodynamic determinants of oxygen consumption of the heart with special reference to the tension-time index. *Am. J. Physiol.* **192,** 148.

Smith, J. J., Bush, J. E., Wiedmeier, V. T., and Tristani, F. E. (1970). Application of impedance cardiography to study postural stress. *J. Appl. Physiol.* **29,** 133–137.

Starling, E. H. (1918). *The Law of the Heart, The Linacre Lecture,* Longmans Green & Co. London.

Stewart, G. N. (1897–1898). Researches on the circulation time and on the influences which affect it. *J. Physiol.* **22,** 158–183.

Stewart, G. N. (1921). The output of the heart in dogs. *Amer. J. Physiol.* **57,** 27–50.

Swan, H., Ganz, W. and Forrester, X. (1970). Catheterization of the heart in man with use of a flow-through balloon-tipped catheter. *N. Engl. J. Med.* **283,** 447–451.

Van De Water, J. M. P., Philips, P. A., Thoun, L. G., Watanabe, L. S., and Lappen, R. S. (1971). Bioelectric impedance. *Arch. Surg.* **102,** 541–547.

Weissler, A. M. (1977). Systolic time intervals. *N. Engl. J. Med.* **296,** 321–324.

Weissel, R. D., Berger, R. L., and Hechtman, H. B. (1975). Measurement of cardiac output by thermodilution. *N. Engl. J. Med.* **292,** 682–684.

Wheeler, H. B. (1973). Impedance testing for venous thrombosis. *Arch. Surg.* **106,** 762–763.

Wheeler, H. B., O'Donnell J. A., Anderson F. A., and Benedict K. (1974). Occlusive impedance phlebography. *Prog. Cardiovasc. Dis.* **17,** 199–203.

Yang, S. S., Bentivoglio, L. G., Maranhao, V., and Goldbert, H. (1972). *From Cardiac Catheterization Data to Hemodynamic Parameters.* F. A. Davis Co., Philadelphia.

CHAPTER 5

Cardiac Valves

Guaranteeing a unidirectional flow of blood are the four cardiac valves: two atrioventricular inflow valves and two ventricular outflow valves. The mitral valve between the left atrium and ventricle prevents reflux of ventricular blood during left-ventricular systole and allows atrial filling of the left ventricle during ventricular diastole. Similarly, the tricuspid valve between the right atrium and ventricle prevents reflux of ventricular blood during right ventricular systole and allows atrial filling of the right ventricle during ventricular diastole. The aortic and pulmonic valves are at the outflow to the left and right ventricles, respectively. Figure 5.1 is a sketch showing the locations of four cardiac valves.

The natural cardiac valves can become stenosed (narrowed) and present a high resistance to blood flow. They can also become incompetent, that is, fail to close and allow retrograde blood flow. In both cases replacement heart valves can be used to restore normal valve function. The decision to intervene therapeutically is based on measurement of valve area, by angiography, and by clinical signs, especially the ability to tolerate exercise. This chapter will present the method used to calculate valve area and will describe the currently used replacement (prosthetic) heart valves.

VALVE AREA

Cardiologists have developed the technique of calculating the areas of the four heart valves from graphically recorded pressure data and cardiac

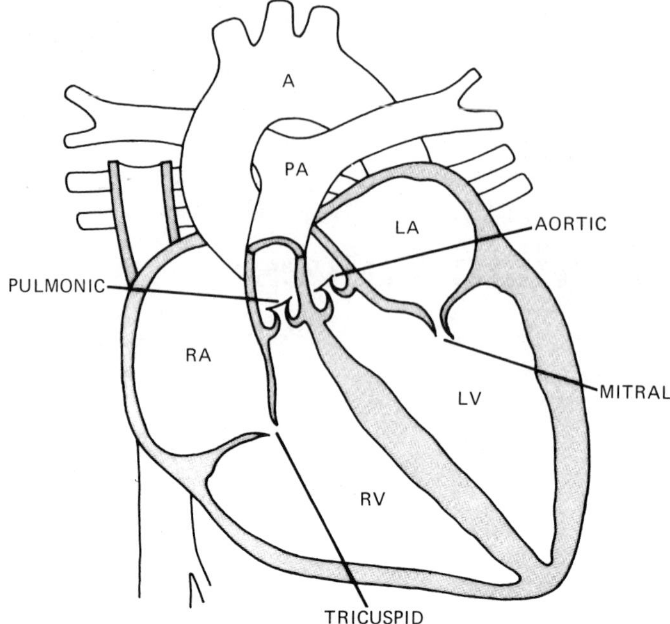

FIGURE 5.1. The four heart valves.

output measurements. Such information is a guide to a decision regarding surgical repair or replacement of a valve. The method of calculating valve area was presented and verified by Gorlin and Gorlin (1951), who pointed out that a cardiac valve resembles an orifice, and by measuring the pressure drop and flow, the area can be calculated. Their derivation of the valve-area expression is as follows.

The flow (ϕ) through an orifice of area A is the product of velocity (V) and area (A):

$$\phi = C_c A V$$

where C_c is the orifice constriction factor, a quantity which is less than unity and, in essence, decreases the area available for flow.

If fluid falls from a height (h) in a tube, it will issue forth with a velocity V, which is given by

$$V = C_v \sqrt{2gh}$$

where g is the gravitational constant (980) and C_V is a friction factor, which is less than unity.

Combining these equations by eliminating velocity (V) gives the following for valve area A:

$$A = \frac{\phi}{C_c C_v \sqrt{2gh}}$$

Since pressure is measured as height in mm Hg (as opposed to cm H_2O), it is necessary to insert the conversion factor 13.6/10, and enter the value for gravity (980) to give

$$A = \frac{\phi}{C_c C_v \sqrt{2665.6\ (P_1 - P_2)}}$$

where P_1 and P_2 are the pressures on either side of the valve in mm Hg. The two orifice coefficients (C_a, C_v) can be combined into a single coefficient (C), and the following is obtained:

$$A = \frac{\phi}{51.6C \sqrt{P_1 - P_2}}$$

This is the general form for the valve-area equation; ϕ is the flow rate through the valve, P_1 and P_2 are the pressures (in mm Hg) across the valve, and C is an empirically derived orifice coefficient, the value of which depends on the valve.

The manner in which the Gorlin formula is applied is peculiar to the physiology of the heart, being slightly different for the inflow (mitral and tricuspid) and outflow (pulmonic and aortic) valves. The following discussion presents illustrative examples for the mitral and aortic valves.

Mitral Valve

The mitral valve between the left atrium and ventricle frequently becomes diseased and its effective area is reduced. Thus the left atrial pressure rises above normal. Measurement of this pressure is not easily accomplished. The only access to the left atrium is via the left ventricle, which can be reached by advancing a catheter into an artery and, during ventricular systole, through the aortic valve. However, advancing beyond this point is extremely difficult. Although the left atrium can be reached via the left ventricle by careful guidance of a catheter under fluoroscopic vision, a simpler technique is used more frequently to obtain left atrial pressure. To apply the method it is first necessary to understand the concept of "wedge pressure."

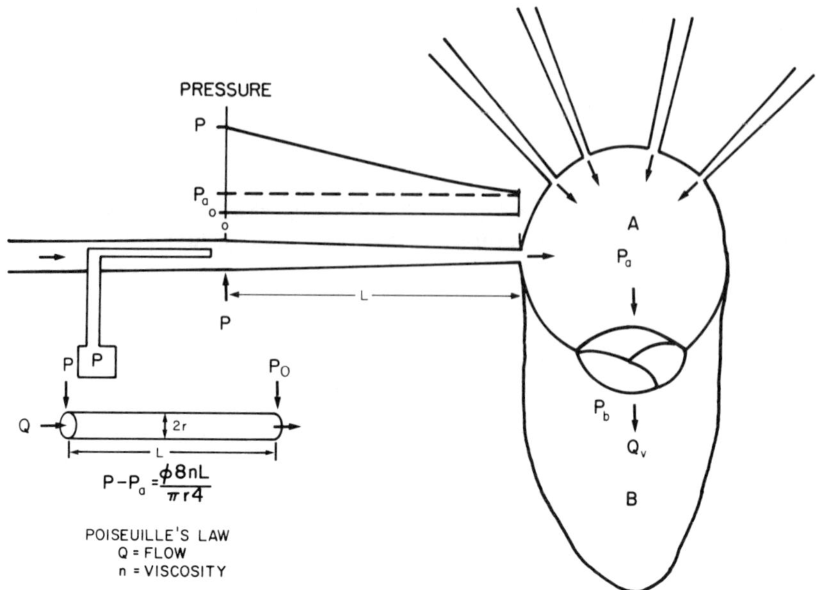

FIGURE 5.2. Pressure drop ($P - P_a$) along a pulmonic vessel with blood flow.

Wedge Pressure. When blood flows along a vessel, there is a pressure drop ($P - P_a$) along it as shown diagrammatically in Figure 5.2, which also illustrates a number of vessels delivering blood into chamber A, the region where it is desired to measure pressure (P_a). If a small fluid-filled catheter connected to a pressure transducer is advanced to point P, blood flows past the catheter tip and the pressure measured is that at point P and is higher than that in the chamber A (P_a). If the catheter is advanced far enough to become wedged in the vessel, flow will cease, as shown in Figure 5.3. The pressure behind the catheter tip will be increased because there is no flow in the vessel; the pressure in front of the catheter will be the pressure P_a in chamber A. Thus, the pressure in an inaccessible chamber can be measured by wedging a catheter into a vessel leading to the chamber and arresting flow in the catheterized vessel. The pressure so obtained is called wedge pressure. Pulmonary capillary wedge (PCW) pressure is obtained in this way by advancing a balloon-tipped (Swan-Ganz) catheter from an arm vein into the right atrium, right ventricle, and pulmonary artery, after which the balloon is deflated slightly. Pressure is recorded continuously to verify the location of the catheter tip. When the catheter is in the pulmonary artery, it is advanced until it can go no further and the balloon is reinflated partially and becomes wedged in a terminal branch of the pulmonary artery. The pressure measured at this site is very nearly equal to left atrial pressure.

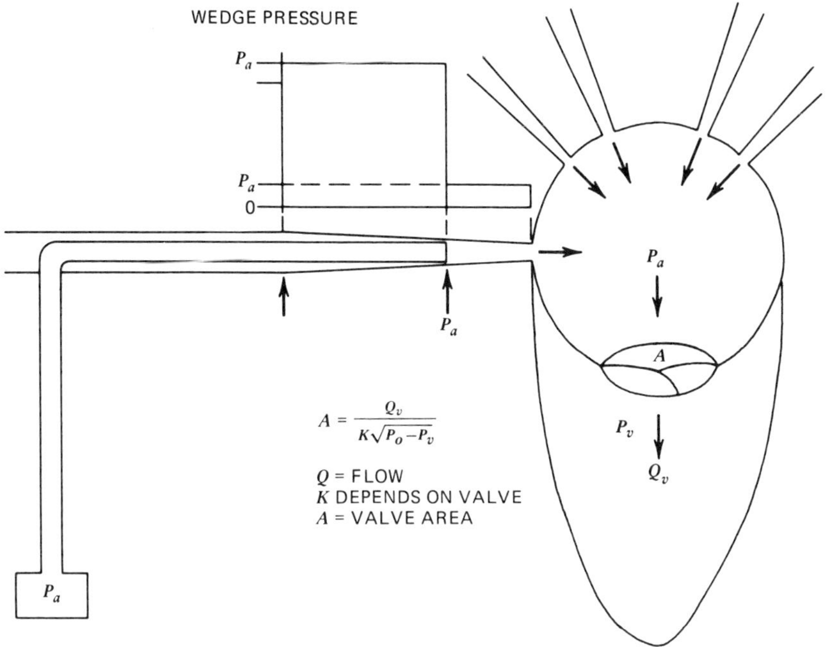

FIGURE 5.3. The concept of wedge pressure.

Area Calculation. The Gorlin formula for mitral valve area A_m can now be written

$$A_m = \frac{\phi_d}{31\sqrt{P_a - P_v}}$$

where 31 includes the conversion factors and C, the orifice coefficient (0.5); ϕ_d is the diastolic blood flow rate through the mitral valve in seconds per minute. P_a is left atrial pressure (which is measured as pulmonary artery wedge pressure) and P_v is left-ventricular end-diastolic pressure. This latter pressure can be measured by left-ventricular catheterization; often it is assumed to be 5 mm Hg.

It is important to recognize that blood flows through the mitral valve only during ventricular diastole. In fact, all of the cardiac output flows through the mitral valve, and the method of calculating ϕ_d for the equation is as follows:

$$\phi_d = \frac{\text{Cardiac output in mL for 1 min}}{\text{Ventricular filling period in sec for 1 min}}$$

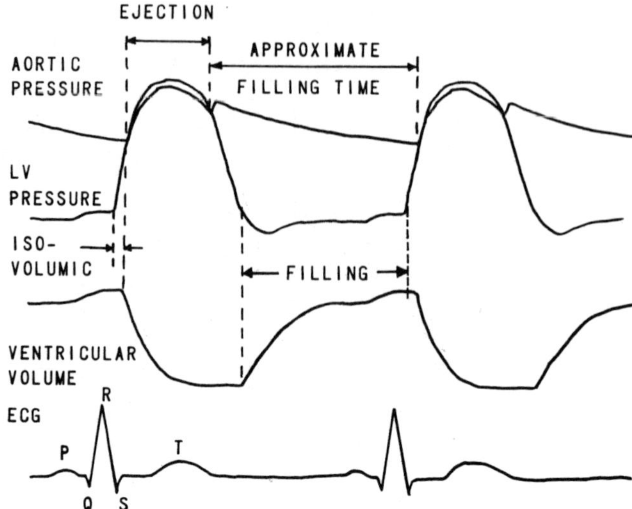

FIGURE 5.4. Pressure and volume relations for the left ventricle.

The diastolic filling period in sec for 1 minute is the diastolic filling period in sec, multiplied by the heart rate in beats per minute. The manner in which the ventricular filling period is estimated will now be described.

Figure 5.4 illustrates aortic and left-ventricular pressures and ventricular volume. The true ventricular filling time is shown on the ventricular volume curve. The ventricular filling period can be estimated from the base of ventricular pressure record. Another approximation of this time can be derived from measurement of the time from the end of ventricular ejection, as signaled by the dicrotic notch, and the beginning of ventricular ejection for the next beat, as signaled by the upstroke of the arterial pressure wave. This latter method was advocated by Gorlin and Gorlin, who used a brachial artery pressure record. These intervals are shown in Figure 5.4.

Thus, the area for the mitral valve can be calculated as

$$A_m = \frac{CO\ (\text{mL/min})}{(\text{Diastolic filling time in sec}) \times (\text{heart rate/min}) \times 31\sqrt{P_a - P_v}}$$

In summary, the items in the expression are derived from the measurement of cardiac output, by the Fick or indicator-dilution method, and recordings obtained from catheterization of the pulmonary artery (to obtain wedge pressure P_a) and catheterization of the left ventricle [to obtain left-ventricular end-diastolic pressure (P_v)] and a value for left-ventricular diastolic filling time. Left-ventricular end-diastolic pressure is sometimes estimated to be 5 mm Hg, and the brachial artery pressure record is often used to estimate the beginning and end of left-ventricular filling time. Heart rate is easily obtained from any of the arterial pressure recordings.

A typical calculation will show the utilitarian value of the expression for calculating mitral-valve area. The following data were presented by Gorlin and Gorlin (1951):

Cardiac output = 5.3 L/min = 5300 mL/min
Diastolic filling time for one heart beat = 0.31 sec
Heart rate = 108 beats per minute
Pulmonary wedge pressure = 39 mm Hg
Left-ventricular end-diastolic pressure = 5 mm Hg

Therefore, the mitral-valve area is

$$A_m = \frac{5300}{0.31 \times 108 \times 31\sqrt{39 - 5}} = 0.876 \text{ cm}^2$$

For a normal adult subject, a valve area of more than 2.5 cm^2 is typical. In a series of autopsy studies, Gorlin and Gorlin were able to show that the expression presented above provided very satisfactory values for mitral-valve area. However, if there is mitral regurgitation, the values are in error. Gorlin and Gorlin reported that this fact can be detected in the wedge pressure recording by the presence of a ventricular pressure pulse.

Pulmonary Valve

The concept just presented lends itself to calculation of the area of the pulmonic, tricuspid, and aortic valves. In using the Gorlin expression for valve area it is necessary to know the time in the cardiac cycle when blood flows through the valve whose area is to be calculated. For example, in calculating mitral-valve area, blood flows through during ventricular diastole, and from cardiac catheterization records and a value for cardiac output, it is possible to calculate mitral-valve area. To apply the expression to calculate the area of the pulmonary valve, it is necessary to recall that flow occurs during the right-ventricular systolic ejection period and the pressures across the pulmonic valve must be determined during ventricular systole. The following will illustrate this concept.

With a narrowing (stenosis) of the pulmonic valve, the resistance to right-ventricular outflow is increased. Hence, during ejection, the right-

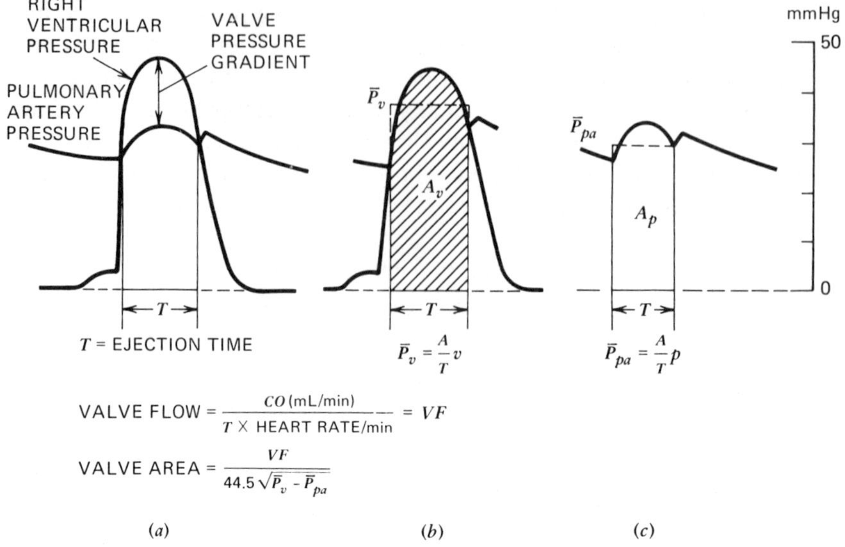

FIGURE 5.5. Computation of aortic valve area from pressure gradient.

ventricular pressure is much higher than pulmonary artery pressure. Figure 5.5*a* illustrates this point. The pressure gradient across the pulmonic valve is identified during ejection. Note that this pressure difference (gradient) varies throughout the ejection period.

The Gorlin expression for the calculation of pulmonary-valve area is

$$A_p = \frac{\text{Valve flow (mL/min)}}{44.5\sqrt{\bar{P}_v - \bar{P}_{pa}}}$$

In this expression the valve flow is calculated by dividing the cardiac output in mL/min by the product of ejection time and the heart rate (this product represents the number of seconds during each minute that blood flows through the valve).

The pressure gradient across the valve, $\bar{P}_v - \bar{P}_{pa}$, is not so easily determined: $\bar{P}_v$ is the mean right-ventricular pressure during the ejection period (Fig. 5.5*b*) and $\bar{P}_{pa}$ is the mean pulmonary artery pressure during the ejection period (Figure 5.5*c*). Mean right-ventricular pressure ($\bar{P}_v$) during the ejection period is determined by measuring the area under the right-ventricular pressure curve during the ejection period (A_v) and dividing this value by the ejection period (T). Similarly, mean pulmonary artery pressure ($\bar{P}_{pa}$) during the ejection period (T) is determined by measuring the area (A_p) under the pulmonary artery pressure recorded during the ejection period and dividing it by T. The method of performing these measurements is shown in Figure 5.4. With these pressures, a value for cardiac output, the ejection time, and heart rate, it is possible to calculate the area of the pulmonic valve. The following example derived from the Gorlin's paper is presented to illustrate a typical calculation:

Pulse rate = 71 beats per minute
Ejection period = 0.35 sec
Cardiac output = 4.6 L/min; 4600 mL/min
$\bar{P}_v$ = 66 mm Hg (mean right-ventricular pressure during ejection)
$\bar{P}_{pa}$ = 12 mm Hg (mean pulmonary artery pressure during ejection)

Valve flow in seconds each minute = 4600/(0.35 × 71) = 185, therefore, pulmonary valve area is

$$A_p = \frac{185}{44.5\sqrt{66 - 12}} = 0.57 \text{ cm}^2$$

Aortic and Tricuspid Valves

In a similar manner, the Gorlin and Gorlin expression can be used to calculate the area of the aortic and tricuspid valves. At present the same expression is used in both cases. There is some uncertainty about the appropriateness of using the same constant 44.5 (which includes the orifice coefficient C, and the conversion factor necessary to satisfy the use of mm Hg for pressure measurement). It is very likely that as experience accumulates, slightly different constants will be used for each of these cardiac valves. In the meantime, however, the Gorlins' formula provides valve areas that are in good agreement with values measured at autopsy.

PROSTHETIC HEART VALVES

Valve Types

The first, and still very popular, cardiac valve prosthesis is the caged-ball valve, which is illustrated in Figure 5.6a. The first valves of this type was introduced by Hufnagel et al. (1954) and Starr and Edwards (1961). Various materials have been used for the ball and cage. The ball has been made of silicone rubber or pyrolytic carbon. Fabric-covered, as well as

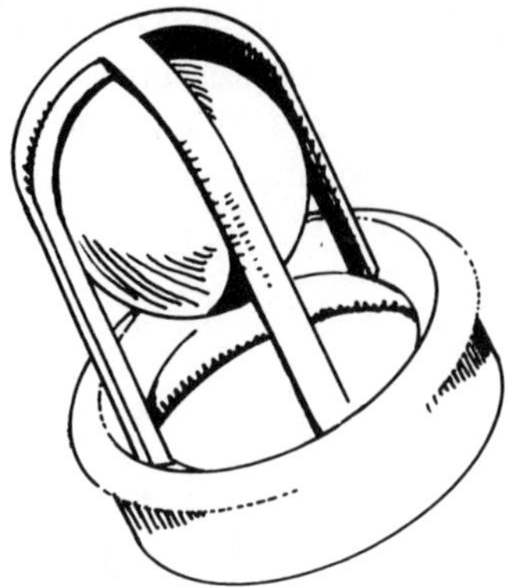

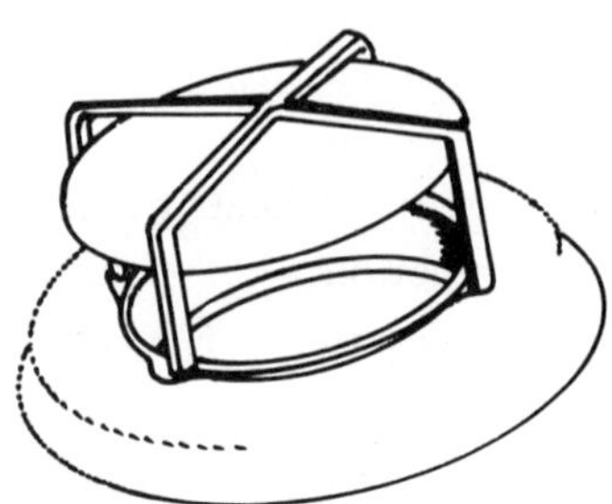

FIGURE 5.6. (*a*) The Starr–Edwards caged-ball valve and (*b*) the disk valve.

bare, balls have been used, the preference apparently going toward the bare silicone-rubber ball. The cage has been made from stellite and alloys of titanium.

Caged-ball valves have been placed in the aortic and mitral positions. In the former site, and with normal cardiac output (5 L/min in the adult), the pressure drop is typically 15 mm Hg. In the mitral position, the pressure drop is on the order of 4 mm Hg.

Several types of disk valves are used, one of which shown in Figure 5.6*b*. The struts are made of a variety of durable alloys and the disks have been made of both hard and soft materials—Teflon seems to be popular at present. Many of the disk types were developed for the mitral site, although many function equally well in the aortic position.

Heart valves removed from cadavers have been used with success. Such valves are processed chemically and stored for later use. However, the logistics of providing valves in the range of sizes and in large numbers makes these homografts unattractive as valve prostheses.

Valves removed from pigs (porcine xenografts) appear to have attractive characteristics. Such valves are readily available and are easily sterilized with gluteraldehyde or irradiation. Porcine valves are mounted in suitable holders and illustrated in Figure 5.7. They are easily installed in the mitral and aortic positions.

Characteristics of Valve Prostheses

Since the early 1960s more than 100,000 mechanical valves have been installed in human subjects. There are over 25 varieties available at present (Morse and Steiner, 1978). Thus a considerable clinical experience

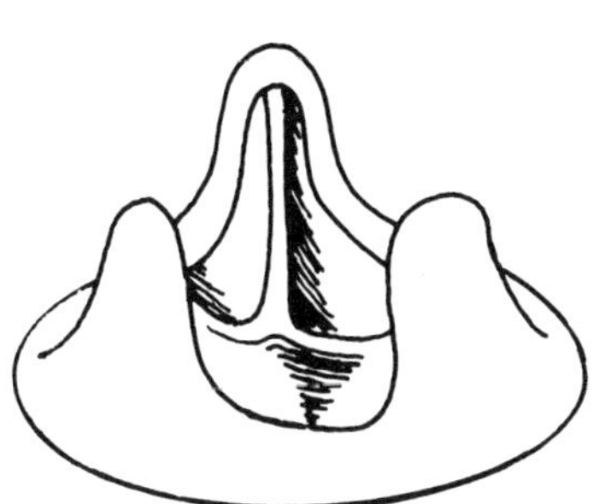
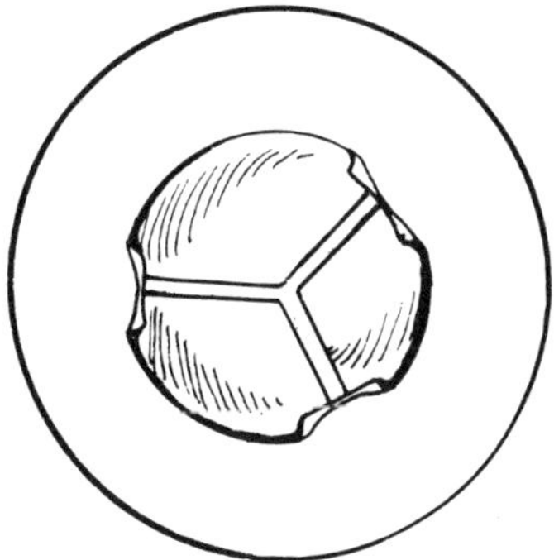

FIGURE 5.7. Porcine prosthetic heart valve for the aortic or mitral position.

has accumulated, and during this period, many important improvements have been made, both in design and in materials. According to Lefrak and Starr (1979), the durability of most mechanical valves is well known, and there are good survival data for mitral and aortic prostheses. It has been found that the use of mechanical valves requires the controlled use of anticoagulants to prevent clot formation and their migration (embolization) to plug the capillaries in vital organs.

The long-term survival associated with bioprostheses is less well known, merely because of their relatively recent introduction. Nonetheless, initial experience is very encouraging. Moreover, it appears that little, if any, anticoagulant therapy is required in most instances.

In order to keep physicians informed about valve prostheses, Morse and Steiner (1978) compiled an atlas of cardiac valves. In it, there is a picture of each valve type and an X-ray of the valve so that the type can be identified easily on a patient's radiograph. The name, address, and telephone number of each manufacturer is also provided so that inquiries about valves can be answered.

HISTORICAL POSTSCRIPT

The event that made cardiovascular surgery and valve replacement possible was introduction of the heart–lung machine by Gibbon in 1954. With this device, the circulation through the heart could be stopped, but the flow of oxygenated blood to vital organs could be maintained. Thus, the surgeons now had time to perform operations in previously inaccessible sites.

In 1954 Hufnagel introduced a caged-ball valve for the mitral position. Starr and Edwards (1961) introduced an improved version that became widely used. Harken et al. (1960) replaced a diseased aortic valve with a caged-ball valve. From this time, valve replacement became an accepted procedure, and the stimulus was at hand to develop valves that produced fewer emboli and offered less resistance to blood flow.

REFERENCES

Gibbon, J. H. (1954). Application of a mechanical heart and lung apparatus in cardiac surgery. *Minnesota Med.* **37,** 171–185.

Gorlin, R. and Gorlin S. G. (1951). Hydraulic formulae for calculating the area of the stenotic mitral valve, other cardiac valves and central circulatory shunts. *Amer. Heart J.,* **11,** 1–28.

Harken, D. E., Soroff, H. S., Taylor, W. J., Lefemine, A. A., Kupta, S. K., and Lunzer, S. (1960). Partial and complete prosthesis in aortic insufficiency. *J. Thor. Cardiovasc. Surg.,* **40,** 744–762.

Hufnagel, C. A., Harvey, C. P., Rabil, P. J. et al. (1954). Surgical correction of aortic insufficiency. *Surgery,* **35,** 673–683.

Lefrak, E. A. and Starr, A. (1979). Current heart valve prostheses. *Amer. Family Pract.,* **20,** 93–99.

Morse D. and Steiner R. M. (1978), *The Pacemaker and Valve Identification Guide,* Medical Examination Publ. Co. Inc., Garden City, N.Y.

Starr, A. and Edwards, M. L. (1961). Mitral replacement: clinical experience with a half-valve prosthesis. *Surgery,* **154,** 726.

CHAPTER 6

Intraaortic Balloon Pump

PRINCIPLE

The intraaortic balloon pump (IABP) is a therapeutic device for increasing coronary artery blood flow during ventricular diastole in patients with a failing heart. It consists of an inflatable cylindrical balloon applied to a catheter placed in the descending aorta via a femoral artery. During ventricular ejection the balloon is actively collapsed and during ventricular relaxation it is suddenly inflated, thereby raising aortic pressure ahead of it, which increases coronary artery blood flow.

APPLICATION

During ventricular systole the coronary arteries are squeezed shut and there is very little blood flow to the heart muscle. During ventricular relaxation, coronary blood flow is at its maximum. In some types of temporary cardiac failure, a slight increase in coronary artery blood flow will cause the ventricles to regain their lost vigor. It is in such situations that the intraaortic balloon pump sees its best service.

Figure 6.1*a* illustrates the arrangement of components used with the IABP. The IABP is placed in the descending thoracic aorta via a femoral artery. Often a graft is applied to the artery and allows placement of the balloon catheter without arresting blood flow in the artery beyond the point of insertion of the IABP. To ensure that the balloon inflates at the

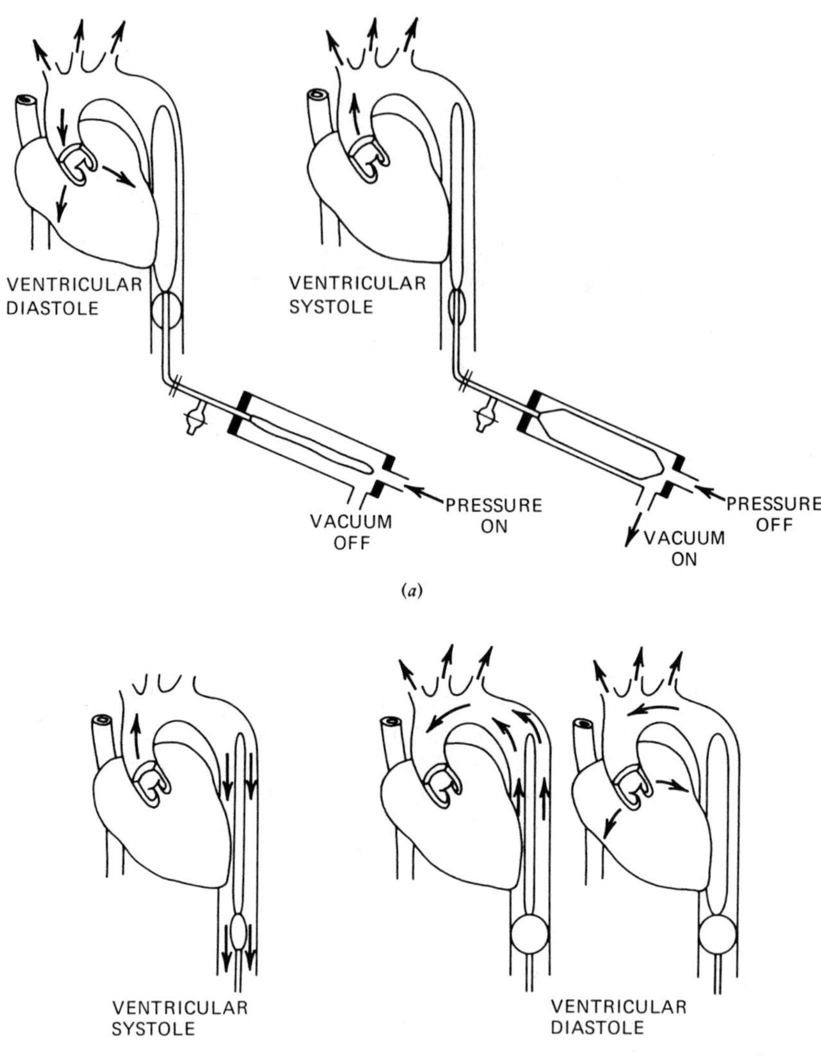

FIGURE 6.1. (*a*) Dual-chambered balloon acting in tandem with slave balloon in safety chamber. *Left,* transfer of CO_2 during diastole from slave balloon in safety chamber to intraaortic balloon. *Right,* complete deflation of intraaortic balloon assisted by vacuum acting on slave balloon. [Redrawn from Bregman, D., Kripke, D. C., and Goetz, R. H. (1970). *Trans. Am. Soc. Artif. Intern. Organs* **16,** 439.] (*b*) Mechanism of action of the dual-chambered intraaortic balloon. The distal spherical balloon inflates slightly earlier in diastole and phasically obstructs aortic flow. The larger cylindrical proximal balloon then pumps the blood unidirectionally toward the aortic root. Both balloons are then completely deflated by an active vacuum just prior to ventricular ejection. [Redrawn from Bregman. D. and Goetz, R. H. (1971). *J. Thorac. Cardiovasc. Surg.* **62,** 577.]

correct time in the cardiac cycle, the *R* wave of the ECG is used to provide the timing signal. Because ventricular contraction starts late in the *R* wave and is not complete until after the *T* wave, the balloon is held deflated during this period. About one-third of a second after the *R* wave, ventricular relaxation has begun and the balloon is quickly inflated with carbon dioxide. It is then quickly deflated so that it does not present the left ventricle with an increased resistance during the next ejection.

There are obvious technical factors that must be heeded in applying an IAPB. For example, there is the risk of balloon rupture, although this has not been encountered frequently. To minimize the side effects of balloon rupture, CO_2, which is very soluble in blood, is used for inflation. Rupture of the balloon merely adds CO_2 to the blood, and the excess CO_2 is eliminated quickly by the respiratory system. In addition, most IABP devices have an automatic shut-off when the balloon ruptures. The maximum volume of CO_2 that can be added to the blood is the volume required to inflate the balloon once, which amounts to about 30 mL, although 20-, 40-, and 60-mL balloons are used.

In routine use, the balloon material is slightly permeable to CO_2. Bregman (1975) reported that the amount of CO_2 that enters the blood by this route is 1–2 mL/hr in routine use of a double-balloon IABP.

Another important consideration in the operation of an IABP is triggering with the ECG, because failure to trigger would not inflate the balloon at the correct time in the cardiac cycle. In some units electronic circuitry has been provided to accommodate the arterial pressure signal for use as a trigger for the IABP. A major practical difficulty in securing adequate assistance from the balloon pump relates to heart rate. Failing hearts usually beat rapidly, and the finite time required to inflate and deflate the balloon can encroach on the times between successive heart beats. Many IABP controllers allow triggering to take place on every second or third *R* wave of the ECG. A relatively high pumping rate is accommodated by placing the CO_2 resevoir close to the exit point of the IABP catheter.

It has been found by Talpins *et al.* (1968) that the use of two balloons on the catheter increases coronary blood flow considerably. The second balloon is spherical and below the first. Inflation of the spherical and cylindrical balloons are synchronized to cause a headward flow of all of the blood moved by inflation of the cylindrical balloon. Figure 6.1*b* illustrates the operating sequence of the double-balloon IABP, and Figure 6.2 illustrates the augmentation in blood flow in the left anterior descending coronary artery when a double-balloon IABP was triggered by every second *R* wave of the ECG. Figure 6.3 presents a tabulation of cardiovascular parameters with single- and double- balloon pumping.

The IABP is clearly designed to temporarily assist the heart by aug-

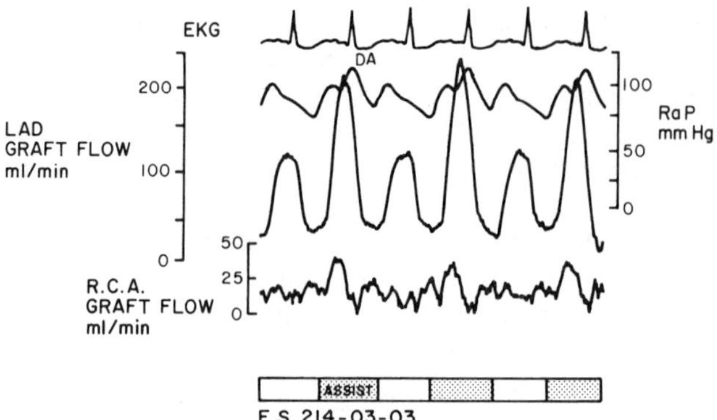

FIGURE 6.2. Dual-chambered IABP in a patient assisted after aortocoronary bypass graft surgery. *RaP,* radial artery pressure: *DA,* diastolic augmentation; *LAD,* left anterior descending coronary artery; *RCA,* right coronary artery. With patient assisted every other beat, note the 100% increase in LAD and RCA graft flows during diastole. Tracing speed 25 mm/sec. [Redrawn from Bregman, D., Parodi, E. N., Edie, R. N., Bowman, F. O. Jr., Reemtsma, K., and Malm, J. R. (1975). *J. Thorac. Cardiovasc. Surg.* **70,** 1010.]

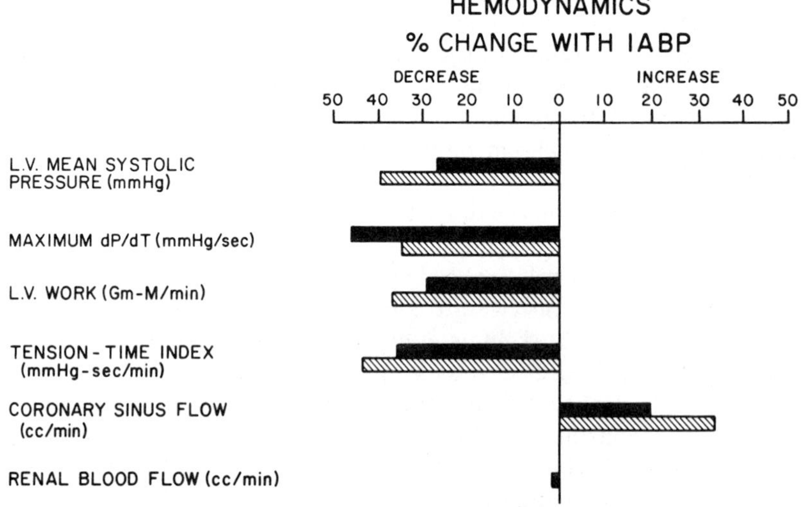

FIGURE 6.3. Effects of IABP on central and peripheral canine hemodynamics. (*Solid bars* represent single-chambered balloon, *shaded bars* dual-chambered.) All parameters of left-ventricular work are diminished while coronary sinus flow is increased. An increase of 66–100% in coronary blood flow is obtained using a dual-chambered balloon, without impairing distal perfusion. [Redrawn from Talpins, N. L., Kripke, D. C., Yellin, E., and Goetz, R. H. (1968). *Surg. Forum* **19,** 122.]

menting coronary artery blood flow. All of the situations in which a temporary increased coronary blood flow is lifesaving have not been defined as yet. However, there appear to be two situations in which the IABP is of value. These situations are cardiogenic shock, that is, failure of the heart to pump an adequate supply of blood, and weaning a patient from the heart–lung machine. Cardiac failure can result from a variety of causes, among which are myocardial infarction (heart attack) and impaired coronary perfusion. An augmentation in coronary blood flow can be provided by an IABP.

When a heart and lungs have been bypassed by a heart–lung machine for several hours, the ventricles are often incapable of resuming their full pumping load. Failing beats and dangerous arrhythmias often develop. Gradual restoration of full pumping can often be achieved by applying the IABP while withdrawing the subject from the heart–lung machine. Later the IABP is withdrawn.

Use of the IABP originated around 1960. To date about 30,000 humans have been treated with the device. Although the maximum pumping time is about 15 days, typical applications extend from 3 to 5 days. It is not known how long the IABP can be used. Although the equipment could function for a very long time, other complications, such as infection or total dependence on the IABP, could develop.

REFERENCES

Bregman, D. (1975), *Mechanical Support of the Failing Heart. Current Problems in Surgery,* Year Book Publishers, Chicago.

Talpins, N. L., Kupke, D. C., and Goetz, R. H. (1968). Counterpulsation and intra-aortic balloon pumping in cardiogenic shock. *Arch. Surg.,* **97,** 991–999.

Talpins, N. L., Kupke, D. C., Yellin, E., et al. (1968). Hemodynamics and coronary blood flow during intra-aortic balloon pumping. *Surg. Forum.,* **19,** 122.

CHAPTER 7

Electrocardiography and the Electrocardiograph

ELECTROCARDIOGRAPH

The electrocardiograph, abbreviated ECG or EKC,* is a recording instrument for graphically displaying the electrical activity of the heart. The recording, called an electrocardiogram, also abbreviated ECG or EKG, is usually produced on a heat-sensitive paper, which moves at 2.5 cm/sec. Newer instruments provide both 2.5 and 5 cm/sec paper speeds. ECGs are also displayed on oscilloscope screens in patient monitors.

An electrocardiogram is a record of the electrical activity of the heart obtained with body-surface electrodes. When both electrodes are placed on or in the heart, the record is called a cardiac electrogram. When one electrode is in or on the heart and the other is on the body surface, the recording is called a semidirect electrocardiogram.

The electrocardiogram permits identification of the sequence of excitation and recovery of the pumping chambers of the heart. Normal and abnormal excitation and rhythm can be identified at a glance. The ECG also provides information on the adequacy of circulation to the heart muscle in exercise and gives instant indication of diminished blood flow,

*Originally EKG, from the German.

as in a heart attack. The ECG also provides evidence of atrial or ventricular enlargement (hypertrophy), pericarditis (inflammation of the membranous sac, the pericardium, that surrounds the heart), the presence of systemic diseases that affect the heart, the effect of some drugs, and the level of potassium in the blood. Despite its ability to display cardiac abnormalities, the ECG should be viewed as another laboratory test and its evidence judged along with other clinical indications. It is possible for a patient to have a normal ECG and a normal subject to show nonspecific ECG abnormalities.

Although the Einthoven silvered quartz-fiber (string) galvonometer ushered in clinical electrocardeography in 1903, such instruments are no longer in use. In their place are vaccuum-tube or transistor-amplifier instruments, which display the electrocardiac potential via a direct-writing heated pen, that records on heat-sensitive paper. Various types of electrosensitive papers are also used. Some recorders eject a fine spray of ink onto a moving paper chart. For clinical electrocardiography, rectilinear recording is essential. In patient monitors two types of oscilloscope displays are employed. In one, the conventional moving spot (bouncing ball) with a long persistance screen is used. In the other, a freeze-display presentation appears on the oscilloscope screen. This latter type of presentation, which employs a digital processing technique, resembles a graphic record moving continuously across the oscilloscope screen.

ELECTRICAL ACTIVITY OF THE HEART

It is traditional to start the process of learning about a new phenomenon by presenting the most fundamental component. However, it is more stimulating to have a knowledge of the phenomenon before dissecting it into its components. For this reason, an overview of the ECG will be presented first, following which there will be a discussion of the electrophysiology that produces it.

The mammalian and many other hearts are two-stage, four-chambered blood pumps. The two auricles, or atria, contract first because the pacemaker (sinoatrial, S-A node) is located therein and has the highest degree of rhythmicity. Atrial contraction pumps blood into the ventricles. Following atrial contraction, the ventricles contract; the right ventricle pumps blood into the pulmonary vascular circuit and the left ventricle pumps blood into the systemic circulation. The trigger for these mechanical events in each of the cardiac chambers is the spread of electrical depolarization of the cardiac muscle fibers that constitute them. Thus, prior to contraction of the atria, electrical excitation is propagated from

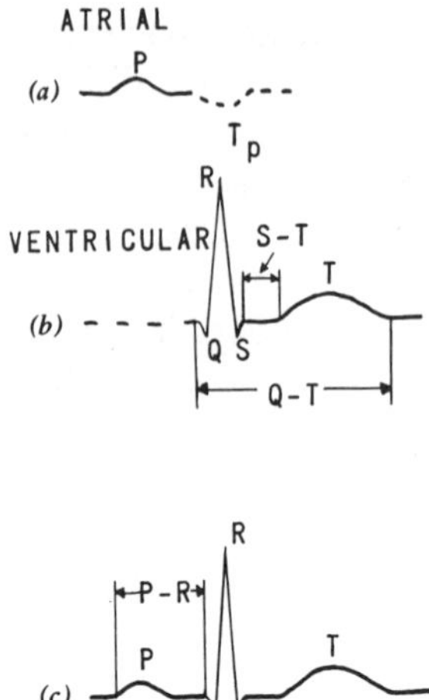

FIGURE 7.1. The atrial and ventricular components of the electrocardiogram.

the pacemaker (S-A node) and travels throughout the atria, giving rise to the *P* wave of the ECG. Then the atrial fibers repolarize, giving rise to an atrial recovery wave, which is designated T_P. The T_P wave is rarely seen in the ECG because it is obscured by the ventricular *QRS* wave which occurs at the same time. The electrical wave of excitation that travels over the atria is transmitted to the ventricles via a specialized conduction (propagating) system consisting of the A-V node, bundle of His, and Purkinje fibers and finally to ventricular muscle. This ventricular conducting system is modified muscle tissue and the spread of excitation over ventricular myocardium gives rise to the *QRS* wave, which triggers contraction of the ventricles. Late in ventricular contraction, the ventricular muscle fibers start to repolarize and give rise to the *T* wave, following which the ventricles relax. Figure 7.1 illustrates a typical mammalian ECG.

In summary, the electrical events of the cardiac cycle start in the pacemaker (S-A node) in the right atrium. Excitation originating here spreads over the atria, giving rise to the *P* wave, which precedes atrial contraction. The rarely seen atrial recovery T_P wave precedes atrial relaxation. The *QRS* wave precedes ventricular contraction, and the *T* wave precedes ventricular relaxation. Electrodes appropriately placed on the body surface can detect all of these waves, with the exception of the T_P wave, signaling recovery of the atria, is rarely seen. Thus, the typical ECG consists of a *P*, *QRS*, and *T* complex as shown in Figure 7.1*c*. It is important to note that the electrocardiogram represents a timing signal of cardiac activity and does not in any way provide information about the force of contraction of any of the cardiac chambers.

To record the ECG, body-surface electrodes are used. There are numerous standard and nonstandard leads for monitoring the ECG. It should be apparent at this point that the elementary description of the ECG just presented will allow the reader to identify the atrial and ventricular components with any lead system. However, to exploit more fully the information contained in the ECG, it is necessary to know some fundamentals of cardiac electrophysiology.

GENESIS OF THE ELECTROCARDIOGRAM

The Transmembrane Potential

The origin of the ECG is the excursion in transmembrane potential that occurs in the atria and ventricles when they become active and recover. In all structures of the heart there is a transmembrane potential, which is the result of a high intracellular and low extracellular concentration of potassium. The net result is that the interior of the cell is negative with respect to the exterior. When stimulated, that is, when a cardiac cell becomes active, it depolarizes; extracellular sodium rushes in and intracellular potassium leaks out owing to a transient change in membrane permeability. Shortly thereafter, the membrane permeability returns to its original state and the cell recovers or repolarizes. Metabolic processes restore the lost potassium and extrude the sodium that entered.

The resting membrane and action potential of cardiac muscle can be measured with transmembrane electrodes. With a (macro) electrode outside the cell and a tiny (micro) electrode also outside a cardiac cell, no potential is registered or shown in Figure 7.2*a*. When the microelectrode is advanced into the cell, the voltage indicator shows that the interior is negative with respect to the exterior by about 90 mV; this is the resting or transmembrane potential as shown in Figure 7.2*b*. The magnitude and stability of the resting transmembrane potential depends on the location of the cell within the heart.

When a cardiac cell becomes active, either spontaneously or by being stimulated by an adjacent cell, there occurs a cyclic change in membrane potential and ion fluxes as stated earlier. Activity is signaled by a sudden depolarization and reverse polarization, that is, the outside becomes negative with respect to the inside. This part of the rapid depolarization process is called phase 0 as shown in Figure 7.2*c*. Immediately, forces are brought into action to start the cell recovering, and the transmembrane

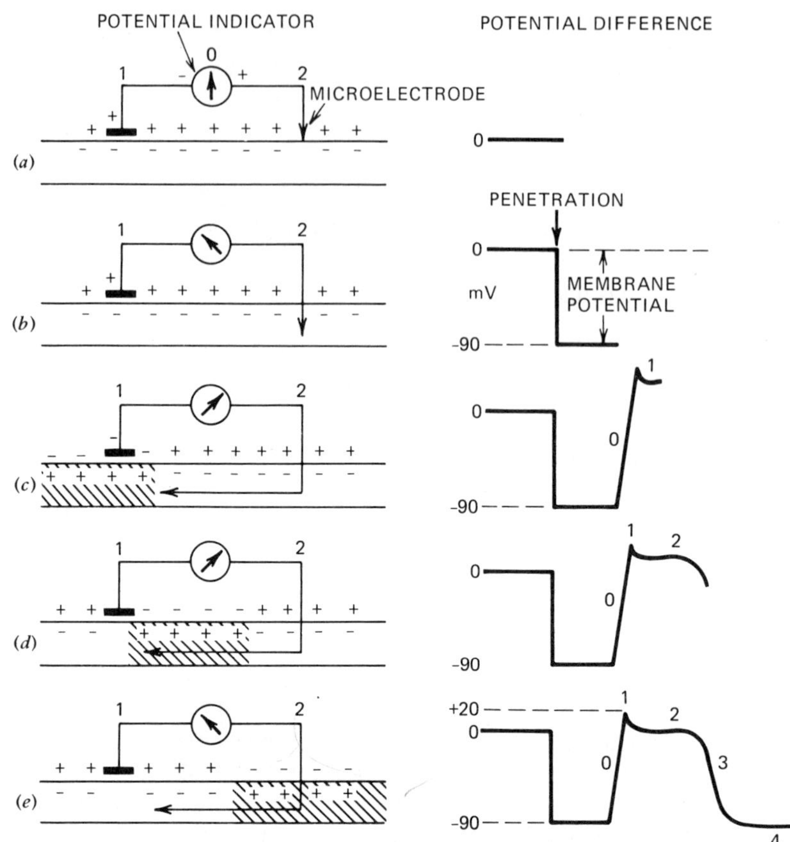

FIGURE 7.2. The transmembrane potential of cardiac muscle.

potential begins to diminish in a characteristic way, as identified by phase 1 in Figure 7.2*c*. During phase 2 of depolarization which follows, mechanical contraction starts. Shortly thereafter, repolarization accelerates to restore the transmembrane potential; this period, shown in Figure 7.2*d*, is called phase 3. Sometime during phase 3 contraction (systole) has ended and relaxtion (diastole) has begun. Throughout phases 0,1,2, and until just beyond the middle of phase 3, the cell cannot respond to a second stimulus and is said to be refractory. Late in phase 3 and throughout phase 4, excitability has recovered and the cell can respond to another stimulus. Figure 7.2*e* summarizes the sequence just described.

The type of action potential, that is, excursion in transmembrane potential, is dependent on the type of cardiac cell. The example just discussed is applicable to ventricular myocardium. The action potentials of

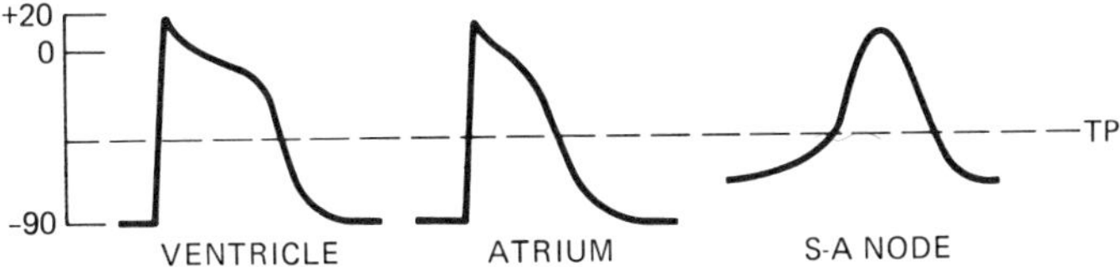

FIGURE 7.3. Action potentials of different parts of the heart.

the conduction system, atrial muscle, and the pacemaker (S-A node) are slightly different as summarized in Figure 7.3. Particularly important about all of these action potentials is the threshold potential (TP), which describes the ability of the cell to be stimulated. If the transmembrane potential is reduced (e.g., by an electrical stimulus) to this level, the cell will spontaneously become active and exhibit the cyclic change in transmembrane potential. The membrane potential of the pacemaker (S-A node) is not stable and decreases spontaneously; when it reaches the threshold potential, the cell fires spontaneously; it is for this reason that the cells in the S-A node are the pacemaker of the heart. Note also that the transmembrane potential of ventricular myocardium is larger and stable. For this reason ventricular muscle rarely becomes a pacemaker. However, the A-V node and the conduction system have less stable membrane potentials and can, and often do, become cardiac pacemakers.

The Electrocardiogram

Examination of the ECG reveals that it has few of the characteristics of the electrical event of cardiac muscle, despite the fact that the excursion in transmembrane potential is what produces the ECG. It is therefore necessary to find a way of explaining the ECG in terms of this basic bioelectric phenomenon. Making this connection has always been difficult for those who write textbooks on electrocardiography and for those who study cardiac transmembrane potentials. In general, however, the link is made by using one of three theories: the membrane theory, the interference theory, or the dipole theory. Brief accounts of each will now be presented.

Membrane Theory. The refractory period is long in cardiac muscle, that is, a cardiac cell cannot be restimulated until nearly the end of the action potential, which is long in duration and occupies almost the same amount of time as mechanical contraction and relaxation. Because the heart is physically small and the refractory period is long, all of the atria and (later) all of the ventricles become active (depolarized) before recovery occurs in each structure. With these facts as a starting point, it is possible to present the membrane theory for genesis of the ECG.

Consider a uniform strip of cardiac muscle as shown in Figure 7.4. On the strip are two electrodes connected to a potential indicator. At rest (Figure 7.4*a*) the indicator shows no potential difference. Now consider excitation advancing into the tissue from the left, as shown in Figure 7.4*b*. Active tissue is negative with respect to resting or inactive tissue; therefore, electrode 1 will be negative with respect to electrode 2. The direction displayed by the potential recorder will depend on how it is connected to the two electrodes. For convenience, let us choose the polarity indication so that 1 negative (or 2 positive) produces an upward indication when excitation occupies the tissue under 1. Now, as excitation advances and appears under electrode 2, the potential under each electrode is the same, that is, the tissue under both electrodes is negative. Therefore the indicator reveals zero potential, as shown in Figure 7.4*c*. At this instant the tissue is totally depolarized (active) and refractory. What happens next depends on the manner in which the tissue recovers. If the tissue is uniform, recovery will follow in the same direction as excitation and the tissue under electrode 1 will recover first, as shown in Figure 7.4*d*. In this case, electrode 1 will be positive with respect to 2 and the indicator will show a downward deflection. As recovery advances toward electrode 2, and finally leaves the region of the recording electrodes, the tissue has recovered and the indicator shows zero deflection, as shown in Figure 7.4*e*. In summary, the first phase of the action potential reflects excitation and the second signals recovery. Between the two phases the tissue is totally depolarized and refractory.

If, in Figure 7.4*c*, when the tissue is fully depolarized, recovery occurs first in the region last to be excited, that is, under electrode 2, the tissue in this region would be positive and the indicator would rise, as shown in Figure 7.4*f*. When recovery occurs under electrode 1, all of the tissue is repolarized and the indicator records zero; Figure 7.4*g* illustrates this situation. In this case, the first and second phases of the two potential changes are upward, indicating that excitation and recovery traveled in opposite directions. It may seem unlikely that such a situation can occur; but it does in the ventricles of most warm-blooded animals, probably due to the rich coronary circulation.

The simplified presentation of the membrane theory permits drawing a number of important conclusions. First, if the polarity indicated by the recording instrument is known, it is possible to identify the direction of the spread of excitation. For example, since excitation is a traveling wave of negativity, an upward deflection will be obtained when excitation passes under the negative electrode (1) on its way to the positive

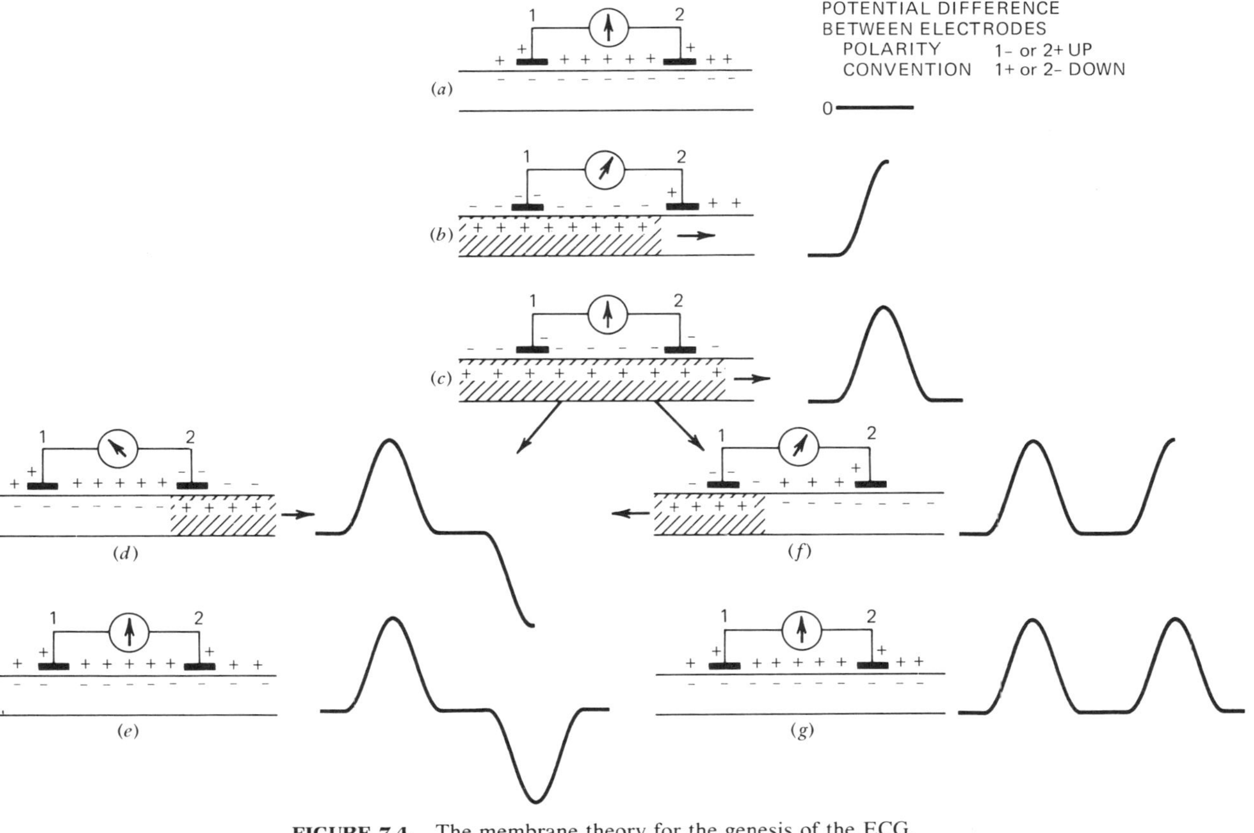

FIGURE 7.4. The membrane theory for the genesis of the ECG.

electrode. If excitation traveled from right to left, the first phase of the action potential would be downward in this example.

The next important conclusion that can be drawn relates to the polarity of the excitation and recovery waves. If they are of the opposite polarity, recovery travels in the same direction as excitation. If they have the same polarity excitation and recovery travel in opposite directions.

If the recording electrodes are placed to encompass the strip of irritable tissue so that excitation (or recovery) travels at right angles to the axis of the electrodes, as shown in Figure 7.5, the potential indicator will show zero potential, because depolarization (or repolarization) will occur simultaneously under both electrodes. Thus, a general rule can be formulated which states that the amplitude of the recording is maximal when excitation or recovery travels parallel to the electrode axis; the amplitude will be a minimum when excitation (or recovery) travels at right angles to the electrode axis. There is, however, one exception to this general rule, which will be presented now.

In Figure 7.6 consider an excitation starting midway between electrodes 1 and 2. Excitation (or recovery) will arrive under electrodes 1 and 2 at the same instant. Therefore, no potential will be recorded. It is to be noted that in this special case excitation (or recovery) travels in the direction of the electrode axis.

At this point it is important to observe that the recorded potential does not resemble the long-duration excursion in transmembrane potential (Figure 7.2*e*) that is known to occur under each electrode. The membrane theory merely permits conceptualization of the genesis of the excitation and recovery waveforms and allows deducing very important facts relative to excitation, recovery, and their directions of progression. The interference theory, which will now be presented, provides a better bridge between the ECG and the excursion in transmembrane potential, which is also called the monophasic action potential.

Interference Theory

The interference theory states that the potential seen by two recording electrodes on the surface of a strip of irritable tissue is the instantaneous algebraic sum of the potential under each electrode. The basic bioelectric event under each electrode is the monophasic action potential, that is, the excursion in transmembrane potential, as shown in Figure 7.7*a*. Consider that excitation progresses from electrode 1 to electrode 2. As before, when the tissue under electrode 1 becomes negative, an upward deflection of the recorder is obtained. When tissue under electrode 2 becomes negative, a downward deflection is obtained. Figure 7.7*b* illustrates these facts

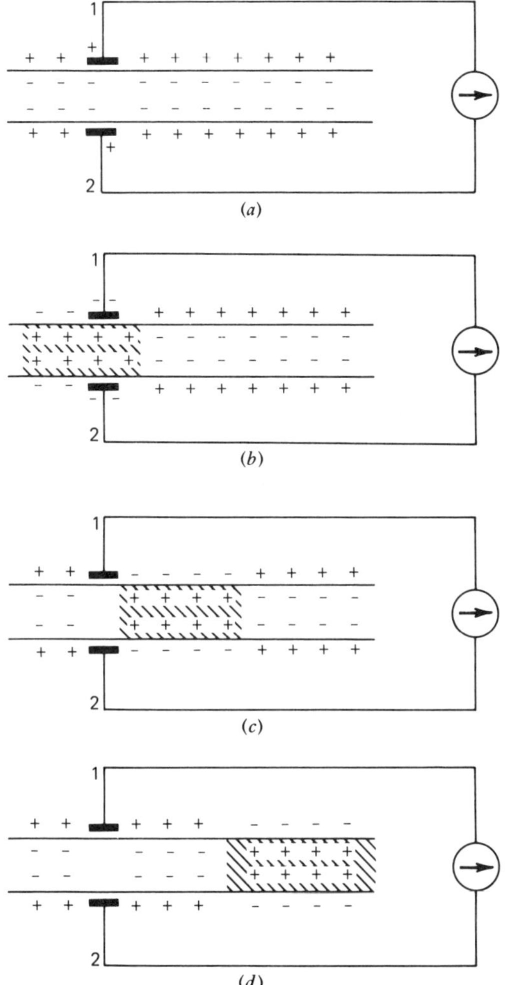

FIGURE 7.5. Excitation (or recovery) traveling at right angles to the electrode axis produces no potential differences measured between electrodes 1 and 2.

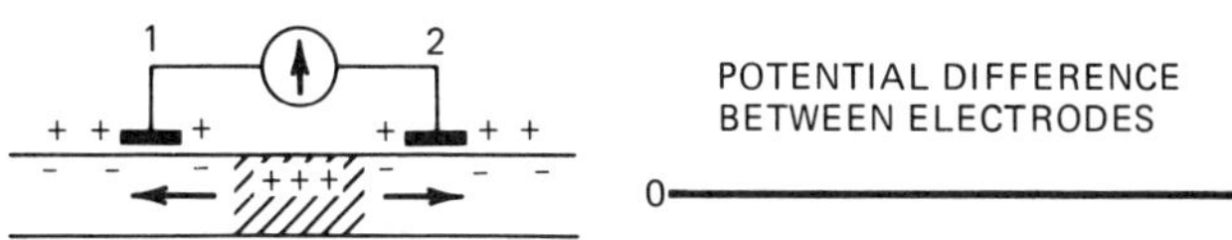

FIGURE 7.6. Simultaneous excitation under both electrodes due to stimulus (x) occurring midway between electrodes 1 and 2.

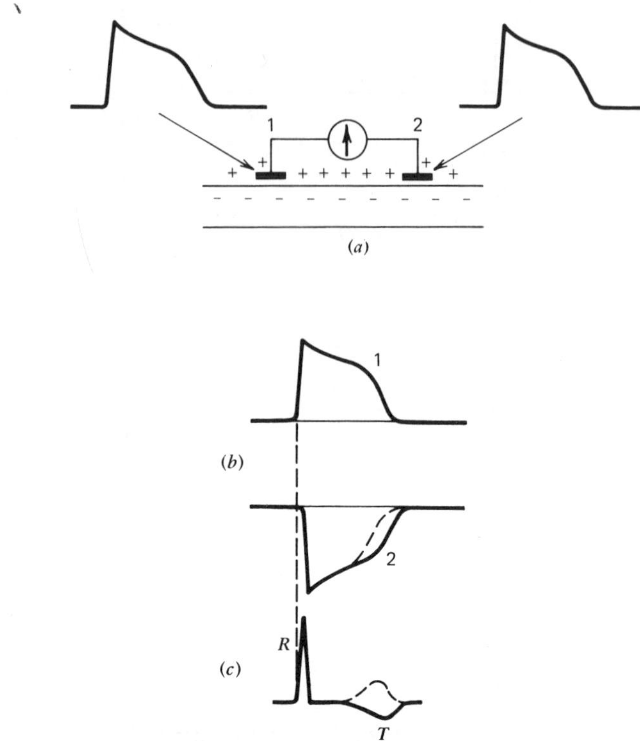

FIGURE 7.7. Genesis of the *R* and *T* waves of the ECG by summation of the excursions in transmembrane potential under electrodes 1 and 2.

and the instantaneous algebraic sum of the potentials seen by the recorder. As stated previously, the refractory period of cardiac muscle is long, and before recovery occurs at electrode 1, excitation is under electrode 2, causing the indicator to move downward. Thus electrode 1 sees excitation first and, slightly later, electrode 2 sees excitation. The potential presented to the recorder will be the instantaneous algebraic sum of two slightly displaced, oppositely directed, monophasic action potentials, as shown in Figure 7.7*b*. Note that since the propagation (conduction) time from 1 to 2 is relatively short, depolarization occurs under 2 before it is complete under 1, the net sum being a spiked wave for excitation. After the spike all of the tissue is depolarized, following which recovery begins. In uniform tissue the monophasic action potentials have the same duration under each electrode and, therefore, recovery occurs sooner under the first electrode. Hence, summation of the monophasic action potentials produces a downward recovery *T* wave as shown in Figure 7.7*c*. If recovery is made to occur earlier under the second electrode, the duration of

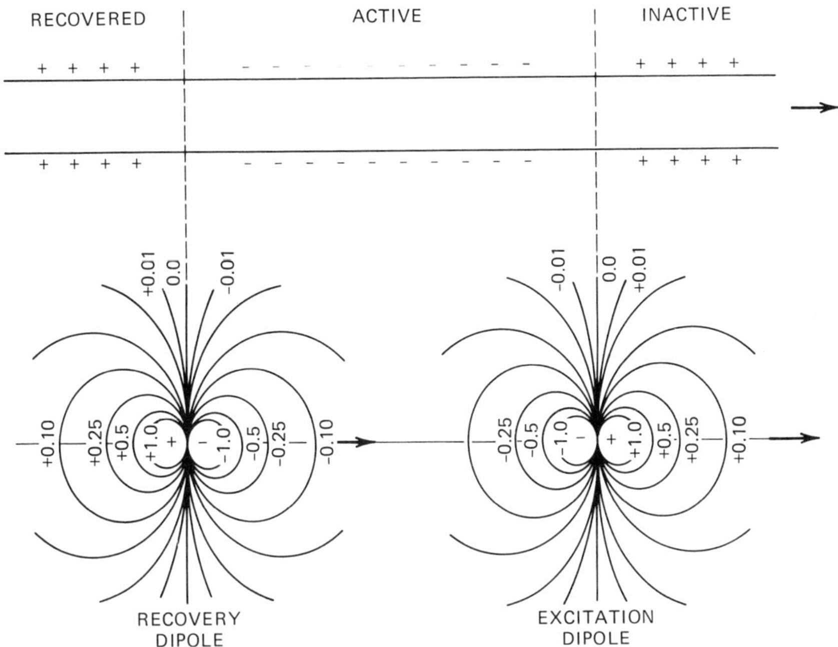

FIGURE 7.8. The dipole representation for the boundary between resting and active tissue.

the (downward) monophasic action potential is shorter, as shown by the dashed line in Figure 7.7*b*. In this situation, the instantaneous sum of the monophasic action potentials will produce an upward recovery wave as shown in Figure 7.7*c* (dashed curve).

It is to be noted that the interference theory provides the same kind of information about excitation and recovery as does the membrane theory. However, it illustrates more clearly how the recorded ECG arises from the temporal sum of two fundamental monophasic action potentials that bear little resemblance to the ECG.

Dipole Theory. When viewed from the surface, excited tissue is electronegative with respect to resting or recovered tissue. Therefore, it is possible to express the boundary between these two regions as an array of dipoles, as shown in Figure 7.8. Because excitation and recovery travel throughout the heart, the dipole of excitation has its positive pole facing the direction of propagation. The dipole of recovery has it negative pole facing the direction of propagation of recovery. This dipole concept is used extensively in explaining the electrocardiographic patterns obtained from body-surface leads.

The heart is contained in conducting body fluids and tissues. The dipoles of excitation and recovery are created when cardiac muscle becomes active. The cardiac dipoles are in reality in a volume conductor and send current through its extent. As a consequence, a potential field is created, as shown in Figure 7.8. The potential distribution surrounding this idealized dipole shows that the voltage presented to an environmental electrode decreases with increasing distance from the dipole and also depends on the electrode orientation with respect to the dipole axis.

The manner in which the dipole concept is applied to generate the excitation and recovery waves of the ECG is not strictly in accordance with the properties of a physical dipole, which is in reality two equal charges of opposite polarity separated by a constant distance. Nonetheless, the physiological application provides very useful information.

Consider a small strip of myocardium in a volume conductor with two measuring electrodes at a considerable distance and in line with the strip as shown in Figure 7.9a. When the tissue is inactive, all of the exterior is positive, and there is no potential difference over the surface. Therefore, there is no dipole, and the voltage appearing between electrodes 1 and 2 is zero. Assume now that a stimulus has been delivered to the myocardial strip at the end nearest to electrode 1. The stimulated point becomes negative with respect to the rest of the myocardial strip. Hence, a dipole of excitation has been created and electrode 1 becomes negative with respect to electrode 2. The recorder is connected to the electrodes so that an upward deflection is indicated. As excitation spreads and travels over the tissue toward electrode 2, the dipole strength increases and the voltage appearing between electrodes 1 and 2 increases. As excitation occupies more of the strip, more of the outside is negative, and when the strip is half excited, the voltage detected by the electrodes is maximal. As excitation proceeds more of the exterior of the strip is negative and finally excitation occupies all of the strip, and there is again no potential differences over the surface. Hence, with the full excitation, the dipole of excitation disappears and the voltage between electrodes 1 and 2 is zero. This sequence of excitation arising and fully occupying the myocardial strip is shown in Figure 9*b*. Note that excitation was represented as a dipole that arose at the point of stimulation, grew in strength as more tissue was occupied by excitation, and decreased as the tissue was fully occupied by excitation. This sequence of events gave rise to an excitation potential, equated to a dipole with its positive pole traveling in the direction of excitation as shown in Figure 7.9*b*.

With the myocardial strip totally depolarized, the entire surface is negative, and no potential difference exists over its surface (Figure 7.9*b*). When recovery starts (Figure 7.9*c*), the recovered area becomes positive with respect to active tissue. The boundary between recovering and ac-

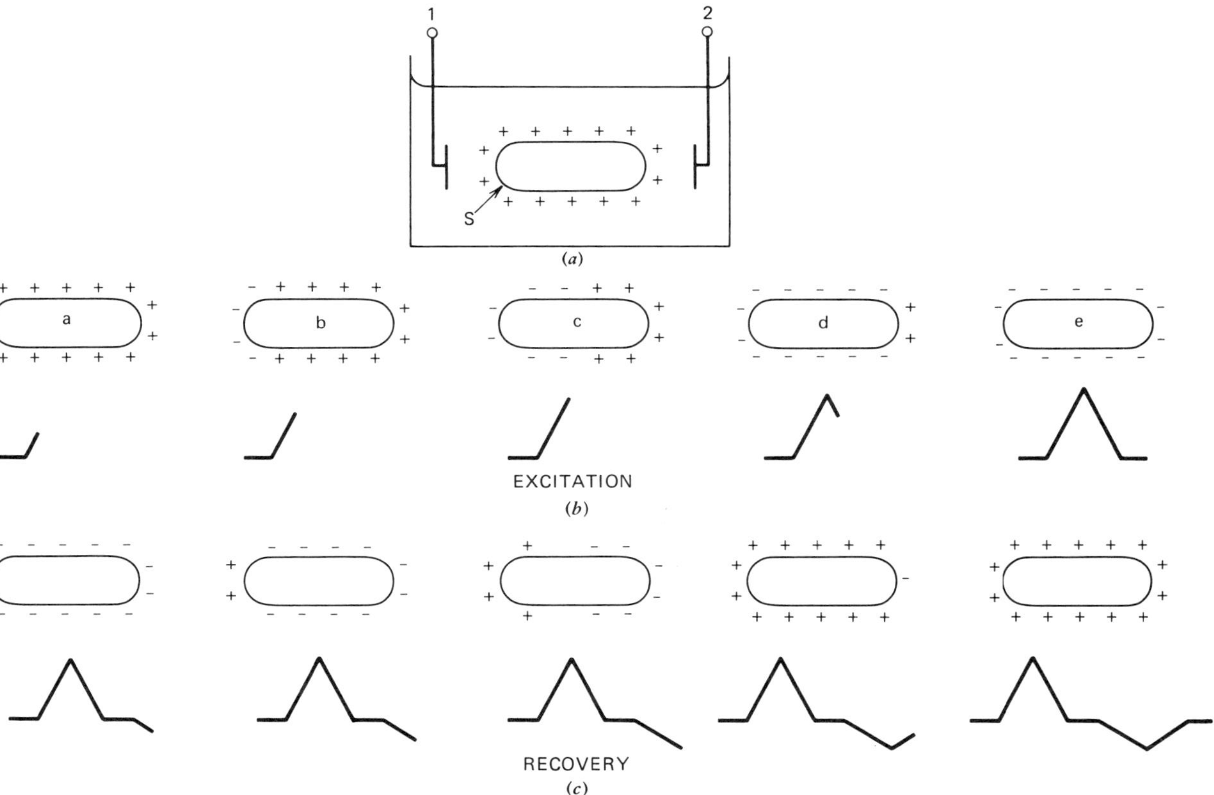

FIGURE 7.9. The cardiac dipole of excitation and recovery.

tive tissue is diffuse; thus, the dipole of recovery is spread over a larger region and produces a potential field that is much more irregular and lower in strength. Assume that recovery advances in the same direction as excitation. Thus, in Figure 7.9*c*, recovery starts in the region nearest to electrode 1 which becomes positive, causing electrode 1 to be positive. The recorder connected to electrodes 1 and 2 will move downward. As more tissue is occupied by recovery progressing toward electrode 2, more recovery dipoles are created and the voltage difference increases. When more than half of the tissue has recovered, the potential difference starts to diminish. When recovery occurs everywhere (Figure 7.9*c*), there is no potential difference and the indicator reads zero. Thus, recovery has been equated to a dipole with its negative pole facing the direction of the propogation of recovery; therefore, the recovery wave is downward as shown in Figure 7.9*c*.

From this discussion it is easy to see that if recovery had progressed in the direction opposite to the excitation, the recovery wave would have the same polarity as the excitation wave. Likewise, if stimulation had occurred near electrode 2, the sequence of events would be the same but the recorded polarities would be inverted. Thus, the dipole theory states that the dipole of excitation travels with its positive pole forward and the recovery dipole has its negative pole forward. During excitation and recovery the strengths of the dipoles increase and decrease.

The dipole theory is extremely useful in interpreting the ECG when analyzed with the various electrode reference frames. Examples will be given to illustrate this point after describing the standard leads.

ELECTROCARDIOGRAPHIC LEADS

To enable others to obtain electrocardiograms for comparison with his own, Einthoven, who developed the first clinically usable ECG in 1903, selected anatomical sites for placing electrodes. He chose the two arms (RA, LA) and left leg (LL), designating the three different recording schemes as lead I (RA − LA), lead II (RA − LL), and lead III (LA − LL). The polarities for an upward deflection of the recording pen are shown in Figure 7.10. Although the electrodes are placed on the members, the latter act as electrolytic conductors and, in reality, the electrodes are electrically at the shoulders and left abdomen.

It was soon recognized that the limb electrodes are quite distant from the heart and in order to examine its electrical activity more accurately, chest leads were introduced. Since physiologists like to be able to examine events under a single electrode, Wilson et al. (1934) introduced the V terminal, which constitutes an "indifferent" electrode. The V lead is

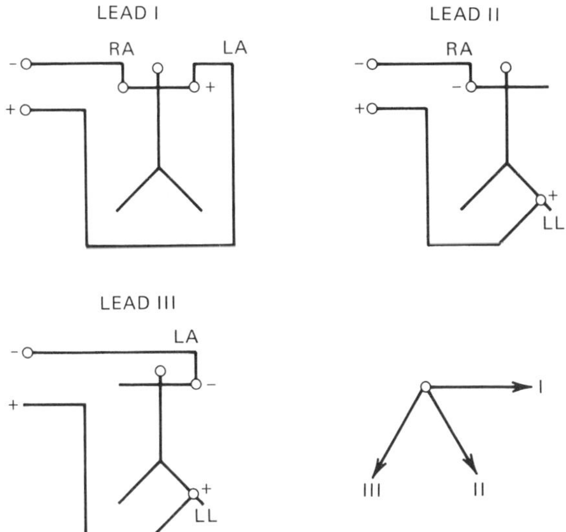

FIGURE 7.10. The standard limb leads introduced by Einthoven. The polarities shown provide an upward deflection on the ECG record.

formed by connecting resistors (5K–100K ohms) from a common point to the right arm, left arm, and left leg electrodes. The "active" exploring electrode is placed on the chest at the sites shown in Figure 7.11. There are six standard V leads. Occasionally, additional sites on the right chest are used (e.g., V_{3R}) as shown in Figure 7.11.

Goldberger (1942) introduced the augmented V leads (aV), which are shown in Figure 7.12. With the three standard, three augmented, and six V leads, the spatial direction of excitation and recovery of the heart chambers can be identified. Figure 7.13 summarizes the directions that correspond to the six frontal plane leads. Such representations are often called reference frames.

At this point it may be thought that there is an excessive number of leads for electrocardiography. From a mathematical viewpoint this is certainly true, since only three leads obtained from mutually perpendicular (orthogonal) axes are required to locate a vector in space. However, each ECG lead "sees" a different part of the heart. For example, the chest (V) leads provide a highly localized examination of the ventricular myocardium, and the activity that is recorded is the projection in the horizontal plane. The limb leads record the frontal-plane projection and are less highly localized. As will be demonstrated later, by recording a large number of leads it is possible to examine the ECG and estimate the axis of excitation and recovery by inspection, rather than by having to plot amplitudes on the reference frames and graphically determine the vectors.

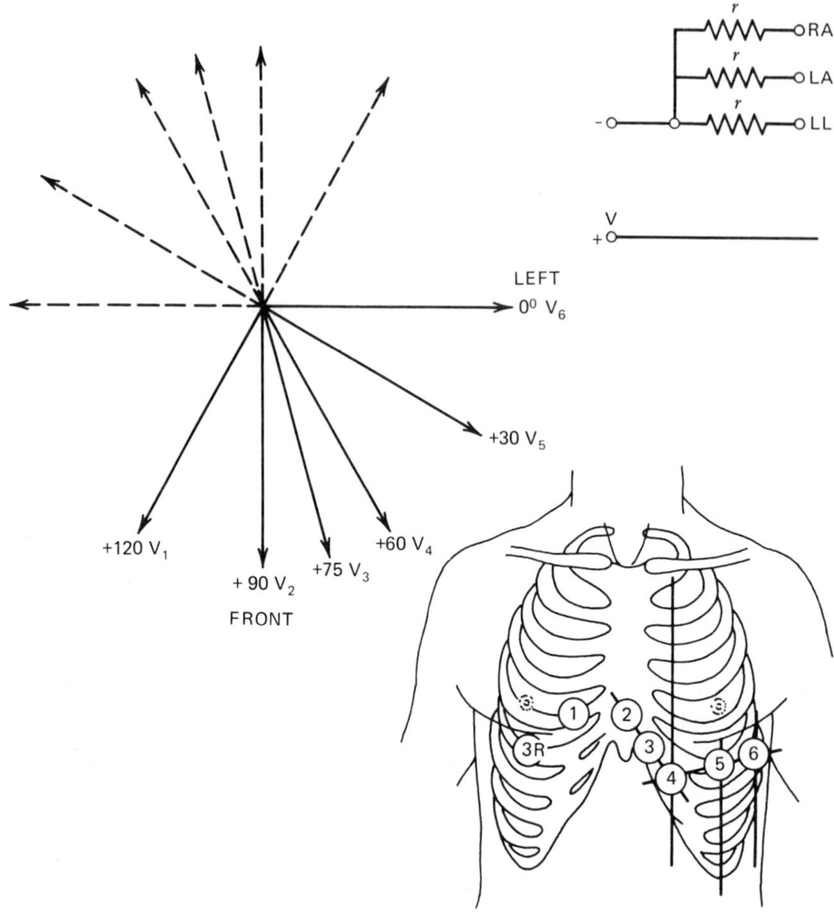

FIGURE 7.11. The V leads of Wilson and the directions that they represent. The polarity shown is for an upward deflection on the ECG.

ELECTROCARDIOGRAPHIC PATTERNS

Normal Excitation and Recovery

To exploit the ECG for the diagnostic information that it contains, it is necessary to know only a few basic facts; these are:

1. The origin of the normal heart beat is in the S-A node which lies in the right atrium. When the S-A node fires, the atria are excited and

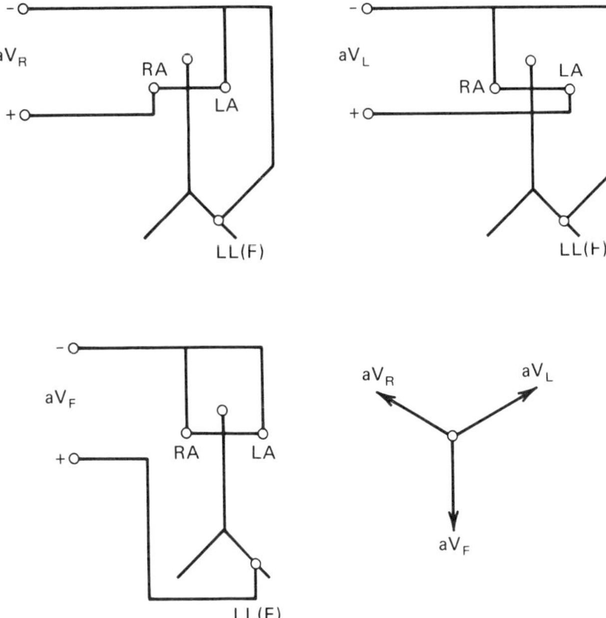

FIGURE 7.12. The augmented (aV) leads of Goldberger. (In many ECG instruments the limb electrodes are joined together with series resistors or after the signal has been passed through a buffer amplifier.)

give rise to the P wave. Recovery of the atria is associated with the T_P wave which is obscured by ventricular excitation.

2. Excitation takes place in an orderly sequence from the atria to the ventricles. Excitation of the atria stimulates the A-V node and conduction system in the ventricles. When the ventricles are excited, the *QRS* wave is generated; when they recover, the *T* wave is developed.
3. When excitation (or recovery) travels parallel to the axis of a lead, the amplitude is maximum. When excitation (or recovery) travels at right angles to the axis of a lead, the amplitude is a minimum.
4. Knowledge of the directions for the various leads allows determination of the direction of excitation and recovery. A heart vector (i.e., spread of excitation or recovery) pointing toward the head of the arrow in the reference frame will cause an upward deflection in that lead. Although seldom pointed out, vectors of excitation and recovery are *represented* with the arrow facing *positive* (recovered) tissue.

LEAD	NEGATIVE	POSITIVE
I	RIGHT ARM	LEFT ARM
II	RIGHT ARM	LEFT LEG
III	LEFT ARM	LEFT LEG
aVR	LA+LL	RIGHT ARM
aVL	RA+LL	LEFT ARM
aVF	RA+LA	LEFT LEG(F)

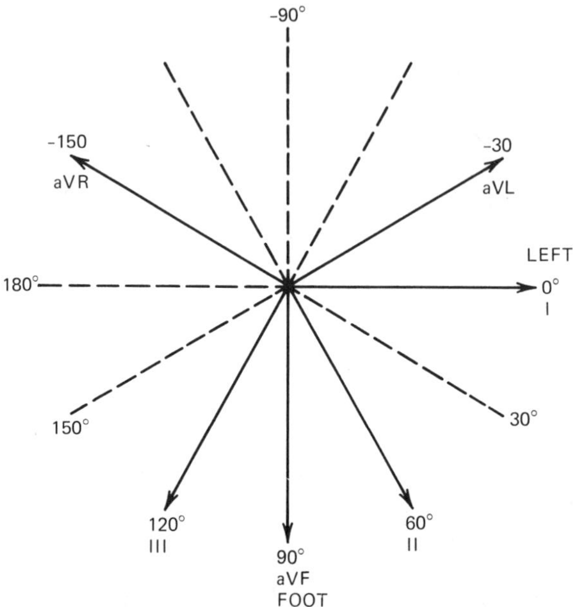

FIGURE 7.13. The frontal-plane leads.

5. All myocardial tissues have the propensity to become a pacemaker; some regions are more likely to than others.
6. There is a normal range of values for the durations and intervals of the ECG (e.g., *P*, *P-R*, *QRS*, and *Q-T*). These values are slightly dependent on heart rate and are shown in Table 7.1.

Figure 7.14 illustrates a standard 12-lead ECG from a normal subject. It is easy to see that the different leads "see" different parts of the heart. The general rule that excitation is represented by a dipole traveling with its positive pole forward, allows concluding that excitation of the atria, as signaled by the *P* wave, traveled in the footward direction in the frontal plane (as indicated by the limb leads), and anteriorly in the horizontal plane (as indicated by the V leads). Note that in aVR, the *P* wave is inverted. Recall that this lead would give an upward deflection only if

TABLE 7.1. Normal Intervals and Durations

P-R, Atrioventricular Conduction Time
(Depends slightly on heart rate)

	Age	*P-R*
Children	1 year	0.11 sec
Children	6 years	0.13 sec
Children	12 years	0.14 sec
Adults	Adult	0.12–0.20 sec (A few normal subjects have a range of 0.12–0.24. Very few normals have an interval extending to 0.39 sec)

QRS: Duration for ventricular depolarization

Adults 0.05–0.10 sec typically
(0.04–0.11 sec is normal limit)

Q-T: Duration for ventricular depolarization and repolarization (depends on heart rate)[a]

			Upper Limits of the Normal	
Heart Rate per Minute	Men and Children (sec)	Women (sec)	Men and Children (sec)	Women (sec)
40.0	0.449	0.461	0.491	0.503
43.0	0.438	0.450	0.479	0.491
46.0	0.426	0.438	0.466	0.478
48.0	0.420	0.432	0.460	0.471
50.0	0.414	0.425	0.453	0.464
52.0	0.407	0.418	0.445	0.456
54.5	0.400	0.411	0.438	0.449
57.0	0.393	0.404	0.430	0.441
60.0	0.386	0.396	0.422	0.432
63.0	0.378	0.388	0.413	0.423
66.5	0.370	0.380	0.404	0.414
70.5	0.361	0.371	0.395	0.405
75.0	0.352	0.362	0.384	0.394
80.0	0.342	0.352	0.374	0.384
86.0	0.332	0.341	0.363	0.372
92.5	0.321	0.330	0.351	0.360
100.0	0.310	0.318	0.338	0.347
109.0	0.297	0.305	0.325	0.333
120.0	0.283	0.291	0.310	0.317
133.0	0.268	0.276	0.294	0.301
150.0	0.252	0.258	0.275	0.282
172.0	0.234	0.240	0.255	0.262

[a] Reproduced with kind permission of the publishers from *Essentials of Electrocardiography* by R. Ashman and E. Hull, The Macmillan Company, New York, 1945.

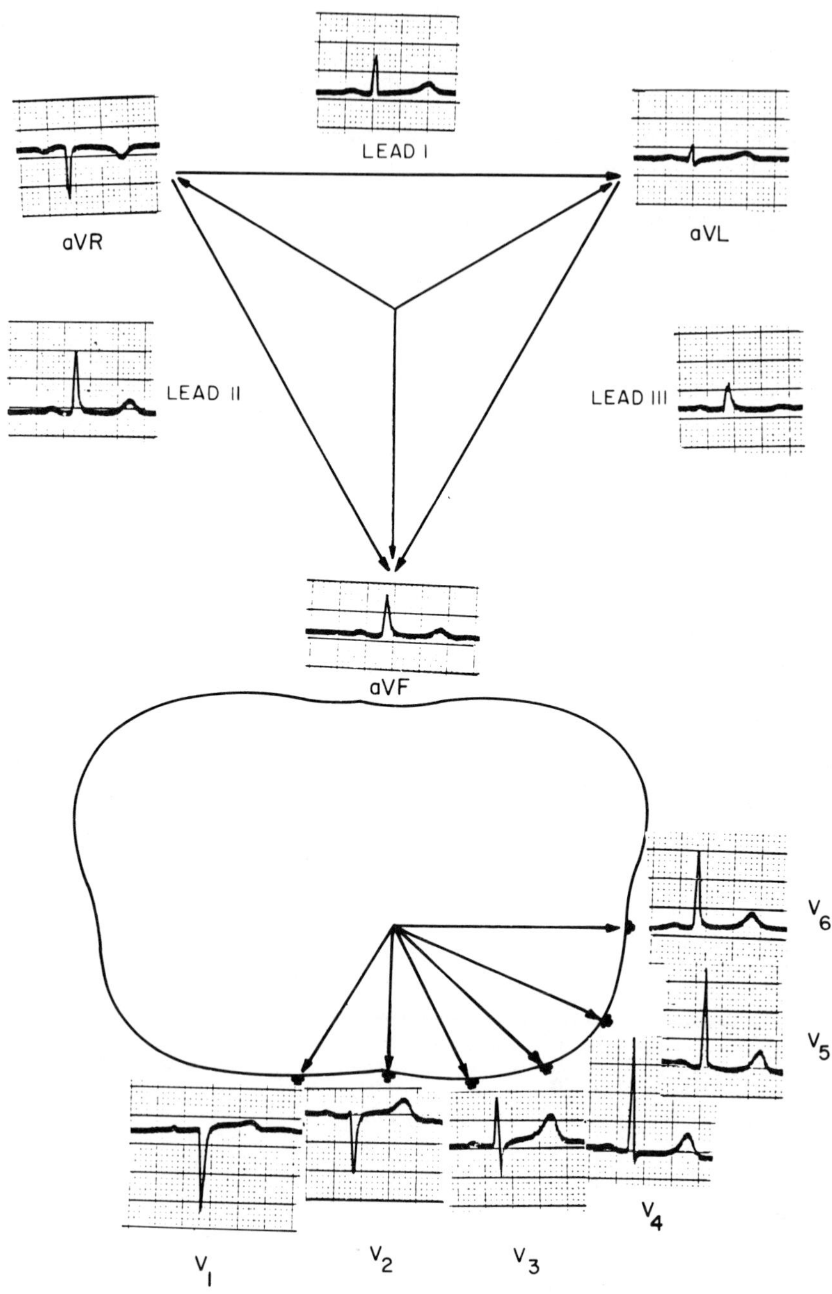

FIGURE 7.14. Typical normal ECG waveforms.

excitation traveled in the opposite direction. The *P* wave is almost equal in amplitude in leads I and II; therefore, excitation traveled in a direction between 0° and 60°.

In Figure 7.14, ventricular excitation, as signaled by the *QRS* wave, is upward in all three limb leads and aVL and aVF, indicating that excitation traveled slightly to the left of footward. The *QRS* wave is large and inverted in aVR because excitation advanced in a direction almost opposite to the right arm. The amplitudes of *QRS* is leads I and aVF are equal, therefore, ventricular excitation traveled at an angle of 45°; this is consistent with the fact that aVL is almost isoelectric, because it is nearly perpendicular to the direction of excitation.

In Figure 7.14, ventricular recovery, as signaled by the *T* wave, is almost zero in lead III and almost equal in I and II, therefore, recovery traveled at about 30°.

Examination of the six V leads in Figure 7.14 indicates that ventricular excitation started first along the axis of V_3 and moved toward V_6. A more complete discussion of this sequence will be presented in the section on vectorcardiography.

A-V Block

A disturbance in the conduction (i.e., propagation) of excitation from the atria to the ventricles is revealed by a prolongation of the P-R interval. Any electrocardiographic lead which shows a P and *QRS* wave can be used to diagnose atrioventricular conduction defects. Prolongation of A-V conduction beyond about 0.20 sec in humans is known as first-degree block by clinicians. A more-severe impairment in atrioventricular conduction can result in intermittent conduction between the atria and ventricles. Thus, only every second, third, etc., atrial excitation may be transmitted to the ventricles. In such a case, called second-degree A-V block by clinicians, the ventricular rate, as identified by the *QRS-T* complexes, has a submultiple of the atrial rate, which is indicated by the number of *P* waves. Physiologists designate this type of block as 2:1, 3:1, etc., A-V block. An example of second-degree (2:1) A-V block is illustrated in Figure 7.15. Just beyond the middle of the record 1:1 conduction was established.

The A-V conduction system can be impaired to such an extent that none of the atrial impulses are conducted from the atria to the ventricles. This condition is known as total A-V or third-degree A-V block. Because the ventricles are capable of beating by themselves, they do so but at a slow rate. The ECG displays normal *P* waves with no fixed relationship to the ventricular excitation and recovery waves. The magnitude and polar-

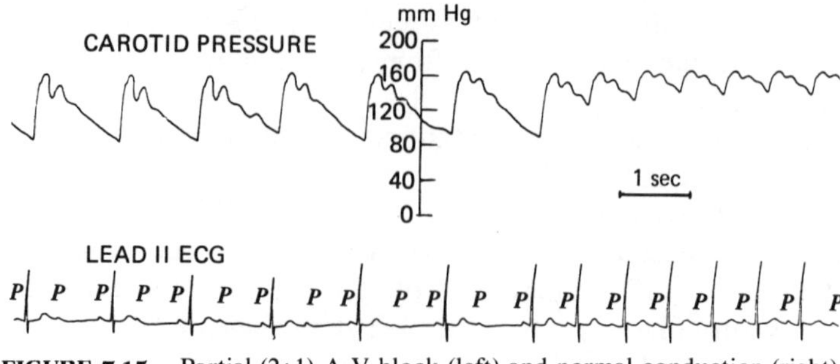

FIGURE 7.15. Partial (2:1) A-V block (left) and normal conduction (right).

ity of the ventricular *QRS* wave depends on the point of excitation in the ventricles. When excitation travels over the A-V node, bundle of His, and Purkinje fibers, the *QRS* wave has a virtually normal configuration and duration. There is a relatively narrow range of duration for the *QRS* wave. If excitation arises in, and travels over, ventricular muscle, the duration of the *QRS* wave is longer. Figure 7.16 illustrates total A-V block with a rhythm that has been established by a ventricular pacemaker toward the apex of the ventricle, as evidenced by the inverted *QRS* complex in lead II.

Atrial Arrhythmias

The metabolism of the atria can be altered in such a way that a high rhythmicity results. This situation is called atrial tachycardia, and in humans, if very rapid (e.g., above 200/min and still organized) it is called atrial flutter. Figure 7.17 illustrates atrial flutter in the dog heart. In such a case the A-V node is bombarded with so many excitations from the atria

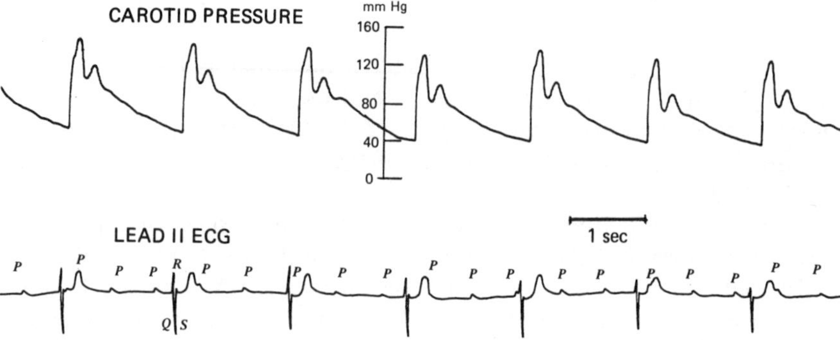

FIGURE 7.16. Total A-V (third-degree) block in which the atria and ventricles beat independently.

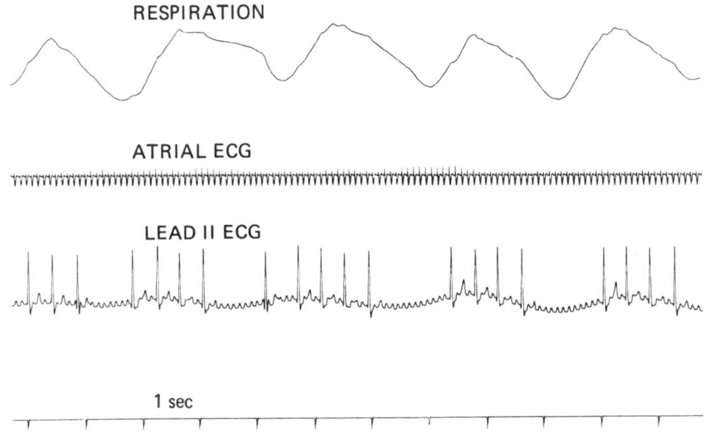

FIGURE 7.17. Atrial flutter in the dog.

that it cannot respond to each. Consequently, the atrial rate is much higher than the ventricular rate, as signaled by the number of *QRS* waves. In addition, the ventricular rate is irregular and in the illustration presented is modulated by respiration, increasing on inspiration.

Atrial metabolism can be altered further to such a degree that fibrillation can occur. In this situation all of the atrial fibers are contracting and relaxing very rapidly and randomly. There are no *P* waves in the ECG, which consists of irregular fibrillation waves (above 500/min). A rapid, irregular ventricular rate results, limited only by the recovery time of the A-V node. Figure 7.18 illustrates the ECG and respiration during atrial fibrillation in the dog. In atrial fibrillation, the pumping action of the atria is lost. However, atrial contribution to ventricular filling is small and atrial fibrillation is compatible with life. The main difficulty is the high ventricular rate, which is controlled by drugs that reduce the number of atrial impulses traveling over the A-V node.

Ventricular Recovery and Injury

Ventricular recovery is indicated by the *T* wave and the position of the baseline between the *QRS* and *T* waves; this region is called the *S-T* segment. In normally nourished ventricles this segment is at the same level as that just before the *P* wave, that is, the isoelectric baseline, and there is no shift in the *S-T* segment. During the *S-T* segment, all of the ventricular muscle is depolarized. If the ventricles do not receive an adequate supply of oxygenated blood, full repolarization may not occur in all of the ventricular muscle and there will be a region with less membrane

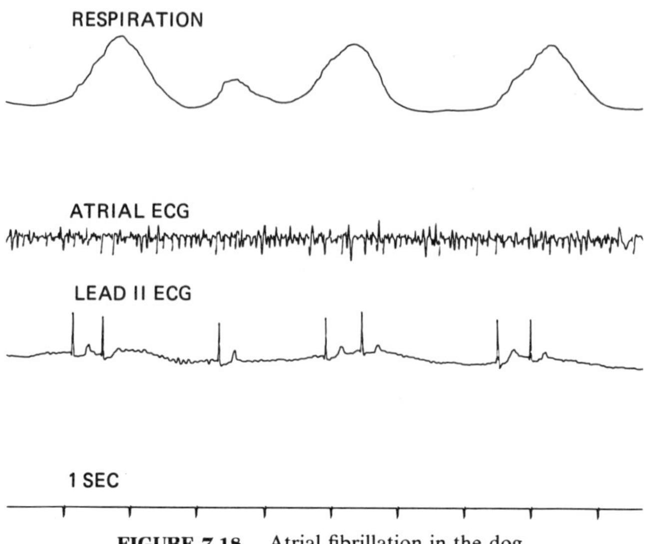

FIGURE 7.18. Atrial fibrillation in the dog.

potential. Because the amplifiers in ECGs are condenser coupled, this persistent hypopolarized does not show up as a shift in the ECG baseline. However, it does show up as an *S-T* segment shift following sudden depolarization of the ventricles, as signaled by the *QRS* wave. In exercise teting on the treadmill, the coronary arterial system is stressed to its limit to deliver a sufficient quantity of oxygenated blood to the ventricles. If coronary circulation is insufficient, full repolarization of all of the ventricles does not occur and there appears a shift in the *S-T* segment. The magnitude of the shift depends on the particular lead used, as well as the insufficiency. Because of their proximity to the ventricles, the precordial leads are used to detect a shift in the *S-T* segment. In exercise stress testing, a displacement of the *S-T* segment of 0.15 mV in lead V_5 is usually the point where the exercise test is discontinued. Obviously the longer the period of exercise required to attain this point, the better the coronary circulation.

If a coronary artery becomes blocked, the region of the heart supplied by it will not receive an adequate amount of blood. Therefore, the myocardial cells cannot sustain normal metabolism and their cell membranes depolarize and remain in this state as the cells die and are replaced by scar tissue. Thus, with a coronary occlusion, there occurs an immediate shift in the *S-T* segment. Its visibility depends, of course, on the site and extent of the occlusion and the particular lead being used to record the ECG. Figure 7.19 illustrates lead III ECG of a myocardial infarction caused by

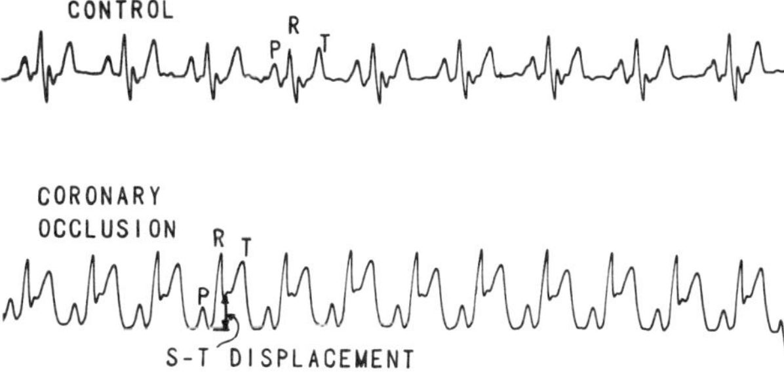

FIGURE 7.19. The *S-T* segment displacement in early coronary artery occlusion in the dog.

closure of a coronary artery branch that serves the apical region of the left ventricle.

In myocardial infarction, the cells that die alter the propagation of excitation through the ventricles. For this reason the *QRS* wave is altered and, in general, the *Q* wave becomes more prominent. Thus, the two changes usually seen in the ECG are an early shift in the *S-T* segment and a change in the magnitude of the *Q* wave. Location of the infarct can be accomplished by considering the *S-T* shift to be similar to other recorded amplitudes and applying the same rules for localization.

Ventricular Fibrillation

Fibrillation in the ventricles results in a loss of pumping and a fall in blood pressure to a near-zero level. Cardiac output is zero, and tissues start to die because they are deprived of oxygenated blood. The *QRS-T* waves of the ECG are replaced by fibrillation waves. Figure 7.20 illustrates the ECG and blood pressure prior to and during ventricular fibrillation. Ventricular defibrillation is an emergency procedure and is usually preceded by cardiopulmonary resuscitation (CPR) in which the chest is rhythmically and forcefully compressed, to squeeze blood out of the heart, and the lungs are inflated rhythmically by mouth-to-mouth breathing. Defibrillation is achieved by passing a pulse of current through the heart by electrodes applied to the chest. Figure 7.21 illustrates delivery of a defibrillating shock with restoration of ventricular pumping and cardiac output.

Bundle-Branch Block

Excitation of the ventricular myocardium develops in an orderly manner because of the conduction system, which consists of the A-V node, the

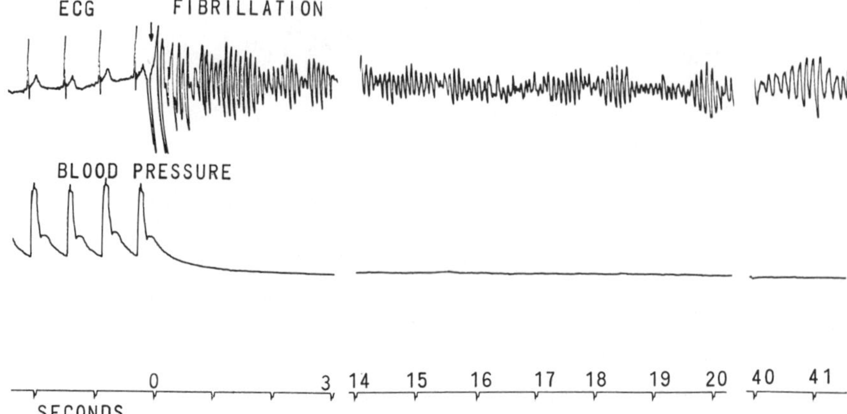

FIGURE 7.20. The ECG and blood pressure prior to and during ventricular fibrillation.

His bundle, with its left and right branches, and the Purkinje fibers. This conduction system has a propagation velocity that is higher than in ventricular muscle. The net result is that both ventricles contract almost simultaneously and the beat that results develops the maximum force. The temporal and spatial spread of excitation in the ventricles is what gives the *QRS* wave its characteristic shape in the various leads. Figure 7.22 diagrams the essentials of the conduction system and the numbers indicate the *QR* times for normal progression of excitation over the ventricles; the numbers (2–6) indicate the general direction of excitation.

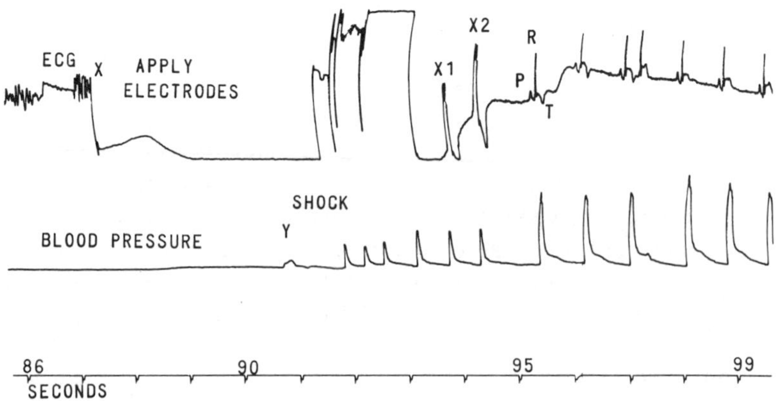

FIGURE 7.21. The ECG and blood pressure prior to and after delivery of a defibrillating shock directly to the ventricles. Note the two ectopic beats (X_1, x_2) prior to restoration of a normal rhythm.

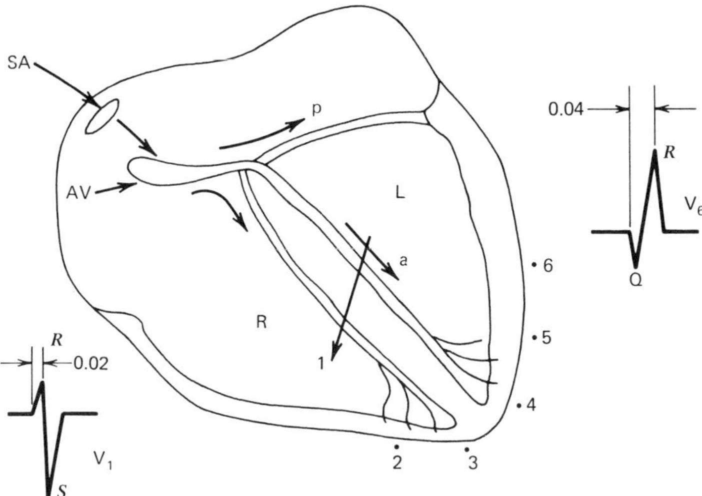

FIGURE 7.22. Essentials of the conduction system of the heart and recordings from V_1 and V_6 in the normal subject.

The conduction system can malfunction due to circulatory impairment or disease. The most common type of disturbance in conduction is block of the left or right branches. The names given to failure of the left bundle branch to transmit excitation is left bundle-branch block (LBBB); the name for block of the right bundle is right bundle-branch block (RBBB). A block of excitation in one of the branches will cause the affected side to be excited, that is, depolarized, late and this fact will be revealed in a prolongation of the duration of the *QRS* complex of the ECG. Thus, in bundle-branch block, the ventricles will be excited serially, the affected side being excited last. To identify electrocardiographically late activation due to block of one of the bundle braches, it is appropriate to use leads that are closest to the ventricles, that is, the chest (V) leads, although evidence of bundle-branch block shows up in the limb leads.

To understand how bundle-branch block alters the ECG, it is first necessary to know the sequence of excitation in normal ventricles. Owing to the nature of the conduction system and the differing thicknesses of the ventricular myocardium, excitation first appears on the surface of the thin-walled right ventricle. Thus, excitation, represented by dipoles with their positive poles facing the direction of excitation, will produce an initial upward wave in V_1 and a downward wave in V_6 (Figure 7.22). Then excitation of the left ventricle takes place and the dipoles of excitation travel toward the left; consequently, a downward wave is recorded in V_1 and an upward wave in V_6. Therefore, normal activation of the ventricles

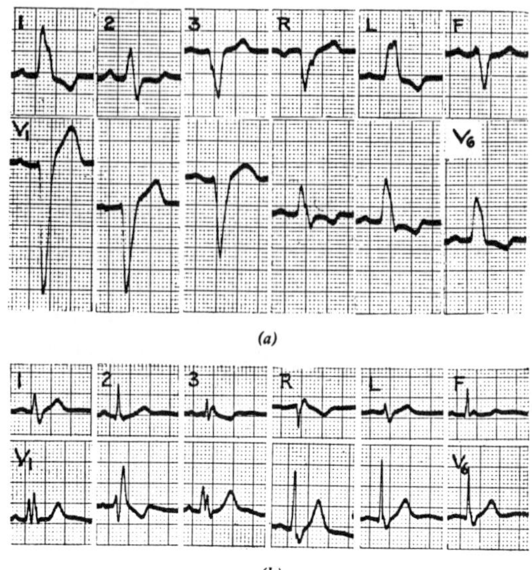

FIGURE 7.23. Bundle-branch block: (*a*) left bundle-branch block and (*b*) right bundle-branch block.

produces an *R-S* wave in V_1 and a *Q-R* wave in V_6. In normal hearts, the start of the downstroke will be no greater than 0.02 sec in lead V_1 (and other leads that see the right ventricle). Similarly, the normal *Q-R* time in V_6 is 0.04 sec.

In left bundle-branch block, excitation of the left ventricle is delayed and excitation travels generally from right to left. The initial *Q* wave in left-sided V leads seen in normals is absent. The right-sided V leads show a large, broad, downward wave. The left-sided V leads show a broad, upward wave, which is notched to the late spread of excitation to the left ventricle.

Figure 7.23*a* illustrates the ECG of a patient with left bundle-branch block. Recall that the affected side (left ventricle) is depolarized late and therefore attention should be focused on the ECG leads that see the left ventricle, for example, V_{5-6} and aV_L. Note that the duration of the *QRS* is prolonged (0.16 sec); there is a slight notching and the downstroke occurs about 0.06 sec after the start of ventricular depolarization. Leads aV_L and I, which also see the left ventricle, provide the same information. Because of the altered pattern of early excitation, *Q* waves are rarely seen in left-chest leads with LBBB. Note that leads V_{1-3} give little evidence of delayed conduction because they see predominantly the right ventricle.

In right bundle-branch block, there is a delay in exciting the right ventricle. The early part of excitation occurs as in a normal heart, with the first part of the *QRS* representing excitation spreading from left to right. However, the delayed excitation of the right ventricle soon appears as a prominent wave occurring late in the complex. When viewed from right-sided V leads, the deflection is upward and in the left-sided V leads, a prominent S wave is seen.

Figure 7.23*b* illustrates the ECG of right-bundle branch block. Note that the duration of the *QRS* wave is prolonged in leads V_{1-3}, which see the right ventricle. Note also that the *QRS* wave is M-shaped, which is often seen in right bundle-branch block. This M-shaped wave is designated *rSR'*, the *R'* wave representing the delayed excitation advancing over the right ventricle.

HIS-BUNDLE ELECTROGRAM (HBE)

By recording the activity of the His bundle with a catheter electrode, it is possible to obtain information on the integrity of the propagation of excitation from the origin of the heart beat in the sinoatrial (S-A) node, to the ultimate excitatory event, ventricular excitation. With the body-surface ECG, it is only possible to obtain information on the time taken for excitation to travel from the atria to the ventricles, the *P-R* interval. With His-bundle recording, this time can be divided into three components, *PA*, *AH*, and *HV*, where *A* refers to atrial, *H* to His-bundle, and *V* to ventricular excitation. The onset of the *A* wave occurs slightly after the onset of the *P* wave; therefore, the *P-A* interval represents conduction through the atria. The *A-H* interval represents the time taken for excitation to travel across the atrioventricular (A-V) node. The *H-V* interval identifies the time taken for excitation to travel from the His bundle to the ventricles, the *V* wave being the analog of the *QRS* wave in the ECG. Figure 7.24 illustrates a typical His-bundle electrogram (HBE) made by passing a catheter electrode through the venous system into the right heart; this technique will be described subsequently. The ECG is shown for comparison and indicates that the His-bundle (*H*) wave occurs between the *P* and *QRS* waves.

There are normal values for the components of the HBE. Roberts (1975) provided the data for normal subjects shown in Table 7.2.

The autonomic nervous system, pharmacologic agents, congenital abnormalities, and disease alter the propagation of excitation over the conducting systems of the heart, changing the *P-A*, *A-H*, and *H-V* intervals. Activation of the parasympathetic division of the autonomic nervous system prolongs the *A-H* interval, while activation of the sympathetic divi-

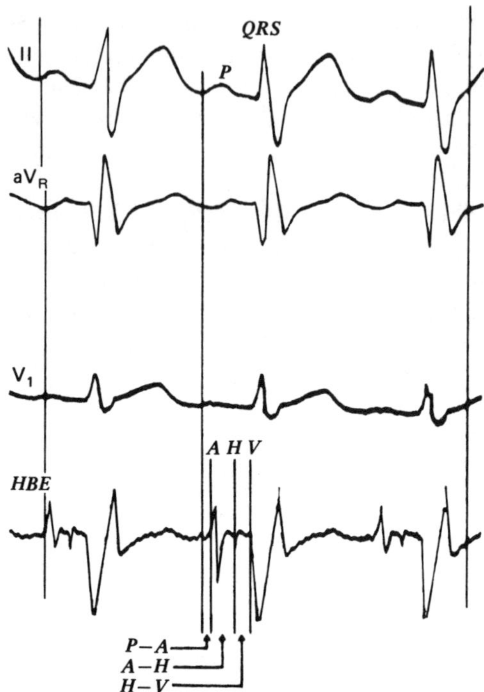

FIGURE 7.24. The His-bundle electrogram in relation to body-surface electrocardiograms. [Redrawn from Roberts (1975).]

sion decreases the *A-H* and *H-V* intervals. There are numerous drugs that either prolong or shorten the propagation of excitation across the A-V node. Disease can depress or block conduction in the A-V node and His bundle, and this effect is not only clearly revealed, but is localizable by the HBE.

Sometimes atrial pacing is used to aid in interpreting the HBE. However, when compared to the normal, the *A-H* interval is increased. The administration of atropine restores the *A-H* interval to normal. Presum-

TABLE 7.2. Normal Values for the His-Bundle Electrogram[a]

	P-R	*P-A*	*A-H*	*H-V*
Adult	155 ± 14	42 ± 11	73 ± 12	40 ± 4
Children (<17 yr)	138 ± 17	21 ± 8.5	86 ± 16	31 ± 5.5

[a]From Roberts (1975).

ably with atrial pacing, some vagal fibers innervating the A-V node are stimulated.

There are many techniques for recording the HBE; with all, a catheter electrode is advanced into the right heart via the venous system. Monopolar, bipolar, and multipolar catheters have been used. However, it is possible to obtain excellent HBEs with the monopolar catheter electrode connected to one terminal of the ECG, with the V terminal constituting the other lead. To obtain a clear HBE, careful adjustment of the catheter electrode is necessary while viewing the recording. Fluoroscopic examination is generally used and the catheter tip is advanced into the right atrium and across the tricuspid valve into the right ventricle. The catheter is slowly withdrawn across the tricuspid valve until the tip electrode is just on the atrial side of the tricuspid valve. At this point the catheter position is adjusted by further withdrawal or advancement or rotation, until a satisfactory HBE is obtained. Although the waveform will vary in contour during this procedure, the intervals will vary little. It is, however, important to note that displacement of the catheter electrode by about a millimeter will dramatically reduce the amplitude of the *H* wave.

VECTORCARDIOGRAPHY

Vectorcardiography deals with the temporal and spatial aspects of the excitation and recovery of the heart. In reality there are two types of vector studies in cardiology. In one the instantaneous vector is displayed, and in the other, the mean vector is reported. Perhaps the best way of illustrating how the cardiac vectors are obtained is to show how they are derived from two limb leads. For simplicity, let us calculate the instantaneous vectors of ventricular excitation (*QRS* vector) using leads 1 and 2, as shown in Figure 7.25*a*. The instantaneous vector is determined by plotting the amplitude (at a given instant) obtained from a lead along the lead direction and erecting a perpendicular at this point. Then the amplitude from another lead is plotted along its lead direction and another perpendicular is erected. The point where the two perpendiculars intersect is joined to the origin of the reference frame and becomes the cardiac vector at that instant in the cardiac cycle. For example, 40 msec after the start of the *QRS* wave, the amplitude in lead I is + 0.75 mV and in lead II it is + 1.3 mV. Plotting these amplitudes and erecting perpendiculars, as shown in Figure 7.25*b* provides an instantaneous cardiac vector of 1.3 mV with a direction of 52° at 40 msec during the *QRS* wave. By carrying out this procedure at each instant in the ventricular cycle, other vectors can be determined as shown in Figure 7.25*b*. By joining the

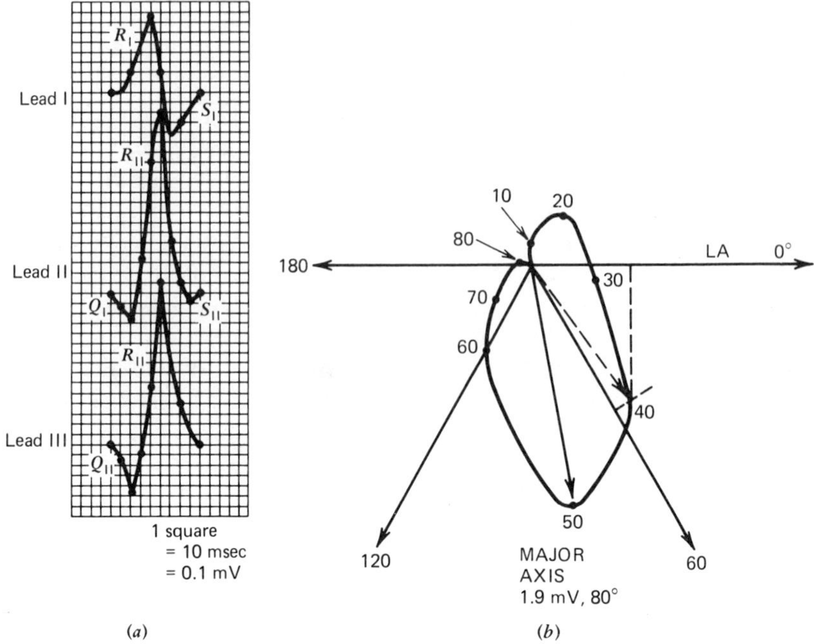

FIGURE 7.25. Instantaneous vectors of the ventricles.

tips of these vectors, a vector loop is obtained, which describes the magnitude and direction of spread of excitation at each instant. Because such vector loops are usually elongated, they are described in terms of the major axis, which in this case is a vector of 1.9 mV at 80°, the left arm being used as the 0° reference direction.

Clinicians find that it is usually simpler, and just as valuable, to estimate the mean cardiac vector by determining the net deflection (i.e., positive minus negative amplitudes) in two leads and plot these amplitudes on the reference frame, as shown in Figure 7.26. For example, in lead I the net amplitude is $+ 0.75 - 0.45 = 0.3$ mV; for lead II the net amplitude is $+ 1.8 - 0.25 = 1.55$ mV. Plotting these amplitudes on the reference frame, as shown in Figure 7.26*b* gives a mean *QRS* vector of 1.68 mV at an angle of 89°. Although the magnitude of the vector is slightly smaller than when calculated accurately, as in Figure 7.25*b*, the direction is quite similar.

It should be apparent that the amplitudes in any two leads will allow calculation of a cardiac vector. Similarly, if the vector is known, the amplitude in any other lead in the same plane can be determined by

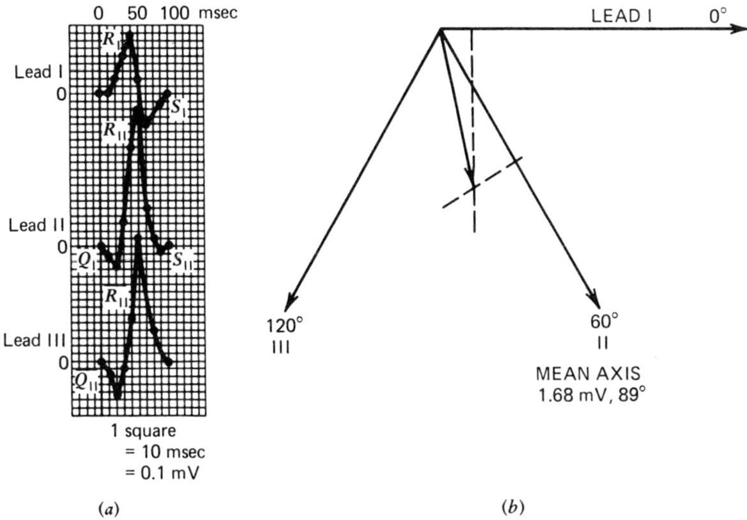

(*a*) (*b*)

FIGURE 7.26. Mean cardiac vector.

dropping a perpendicular from the tip of the vector to the line on the reference frame that identifies the lead of interest.

There is yet another, even simpler, way to establish the direction and magnitude of a cardiac vector. The method employs mere inspection of the 12-lead electrocardiogram. As will be recalled, the six limb leads provide a reference frame that has 30° between the lead axes (Figure 7.14). The six V leads (Figure 8.13) provide about 15° resolution between the axis of two adjacent leads. With simple rules that state (1) the magnitude recorded is zero when excitation and/or recovery travel at right angles to a lead axis and (2) the amplitude is a maximum when excitation and/or recovery travel parallel to the lead axis, it is possible to estimate the cardiac vectors with considerable accuracy by mere inspection. These two rules will now be used to illustrate how simple inspection can be used to determine the mean electrical axes.

Referring to Figure 7.14, the net amplitude of *QRS* is nearly zero in lead aVL; this means that the major axis for excitation is nearly at right angles to lead aVL. Note that the amplitudes in leads I and aVF are almost identical and upward; this means that excitation travels at an angle that is midway between these leads, that is, about 45°. Note that the *T* wave has almost zero amplitude in lead III; therefore recovery moves at right angles to lead III. Because the *T* wave is upward in leads I and aVF, the recovery (*T*-wave) axis is 30°.

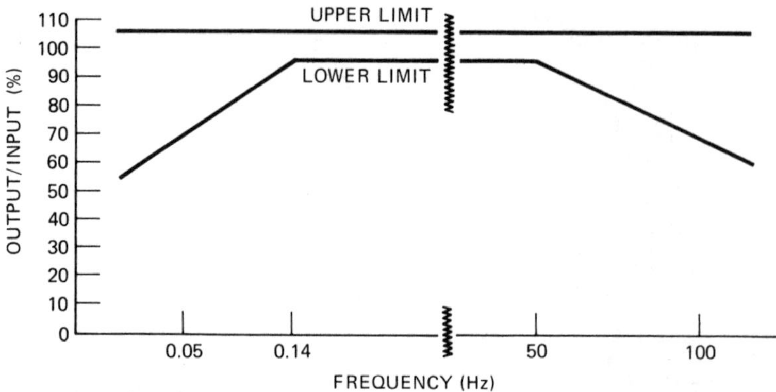

FIGURE 7.27. Frequency response recommendations for clinical electrocardiographs. [From *Circulation* (1975), **52**, 11–31.]

THE INSTRUMENT AND ITS CHARACTERISTICS

The clinical electrocardiograph is a capacitively coupled recording voltmeter with an input impedance in excess of 500,000 ohms. The low-frequency response is limited by the time constant of the amplifier. The high-frequency response is limited by the graphic recording pen. These operating characteristics have been specified on several occasions by committees of the American Heart Association (1954, 1967, 1972) and the Council of Physical Medicine of the American Medical Association (1947, 50). The most recent American Heart Association (1975) recommendations are as follows: The frequency response shall fall within the limits shown in Figure 7.27.

1. With an amplitude response of 20 mm peak-to-peak at 25 Hz, the response to constant-amplitude sinusoidal input signals in the range from 0.14 to 25 Hz shall be flat to within 6% (0.5 dB). The response to 0.05 Hz shall not be reduced by more than 30% (−3 dB) from the response at 0.14 Hz.
2. With an amplitude response of 10 mm peak-to-peak at 25 Hz, the response to constant amplitude sinusoidal input signals up to 50 Hz shall be flat to within ±6% (±0.5 dB).
3. With an amplitude response of 5 mm peak-to-peak at 25 Hz, the response to constant amplitude sinusoidal input signals up to 100 Hz shall not be reduced by more than 30% (−3 dB), leaving an amplitude of at least 3.5 mm at 100 Hz.
4. At no frequency within the band shall the response exceed the upper limits specified for the range of 0.14–50 Hz.

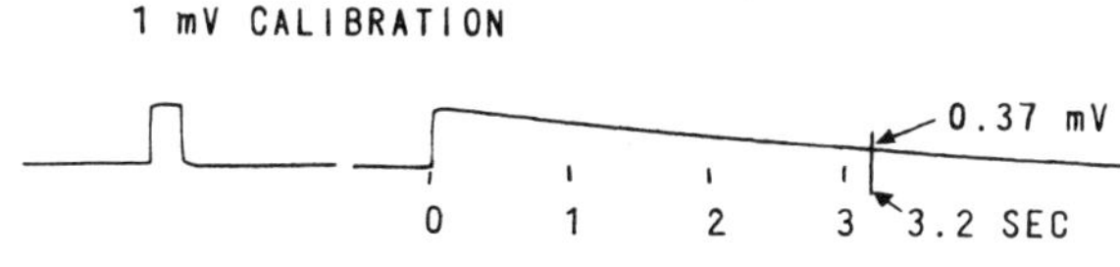

FIGURE 7.28. Typical colibration for an ECG.

5. Provisions to degrade the performance of the instrument for special-purpose recording shall not be incorporated unless a distinct marking on the record is made whenever this alternative is employed. Any such control shall require continuous action on the part of the operator and shall automatically return to the standard (nondegraded) mode of operation.

Perhaps the best way of determining the operating characteristics of an electrocardiograph is to use the 1 mV calibration signal as an input. As stated previously, the standard chart speed is 2.5 cm/sec and the standard calibration is 1 mV for 1 cm of pen deflection. This calibration signal is applied by momentary depression of the calibrate button while the chart is running. This maneuver provides a rectangular pulse as shown in Figure 7.28 (left). On viewing such a pulse, it might be concluded that it was reproduced by a direct-coupled system; that this is not so is easily shown by depressing the calibration button and holding it down to reveal the exponential-decay characteristic of the time constant of the instrument as shown in Figure 7.28 (right). This time constant describes the sinusoidal low-frequency response (f_L) for 70% amplitude. In Figure 7.28 the time constant T is 3.2 sec. Because $T = 1/2\pi f_L$; therefore, $f_L = 0.05$ Hz for 70.7% amplitude.

The sinusoidal high-frequency response can be estimated by measuring the rise time (10–90%) of the calibrating pulse. With standard chart speed (25 mm/sec), the rise time t (10–90% amplitude) can be estimated, and usually amounts to about one-quarter of one division (40 msec), namely, 10 msec. Therefore, the sinusoidal frequency f_h for 70% amplitude is very nearly equal to $1/2t$ and the sinusoidal high-frequency response (70% amplitude) extends to $1/(20 \times 10^{-3}) = 50$ Hz.

The foregoing demonstrates that from careful measurement of the decay and rise times for the 1 mV calibration pulse, it is possible to estimate the sinusoidal frequency response.

It is important to recognize that there is a difference between the operating characteristics of diagnostic and monitoring electrocardiographs. In monitoring electrocardiographs, the time constant is reduced to about 0.2 sec rather than the 3.2 sec recommended. This reduced time

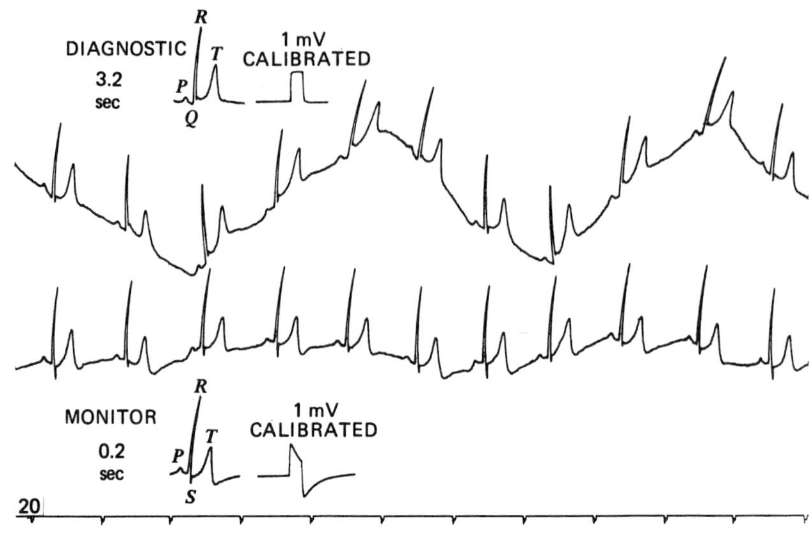

FIGURE 7.29. Sine-wave frequency response and rise time.

constant makes the instrument incapable of responding to low-frequency signals and is useful when electrode-movement artifacts are present. Such artifacts appear as a wandering baseline in clinical ECG recordings. Although the use of a shorter time constant eliminates this type of artifact, it also changes the ECG slightly. The monitor type of ECG is therefore best suited to identify arrhythmias and changes in the ECG, rather than to obtain accurate diagnostic information. Figure 7.29 illustrates a typical ECG recorded with diagnostic (3.2 sec) and monitor (0.2 sec) time constants.

The type of waveform distortion obtained with a system having an excessively short time constant is of clinical concern. This point was made by Swarzschild and Kissin (1934) who recorded the ECG with a string galvanometer and then with various time constants between it and the subject. They found that a noticeable *S-T* segment depression occurred with a 2-sec time constant. When a time constant of 0.1 sec was used, the *S-T* segment depression was 0.65 mV, amounting to 35% of the *R*-wave amplitude. Figure 7.30 illustrates this type of distortion. Thus, the use of a time constant that is too short can simultate myocardial ischemia or injury, as evidenced by an *S-T* segment shift.

HISTORICAL POSTSCRIPT

The discovery that contraction of the cardiac ventricles was accompanied by an electrical signal is due to Kolliker and Mueller (1856) and Donders

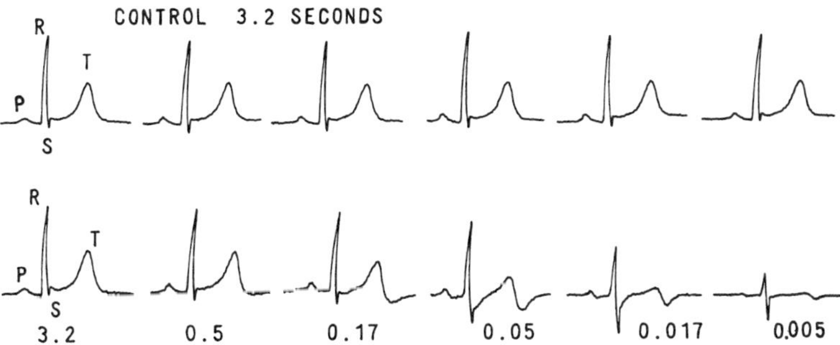

FIGURE 7.30. (*a*) ECG tracing with electrode artifact recorded with the diagnostic (3.2 sec) time constant (upper) and the 0.2 sec monitoring time constant (lower). (*b*) The control ECG (upper) recorded with the diagnostic (3.2 sec) time constant and with time constants of 0.5, 0.17, 0.05, 0.017 and 0.005 sec (lower). Note the *S-T* segment shift as the time constant is reduced.

(1872). At that time there were no rapidly responding indicators for current or voltage. There was, however, the rheoscope, which consisted of a frog sciatic nerve and its attached gastrocnemius muscle. A stimulus applied to the sciatic nerve caused the muscle to twitch. Kolliker and Mueller and Donders laid the sciatic nerve over the surface of a beating frog heart, the electrical activity of which stimulated the nerve and caused the muscle to twitch. Sometimes two twitches were obtained for each beat. We now know that it was the *R* and *T* wave signals that stimulated the sciatic nerve. Figure 7.31 is a sketch of this history-making experiment.

The muscular twitches observed by Kolliker and Mueller and Donders

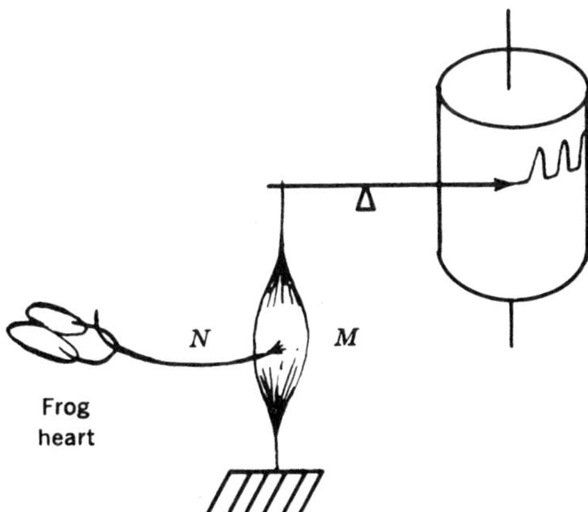

FIGURE 7.31. Method first used to demonstrate the electrical activity of the heart. The sciatic nerve (*N*) was laid across the beating frog ventricle. The cardioelectric signals stimulated the nerve and caused the gastrocnemius muscle to twitch and operate a writing lever, which scratched soot from a rotating drum.

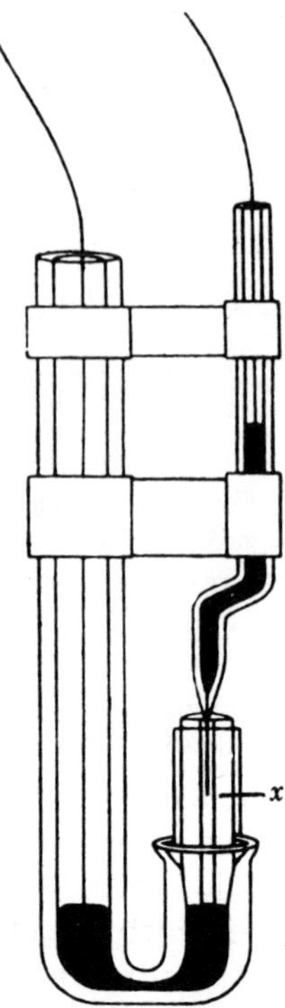

FIGURE 7.32. The Marey-Lippmann capillary electrometer for recording bioelectric events. Passage of current through the mercury–sulfuric-acid interface (*X*) altered the contour of the meniscus. When transilluminated and photographed on a moving chart, the contour changes represented the variation in current flow.

provided no information on the time course of the cardioelectric event; they only signaled presence of the bioelectric event. Measurement of the time course of the electrical signal from the heart preoccupied physiologists for the next half century. Using the rheotome, a current-sampling device, and a slowly responding galvanometer, Burdon-Sanderson (1879), plotted the waveform of the *R* and *T* waves of the frog ventricle (see Hoff and Geddes, 1957). The first instrument to record the waveform of the spontaneously beating heart was the capillary electrometer, which is shown in Figure 7.32. The essential component of this device is a mercury–sulfuric-acid interface (*X*). When current is caused to pass through this interface, the surface charge distribution is altered, which in turn alters the surface tension, thereby changing the contour of the mercury meniscus. By illuminating the meniscus with a bright light and photographing the contour via a cylindrical lens and moving photographic surface, the time course of an applied current could be recorded.

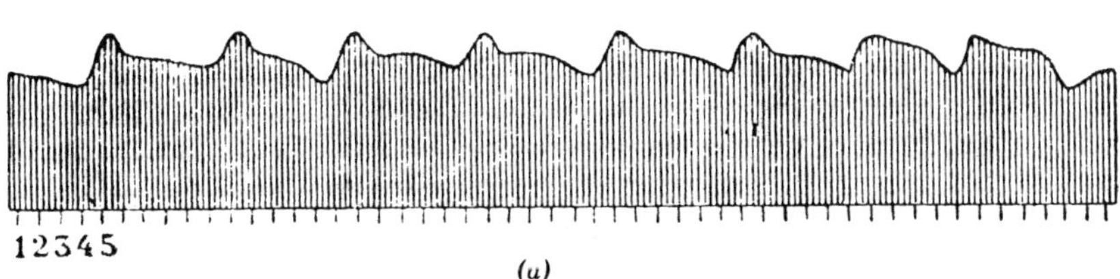

(a)

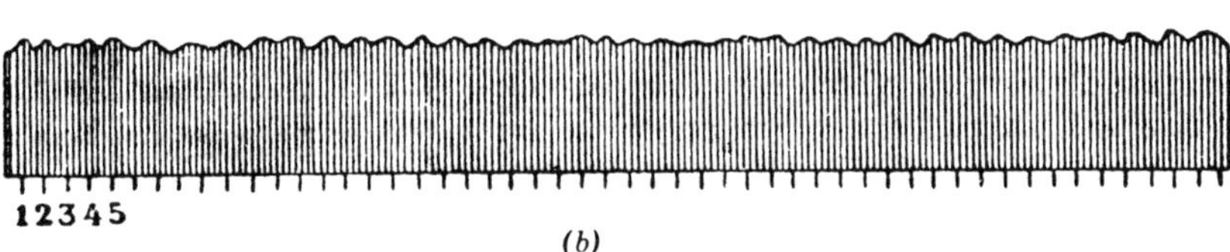

(b)

FIGURE 7.33. (*a*) Marey and Lippmann's tortoise electrocardiogram (T). It is difficult to be certain of the identity of the waves because the authors did not provide enough information on the location of the electrodes. Quite probably the waves shown here are the *R* and *T* waves. (*b*) Marey and Lippmann's frog auricular electrogram (G). If as the authors say the time divisions are 1/25 sec, the auricular rate was 5 per second or 300 per minute, which is excessively fast for a frog heart. Very possibly the auricles were in a state of fibrillation, and if so, this is one of the earliest records of auricular fibrillation.

Marey and Lippmann (1876) in France connected electrodes to the tortoise ventricle and frog atrium and recorded the first cardiac electrograms. Figure 7.33 is a reproduction from Marey's study.

Marey and Lippmann gave physiologists the capillary electrometer, the essential tool for electrophysiological studies. Although it lacked an adequately short response time for recording nerve action potentials, it did demonstrate their presence as it did those of skeletal muscle. Perhaps the most important use for the capillary electrometer was in a study of the mammalian electrocardiogram. Waller (1889) in England employed it to record the electrocardiogram of his bulldog by using bucket electrodes into which the animal placed its paws. Figure 7.34 illustrates Waller's dog and the bucket electrodes. Waller (1889) then used the capillary electrometer to record cardiac action potentials in humans: Figure 7.35 illustrates a record (along with the apex cardiogram). He called those leads that produced the largest amplitude "favorable" and those which provided the smallest amplitude "unfavorable." Table 7.3 summarizes his results.

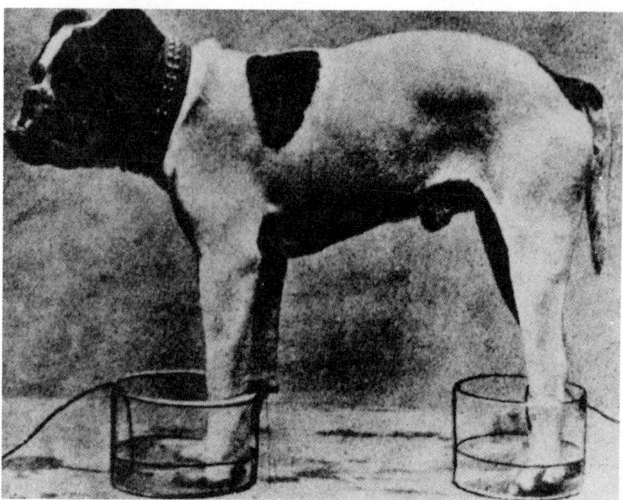

FIGURE 7.34. The method used by Waller to obtain electrocardiogram on his bulldog. The electrodes were connected to the capillary electrometer.

Waller's report indicates that he recognized the importance of standardizing leads to anatomical sites and he clearly understood the vector concept of the electrical activity of the heart. For example, by studying the amplitudes obtained with the various leads, he postulated the existence of a cardiac axis by presenting a sketch showing the potential field surrounding the heart. Figure 7.36 illustrates Waller's concept of the electrical axis of the heart.

Not all who constructed capillary electrometers for electrophysiological studies were satisfied with the performance of this new instrument. Among these was Einthoven in Holland, who constructed several instruments for his own use in furthering Waller's studies. It would appear that the English could build better capillary electrometers than the Dutch.

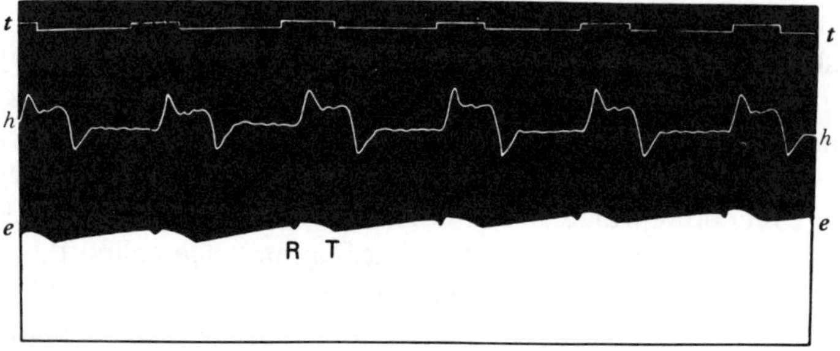

FIGURE 7.35. The first human electrocardiogram (e-e) obtained by Waller (1889) along with the apex cardiogram (h-h).

TABLE 7.3. Waller's Favorable and Unfavorable ECG Leads

Favorable	Unfavorable
Front of chest and back of chest	Left hand and left foot
Left hand and right hand	Left hand and right foot
Right hand and right foot	Right foot and left foot
Right hand and left foot	Mouth and right hand
Mouth and left hand	
Mouth and right foot	
Mouth and left foot	

Correspondence in various journals at that time both praised and bitterly denounced the capillary electrometer. Fortunately, Einthoven had discovered the Ader string telegraphic recorder (1897), and decided to modify it to make an electrocardiographic recorder.

Ader's telegraphic recorder consisted of a slender taut wire suspended between the poles of a permanent magnet. A hole was drilled through the poles of the magnet and a bright light was shone through the holes. The wire (string) was placed so that it blocked passage of the light through the holes in the poles. When telegraphic current was applied to the slender wire, it moved sideways and allowed the light to pass through the poles

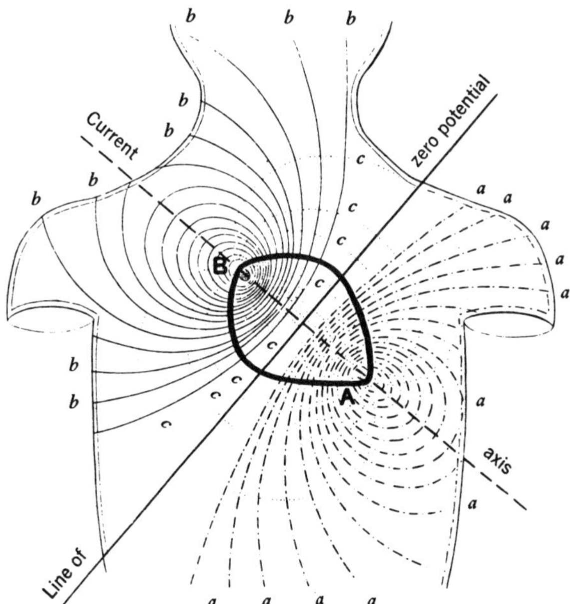

FIGURE 7.36. Waller's concept of the electrical axis of the human heart, derived from studies with the capillary electrometer. [From Waller (1889).]

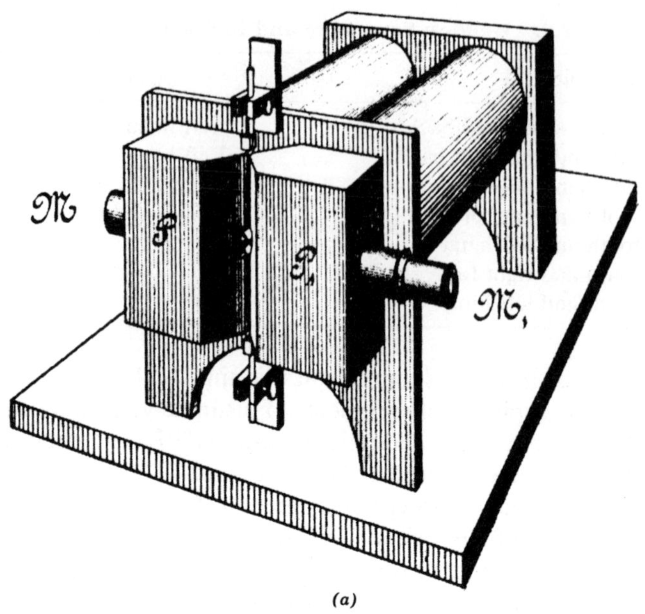

(a)

FIGURE 7.37. Einthoven's string galvanometer (1903). The string, a silvered quartz filament, was mounted between the pole-faces (PP) of an electromagnet. Light was passed through the lenses (MM) to transilluminate the string, the shadow of which was recorded photographically.

and strike a moving photographic paper. In this way the dots and dashes of telegraphic code were recorded photographically.

Einthoven immediately improved Ader's instrument by using a silvered quartz filament as the conductor. He increased the field strength surrounding the filament by using an electromagnet. He added a lens to focus the image of the filament onto a moving photographic surface. Thus, the thick baseline of the string galvanometer recording was the image of the "string" (quartz filament). Electrocardiac current caused the silvered filament (string) to be deflected and its excursions, when recorded photographically, constituted the electrocardiogram. Figure 7.37 illustrates Einthoven's string galvanometer.

Einthoven borrowed handsomely from previous work. He used Marey's recording chart speed (25 mm/sec). He used Waller's bucket electrodes and some of his leads; an electrocardiogram is shown in Figure 7.38.

Einthoven's string galvanometer ushered in clinical electrocardiography in 1903. Soon the string galvanometer was used worldwide, being retarded in its adoption by World War I (1914–1918). The first string galvanometer appeared in the United States in 1912 when it was used at

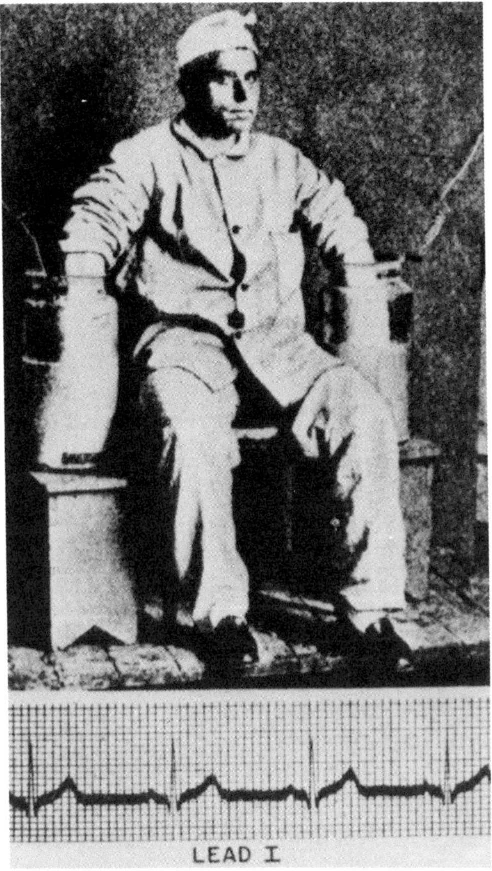

FIGURE 7.38. Einthoven's method of obtaining human electrocardiograms, and a typical record obtained with the string galvanometer.

the Rockefeller Institute Hospital, NY, from 1912 to 1959. This instrument, which is now in the Smithsonian Institution, Washington, DC, was designed by Horatio B. Williams, professor of physiology at the College of Physicians and Surgeons, Columbia University, NY. Williams had spent some time with Einthoven in Leiden in 1910 and 1911. On his return to New York, Williams had Charles F. Hindle, a machinist at Columbia, construct the first American string galvanometer. Soon thereafter, the Cambridge Instrument Co., NY, took over manufacture of the Hindle instrument and made them available for sale in the United States.

Although it is clear that the concept of an electrical axis, that is, cardiac vector, was demonstrated by Waller's studies, it remained for Einthoven to make practical use of the concept. In 1913 Einthoven postulated that the heart was at the center of an equilateral triangle, the apices of which were the right and left shoulders and the point where both legs joined the trunk. In his early studies, Einthoven used the right and left arms and both feet in saline-filled buckets as three electrodes. He found that the electrocardiogram was negligibly altered if the right foot was removed from the bucket electrode. Thus he adopted three standard leads: right and left arms and left leg (foot). He postulated that if the amplitudes of the electrocardiographic waves are plotted on this triaxial (60°) reference frame, it is possible to calculate the magnitude and direction of an electric vector that produces these same voltages in leads I, II, and III, corresponding to the limb electrodes. He further stated that the arithmetic sum of the amplitudes in leads I plus lead III equals the amplitude in lead II. This is Einthoven's law and the relationship is true only for an equilateral triangle reference frame.

Einthoven recorded the amplitudes in three leads and calculated the cardiac vector for ventricular excitation. The electrocardiograms illustrated in Figure 7-25 were taken from a paper by Einthoven et al. (1913). Later, the augmented limb leads were added to allow better resolution in identifying the cardiac axis in the frontal plane. The V leads permitted locating the cardiac vector in the horizontal plane.

Not long after Einthoven described his string galvanometer, efforts were begun to create an electrocardiograph that used vacuum tubes. At this time, there were rapidly responding mirror galvanometers, as well as a limited number of vacuum tubes, despite the fact that they had been invented only a few years earlier by Lee De Forest. According to Marvin (1954), the first discussions relative to such an instrument were held in 1917 between Steinmetz, Neuman, and Robinson of the General Electric Engineering Laboratory. The task of establishing feasibility fell to W.R.G. Baker, who assembled a unit and demonstrated its operation to those just identified. However, because of urgent wartime priorities, the project was shelved.

In about 1921, General Electric reopened the issue of a vacuum-tube ECG. A prototype was built and demonstrated to the Schenectady County Medical Association sometime in 1924 by Robinson and Marvin. The instrument was used by Drs. Neuman, Pardee, Mann, and Oppenheim, all physicians in New York City. Subsequently, six commercial models were made. One instrument was sent to each of the four physicians just identified; the fifth was sent to the General Electric Co. Hospital; and the sixth was sent to the AMA Convention in Atlantic City in 1925. This latter instrument became a prototype for future models provided by the G.E. X-ray Division. The instrument was described by Mann (1930).

REFERENCES

Ader, M. (1897). Sur un mouvel apparareil pour cables sous-marins *Comptes Rendus* **124,** 1440–1442.

AMA Council on Physical Medicine and Rehabilitation (1947). Minimum requirements for acceptable electrocardiographs. *JAMA* **134,** 134–155 (1950) **143,** 654–655.

American Heart Association (1954). Recommendations for standardization of electrocardiographic and vectorcardiographic leads. *Circulation* **10,** 564–573.

American Heart Association (1972). Report on electrocardiography. (Amendment). *Circulation* **46,** 1–2.

American Heart Association (1967). Report on electrocardiography. *Circulation,* **35,** 583–602; *IEEE Trans. on Bio Med. Eng.* **BME 14,** 60–68.

American Heart Association (1975). Recommendations for standardization of leads and specifications for instruments in electrocardiography and vectocardiography. *Circulation* **52,** 11–31.

Burdon-Sanderson, J. S. and Page, F. J. M. (1879). On the time relations of the excitatory process of the ventricle of the heart of the frog. *J. Physiol.* **2,** 384–435.

Donders F. C. (1872). De secundaire contracties onder den inveded der systoles van het hart. *Utrecht Rijksuniversiteit. Physiol. Lab. S3* **1,** 246–255.

Einthoven, W. (1903). Ein neues Galvanometer. *Ann. Phys.* **12**(Supp 4), 1059–1071.

Einthoven W., Fahr G., and de Waart, A. (1913). On the direction and manifest size of the variations of potential in the human heart. *Arch. ges. Physiol.* **150,** 275–315. [See translation by Sekelj, P., and Hoff, H. E. (1950). *Am. Heart J.* **40,** 163–211.]

Goldberger, F. (1942). A simple indifferent electrocardiographic electrode of zero potential and a technique for obtaining augmented, unipolar, extremity leads. *Amer. Heart J.* **13,** 483–492.

Hoff, H. E. and Geddes, L. A. (1957). The rheotome and its prehistory. *Bull. Hist. Med.* **31**(3), 212–347.

Kolliker, R. A. and Mueller, J. (1856). Nachweis der negativen Schwankung des Musketstroms am naturlich sich contrahirenden Muskel. *Verhandl. Phys. Med. Gaz. Wurzburg* **6,** 528–533.

Mann H. (1930–31). A light weight portable EKG. *Am. Heart J.* **7,** 796.

Marey E. J. (1876). Des variations electriques des muscles du coeur en particulier etudies du moyens de l'ectrometre de M. Lippmann. *Comptes Rendus Acad. Sci.* **82,** 975–977. [See translation by Geddes, L. A. and Hoff, H. E. (1961). *Arch. Int. d'Hist. des Sci.* **56–57,** 275–290.]

Marvin, H. B. (1954). Electronics Lab. G.E. Co. Schenectady, N.Y. Personal communication.

Roberts, N. K. (1975). *The Cardiac Conducting System and His Bundle Electrogram,* Appleton-Century-Crofts, New York.

Schwarzschild, M. and Kissen, M. (1934). The effects of condensers in the electrocardiograph. *Amer. Heart J.* **9,** 517–525.

Waller A. D. (1889). On the electromotive changes in the beat of the mammalian heart, and of the human heart in particular. *Phil. Trans. Roy. Soc.* **180B,** 169–194.

Wilson, F. N., Johnston, F. D., MacLeod, G., and Barker, P. S. (1934). Electrocardiograms that represent the potential variations of a single electrode. *Am. Heart J.* **9,** 447–458.

CHAPTER 8

Pacemakers and Cardiac Pacemaking

A cardiac pacemaker is an electrical stimulator that produces repetitive pulses of current designed to elicit contractions in the atria or ventricles of the heart.

ORIGIN OF THE HEART BEAT

In the normal mammalian heart the beat originates in the pacemaker that is the sinoatrial (S-A) node, located in the right atrium (Figure 8.1). This region of modified cardiac muscle is really a chemical oscillator that has the interesting property of developing rhythmic electrical activity which is propagated to the atria causing them to contract and pump blood into the ventricles. The wave of propagated excitation traveling over the atria reaches the atrioventicular (A-V) node in the base of the right ventricle (Figure 8.1). The propagation velocity of excitation through the A-V node is slow; therefore, there is a delay in propagating excitation to the ventricles. Excitation leaving the A-V node is propagated along the bundle of His and Purkinje fibers, ultimately arriving at the ventricular muscle which then contracts. This arborizing network of fibers is called the conduction system, which serves to coordinate the spread of excitation so that a forceful ventricular beat ensues, thereby pumping blood from the ventricles.

Normally the rate of the heart is determined by the rhythmicity of the

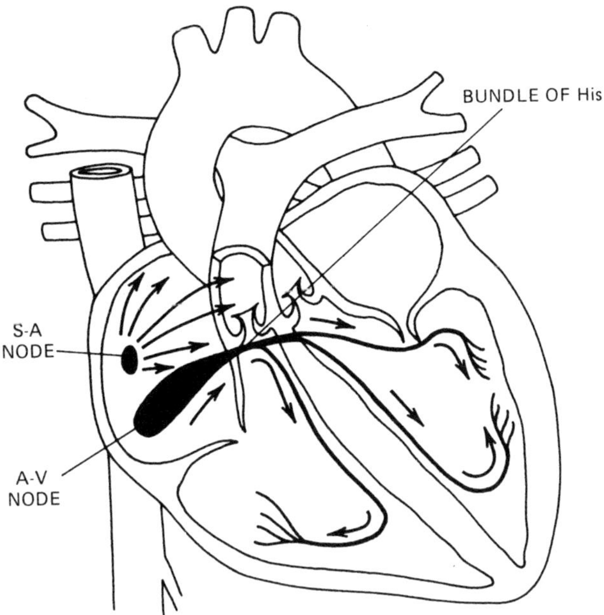

FIGURE 8.1. The pathways traversed by excitation that gives rise to atrial contraction and then ventricular contraction. In the normal heart, the sinoatrial (S-A) node is the pacemaker; the atrioventricular (A-V) node propagates excitation via the bundle of His and Purkinje fibers to the ventricular muscle.

S-A node. It is important to emphasize that the S-A node is spontaneously rhythmic. An excised heart will continue to beat for some time. The rhythmicity of the S-A node is influenced by temperature, nervous, and chemical (humoral) activity. Increasing temperature and an increased activity of the sympathetic nervous system increase the heart rate and force of ventricular contraction, thereby increasing blood pressure and cardiac output. Increased activity of the parasympathetic nervous system decreases the heart rate, thereby decreasing blood pressure and cardiac output. These two branches of the autonomic nervous system are controlled by centers in the medulla and hypothalamus.

While it is true that under normal circumstances the heart rate is dependent on the activity of the S-A node, other areas in the heart can become pacemakers and originate a heart beat. Atrial muscle fibers, the A-V node, the ventricular conducting system, and ventricular muscle fibers all have the capability of becoming rhythmic and acting as pacemakers. For this reason, it is possible that the heart beat may not always consist of an orderly sequence of atrial contraction followed by ventricular contraction. In A-V block, the ventricles can become spontaneously active and beat rhythmically with no relation to atrial contractions. However, when this situation arises, the ventricular rate is usually so slow that an inadequate cardiac output results.

Advancing age and disease can disrupt the organization of the heart beat. One of the most important cardiac impairments is atrioventricular (A-V) block. In this situation, the rhythmic excitations of the atria are not propagated through the A-V node. Sometimes two, three, or more atrial excitations occur before one ventricular beat occurs; this situation is called partial or second-degree A-V block. In many circumstances, none of the atrial excitations pass beyond the A-V node and the ventricles are thereby deprived of their normal pacemaker drive. In this situation, which is called total or third-degree A-V block, the most rhythmic region in the ventricles will start pacemaking and develop propagated excitation that will travel throughout both ventricles. However, in such a case the ventricular rate is often too slow to provide adequate cardiac output for consciousness or normal activity. Rhythmic stimulation of the ventricles by a cardiac pacemaker can provide adequate cardiac output.

The rhythmic excitations arising normally in the S-A node can fail completely, or they can be blocked from entering the atrial muscle. In such a situation the atria will not contract. However, atrial fibers are capable of pacemaking activity, and an atrial rhythm may develop and be propagated to the A-V node and ventricles to provide an adequate cardiac output. However, a physiological atrial pacemaker may not develop and a cardiac pacemaker can be used to rhythmically stimulate the atria or the ventricles.

From the foregoing it can be seen that although the atria and ventricles may lose their pacemaking drive, they can be made to contract by an electrical stimulus provided by a cardiac pacemaker. Thus, atrial or ventricular, or atrial and ventricular stimulation can be applied to restore cardiac output to a level compatible with the maintenance of a reasonable quality of life.

CARDIAC PACEMAKING

Cardiac pacemakers were first introduced for patients with Stokes–Adams disease, a condition in which total A-V block occurs. Rhythmic stimulation of the ventricles at a rate of about 70/minute elicits contractions that increase the cardiac output to a level compatible with the physical needs of the subject. To illustrate cardiac pacemaking, Figure 8.2 is presented. In this animal total A-V block was created surgically and the ventricular rate was 50 beats per minute. Note that the atrial *P* waves in

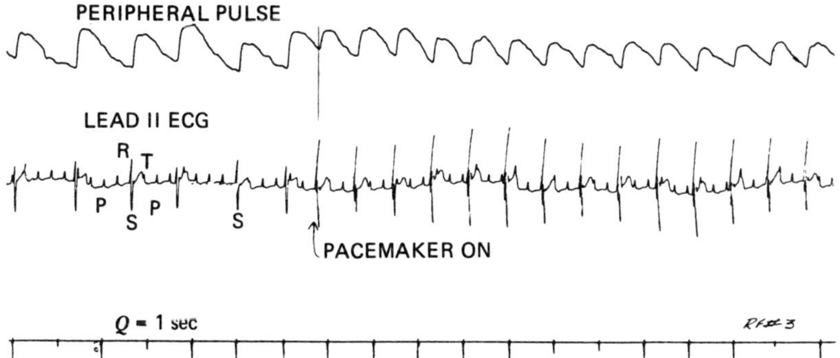

FIGURE 8.2. Total A-V block (left) in a dog showing no fixed relation between the *P* and *RS-T* waves. A cardiac pacemaker was turned on just before the middle of the record; note the increase in pulse rate, as shown by the volume pulse (top channel). [From Hickman et al. (1961).]

the ECG continue at a rate of 180 per minute and the ventricles beat without relation to the atrial impulses. In this animal a radiofrequency-energized receiver (Hickman et al., 1961) had been implanted and its output was connected to two ventricular electrodes. At the point indicated on the record, the transmitting pacemaker was turned on and stimulated the ventricles at a rate of 70 beats per minute. Note the increase in pulse rate and increase in diastolic pressure.

EXCITABILITY OF THE HEART

Before describing the various types of atrial and ventricular pacemakers, it is of value to understand the characteristics of a stimulus that is required to initiate a muscular contraction in the cardiac chambers. The essential requirements for an electrical stimulus to excite irritable tissue are (1) the stimulus must have an abrupt onset, (2) it must be intense enough and (3) it must last long enough, that is, it must have an adequate duration. These features of a single stimulus are embodied in what is known as the strength-duration curve, which is a plot of the minimum current required for a response (with a given electrode system), versus the duration of the stimulus. To illustrate the nature of the excitability of cardiac muscle with a rectangular-wave stimulus, Figure 8.3 is presented. Since stimulation occurs at the cathode, strength-duration curves are usually presented for cathodal stimulation, that is, the negative electrode is placed on the myocardium and a large area (indifferent) distant electrode is used to complete the stimulating circuit. Figure 8.3 shows that as the

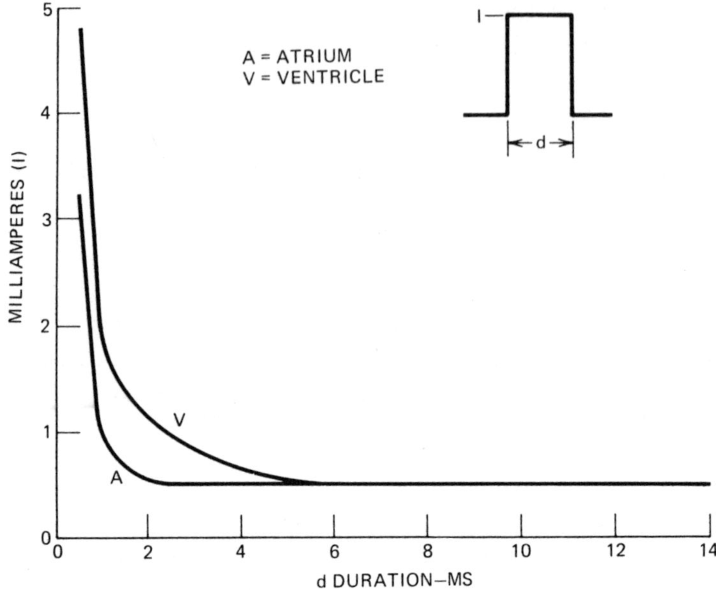

FIGURE 8.3. The strength (I)-duration (d) curve for canine cardiac muscle: A = atrium, V = ventricle.

duration (d) of the stimulus is decreased, the current (I) must be increased to evoke a contraction in the atria or ventricles.

Properties of the Strength–Duration Curve

The nature of the experimentally obtained strength–duration curve shown in Figure 8.3 can be derived mathematically from our present knowledge of the electrical nature of cell membranes. A typical cell membrane consists of a capacitance (C) and a resistance (R), as shown in Figures 8.4*a* and 8.4*b*. Values for R and C have been measured for a variety of cell types. Figure 8.4*a* illustrates a typical resting cell membrane, which is positively charged outside and negatively charged inside. When a stimulating current (I) is delivered, it flows through the membrane capacitance and resistance, as shown in Figure 8.4*b*. This current flow decreases the membrane potential to a value that results in excitation. In Figure 8.4*c*, the stimulus of duration d caused a reduction in resting membrane potential (RMP) by an amount ΔV, which brought the membrane potential to the threshold potential (TP), thereby evoking a propagated excitation revealed by the ensuing cardiac action potential.

The sum of the capacitive and resistive currents, I_C and I_R, is the

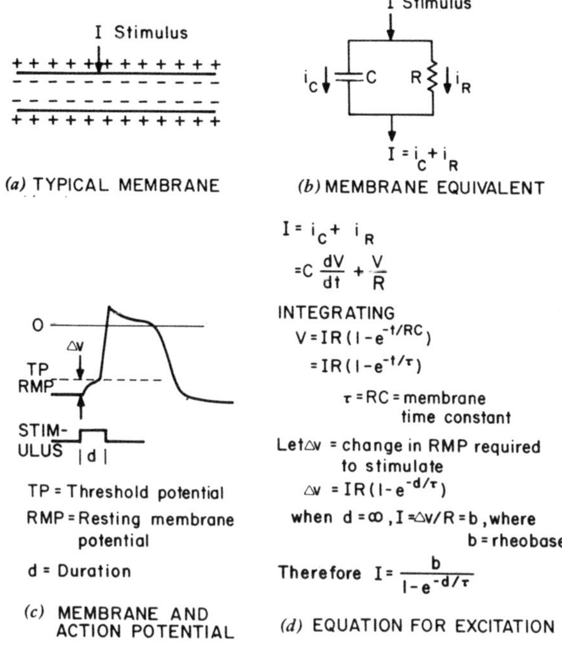

FIGURE 8.4. Stimulation of excitable tissue.

stimulus current (I). Figure 8.4*d* illustrates how these currents, when summed, produce a differential equation which is easily solved to obtain the expression which relates the current (I), duration (d), membrane time constant ($\tau = RC$) and rheobasic current (b). A log-log plot of this expression is shown in Figure 8.5.

Charge and Energy Parameters

Two other useful electrical parameters—charge and energy—can be derived from the expression for the strength-duration curve for current. For a square pulse, charge (Q) is the product of current and duration, that is, $Q = Id$, having the units of coulombs (Q). Charge is of importance because pacemaker batteries are rated in units of charge (ampere-hours). Therefore, for maximum battery life it is desirable to choose a stimulus duration that is associated with the least delivered charge.

Often it is desired to identify the energy content of a stimulus. For a square pulse, energy (U) is the product of current squared, the resistance (R) through which it flows, and the duration (d) of the stimulus. Therefore $U = I^2 Rd$, the units being joules (J) or watt-seconds (W-sec).

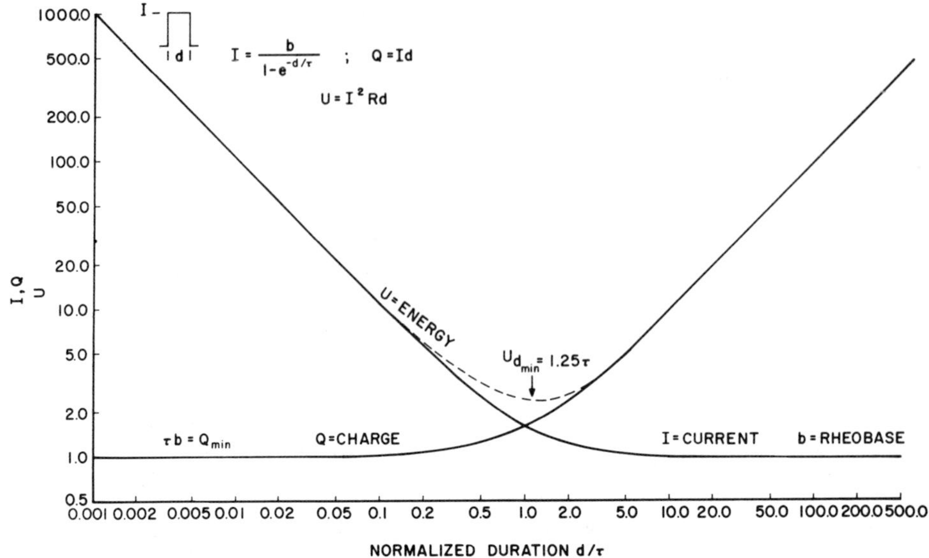

FIGURE 8.5. The strength-duration curve.

Figure 8.5 also presents the charge-versus-duration and energy-versus-duration relationships for a stimulus. Note that the charge asymptotes to a value τb, where τ is the membrane time constant and b is the rheobase or minimum-current asymptote. The energy-duration curve exhibits a minimum for a duration equal to 1.25 times the membrane time constant.

The data in Figure 8.5 clearly illustrate the three electrical parameters of a stimulus—current, charge, and energy—and how they vary with duration. It is clear that for pacemaking the duration of a stimulus should be chosen on the basis minimum charge, which occurs when the duration is about one-tenth of the membrane time constant. For normal mammalian cardiac muscle, Pearce et al. (1982) reported a time constant of about 2 msec; therefore, the duration for minimum charge is on the order of 0.2 msec.

Probably the two most important discoveries that altered pacemaking technology relate to the advantage of using a short-duration stimulus to prolong pacemaker battery life and the use of small-area electrodes which provide the current density needed for stimulation with low stimulating current. Furman *et al.* (1966, 1975) demonstrated that shorter duration pacing stimuli were as effective as longer duration pulses. In 1971, Furman *et al.* demonstrated the practical advantage of small-area electrodes in prolonging the life of the pacemaker battery. Modern pacemakers and electrodes take advantage of both important discoveries.

At present, the majority of cardiac pacemakers provide a stimulus that ranges from 0.1 to 1 msec in duration. The output is typically 5 V and the current delivered to a 500-ohm resistor is 10 mA. This resistance value is approximately the impedance of many pacemaking leads when implanted. However, pacemakers are available with higher output voltage and current.

TYPES OF PACEMAKERS

Since introduction of the first implantable pacemakers, advances in technology have permitted the creation of pacers with increasing sophistication. However, it is useful to recognize that there are only two cardiac chambers that can be paced, and there are three modes of operation: freerunning (fixed rate or asynchronous), inhibited, and triggered. The free-running type is insensitive to any rhythm that may develop in the paced chamber. The inhibited types sense cardiac activity and do nothing if present, but deliver a stimulus after an elapsed time if no further cardiac activity occurs to inhibit operation. The triggered type senses activity and delivers a stimulus in a desired way, as will be shown subsequently. As can be expected these three types of operation can be combined to provide a wide variety of pacemaker function. The classification scheme used to describe these types will be discussed following descriptions of the most commonly encountered pacemaker types.

Fixed Rate (Asynchronous)

A fixed-rate, asynchronous or nontriggered pacemaker is a device that delivers rhythmic stimuli to the ventricles at a constant rate. Such a pacemaker is applicable to patients with permanent atrioventricular (A-V) block. The rate may be fixed or, in some models, it can be altered by an external device such as a magnet or programmer. Since this type of pacemaker continues at its own rate, it does not respond to physiological needs and is oblivious to any rhythm that develops in the ventricles. For example, if the A-V node and conducting system regain their function, the normal pacemaker (S-A node) and the fixed-rate pacemaker will both excite the ventricles. Such a situation is called competitive pacing and is not without the risk of ventricular fibrillation owing to vulnerable-period stimulation. Vulnerable-period stimulation can also occur if pacemaker stimulus is delivered during a ventricular ectopic beat.

Figure 8.6 illustrates schematically the electrical activity of the atria (*a*), and ventricles (*b*) and what could be seen in the ECG (*c*) of a patient

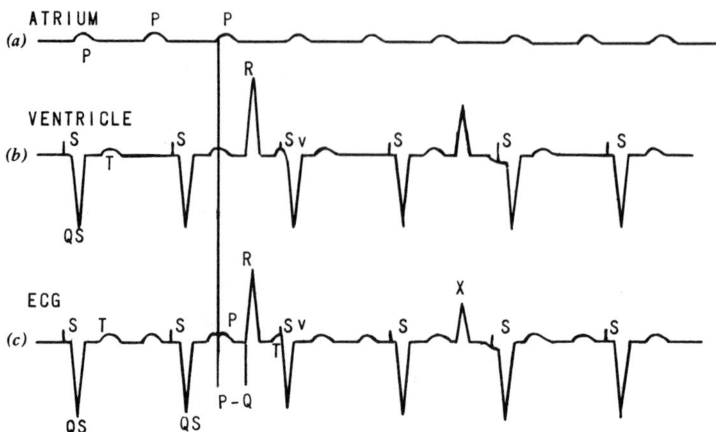

FIGURE 8.6. Diagrammatic representation of the electrical activity of the (*a*) atria and (*b*) ventricles in a subject with a fixed-rate pacemaker; (*c*) illustrates the ECG. Total A-V block is present when the first two *P* waves occurred, and the fixed rate pacemaker stimulated (*S*) the ventricles and produced beats (*QS*). The third *P* wave excited the ventricles and produced a normal beat (*R*). However, during ventricular recovery, stimulus (*Sv*) occurred in the vulnerable period and could have caused ventricular tachycardia or fibrillation.

to whom a fixed-rate ventricular pacemaker had been applied. Figure 8.6*a* shows that the atrial *P* waves are occurring at a regular rate and since there is total A-V block, the ventricles respond only to the fixed-rate pacemaking stimuli (*S*), as shown in Figure 8.6*b*. Note that after the second ventricular beat, conduction from the atria was reestablished (*P-Q*) and a normal beat (*R*) ensued. Note also that the pacemaker delivered its stimulus (*SV*) during the *T* wave of the normally conducted beat and produced a ventricular excitation. The pacemaker pulse occurring at this instant could have produced a ventricular tachycardia or fibrillation because of vulnerable-period stimulation. Note also in Figure 8.6 that an ectopic beat (*X*) occurred, and during its *T* wave, the pacemaker delivered a stimulus evoking a response. This stimulus could also have evoked a tachycardia or fibrillation because it was delivered in the vulnerable period, which will now be described.

Vulnerable-Period Stimulation

The vulnerable period is that time in the ventricular cycle (during the *T* wave of the ECG) when a single stimulus will precipitate ventricular fibrillation, as shown in Figure 8.7*a*. Figure 8.7*b* illustrates the extent of

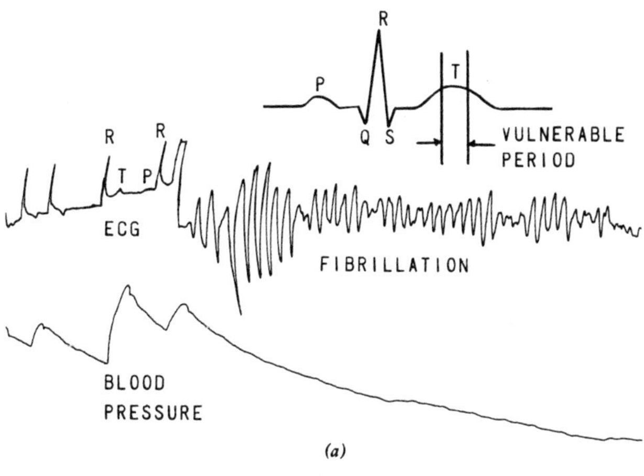

(a)

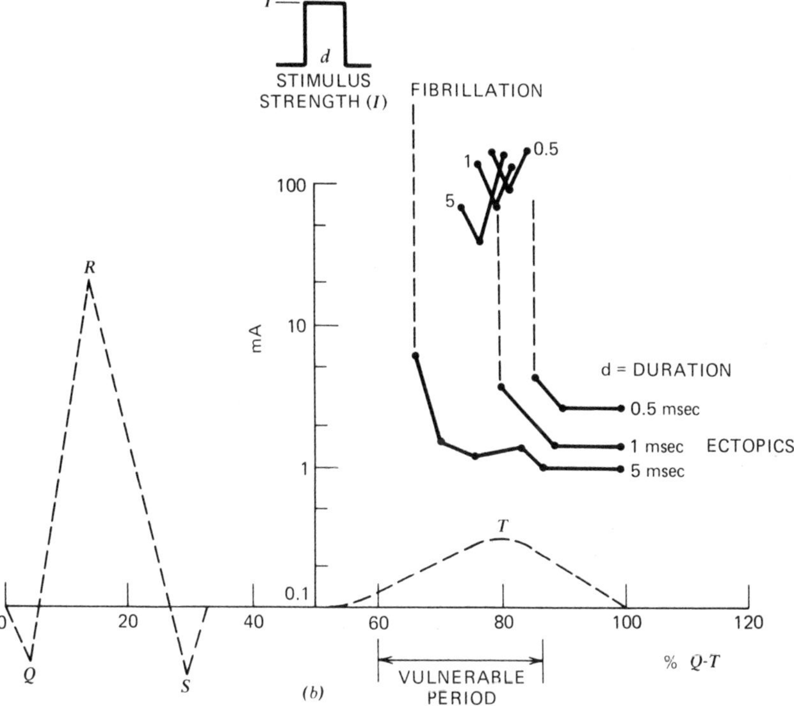

(b)

FIGURE 8.7. (*a*) Ventricular fibrillation by vulnerable-period stimulation. (*b*) Strength-interval curves for inducing ectopic beats and ventricular fibrillation with single stimuli of 0.5, 1, and 5 msec delivered at different instants in the ventricular cycle. The *R* and *T* waves are shown to identify the temporal extent of the vulnerable period of the ventricles.

the vulnerable period in the cardiac cycle. The threshold for fibrillation for 0.5, 1, and 5 msec stimuli are shown, along with the threshold for evoking ectopic beats. It is clear that in the normal heart, the stimulus strength for fibrillation must be considerably higher than the threshold for pacemaking. However, in the ischemic or hypoxic heart, the threshold is reduced for fibrillation by vulnerable-period stimulation. There is no doubt that competitive pacing has resulted in ventricular fibrillation. A review of the literature and the conditions that are required have been described by Jones and Geddes (1977).

Triggered Pacemakers

Pacemakers in this category are responsive to cardiac activity in several different and important ways. Such pacemakers can be triggered by atrial or ventricular action potentials, and the resulting signals can be used to create several types of cardiac pacemakers.

Atrial Triggered

Pacemakers that are triggered by the electrical activity of the atria are called *P*-wave or atrial triggered. The electrical activity of the atria is sensed by an atrial electrode, and after a delay of about 0.15 sec, which corresponds to the A-V conduction time, a stimulus is delivered to the ventricles. The preset delay allows atrial systole to complete filling of the ventricles before they are stimulated to contract by the pacemaker.

Figure 8.8 illustrates schematically the electrical activity of the atria (*a*), ventricles (*b*), and the ECG (*c*) for a subject with an atrial-triggered pacemaker. The atrial *P* waves are sensed and, after a delay, the ventricular stimulus (*S*) is delivered. Note that the pacemaker does not fail if the *P* waves cease, because the pacemaker will deliver a stimulus after an elapsed time (*E*) that is established by the pacemaker circuit. If all *P* waves disappear, the atrial-triggered pacemaker will operate as a fixed-rate (or even a demand) pacemaker.

In theory, the *P*-wave-triggered pacemaker is ideal because the atrial beat determines the pacemaker rate and normally the atrial rate reflects the physiological needs for cardiac output. However, if the atrial rate becomes very high, as in the case of flutter or fibrillation, electronic circuitry in the pacemaker places a limit on the ventricular pacing rate. In such a situation the ventricles are usually driven at a submultiple of the atrial rate. In the absence of atrial activity, the papcemaker reverts to a fixed-rate ventricular pacemaker. If ventricular ectopic beats occur, there is the risk of competitive pacing unless the pacemaker has been designed to sense ventricular activity and be inhibited by it.

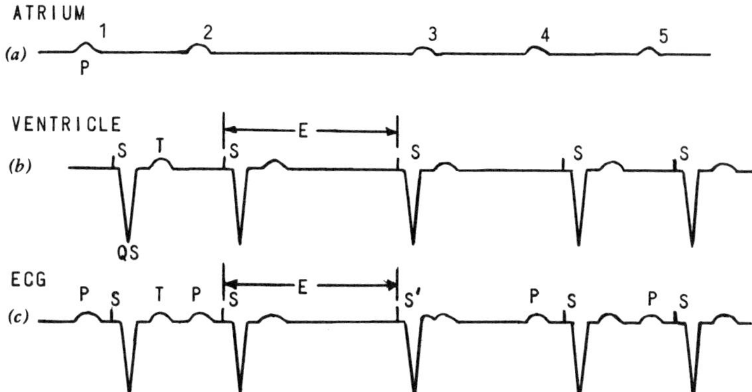

FIGURE 8.8. Operating characteristics of the atrial- or P-wave-triggered ventricular pacemaker are illustrated diagrammatically. The first two P waves were detected, delayed, and used to develop stimuli (S), which excited the ventricles. However, no P wave occurred thereafter and the elapsed time (E) caused the pacemaker to produce a stimulus S'.

Despite the attractiveness of the atrial-triggered ventricular pacemaker, it is not widely used. The main difficulty lies in the relatively high incidence of atrial arrythmias in patients with A-V conduction defects.

Ventricular Triggered. To eliminate competitive pacing with its risk of ventricular fibrillation, two types of demand pacemaker have been developed; one is called the ventricular-synchronous and the other is called the ventricular or R-wave inhibited pacemaker.

1. *Ventricular Synchronous Pacemaker.* The ventricular triggered (synchronous) pacemaker senses the R wave of the ventricles and delivers a stimulus which obviously falls in the refractory period of the ventricles and is therefore ineffective; Figure 8.9 illustrates this mode of operation. At X a ventricular ectopic beat occurred and the pacemaker delivered its stimulus (S) in the refractory period of the ventricles. A normally conducted beat (R) then occurred and again the pacemaker stimulus (S') was delivered during the ventricular refractory period. Following this event, no ventricular beat occurred and the pacemaker waited for an elapsed time (E), then delivered a stimulus (S''); the sequence was repeated for the next beat. Normal A-V conduction was restored and a normal ventricular beat (R) occurred, with the pacemaker stimulus being delivered in the ventricular refractory period.

The ventricular-synchronous pacemaker is obviously wasteful of bat-

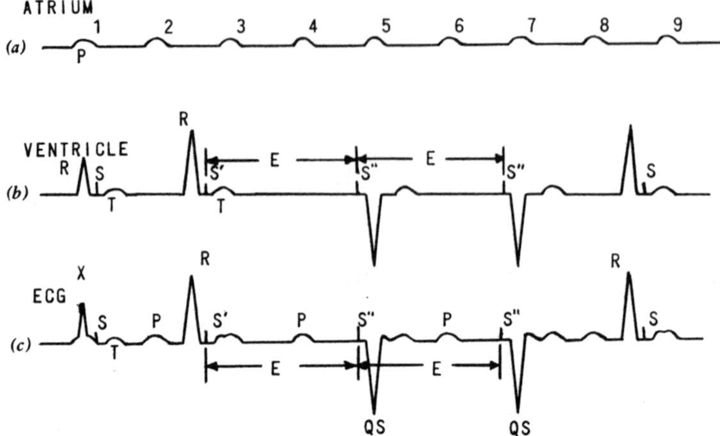

FIGURE 8.9. Diagrammatic illustration of the operating mode of the *R*-wave or ventricular-synchronous pacemaker. (*a*) identifies atrial and (*b*) identifies ventricular activity. The ECG is shown in (*c*). During the first *P* wave a ventricular ectopic beat occurred (*X*) and caused the pacemaker to deliver a stimulus (*S*) during the ventricular refractory period. The second *P* wave conducted excitation to the ventricles and produced a large upright *R* wave, followed by a pacemaker stimulus (*S'*). The next two atrial excitations ($P_{3\text{-}4}$) did not excite the ventricles. Meanwhile, the elapsed time circuit in the pacemaker timed out and delivered a stimulus at *E* sec after the last stimulus.

tery energy because an ineffective stimulus is delivered in response to a ventricular beat. Although this type of pacemaker solves the competitive pacing problem, the reduced battery life is diminishing its popularity. However, it does have two important attributes. For example, the pacemaker stimulus is always identifiable in the electrocardiogram following an *R* wave, indicating that the pacemaker is functional, although it does not evoke a ventricular contraction. The *R*-wave synchronous pacemaker responds to electromagnetic interference by increasing its pacing rate. A refractory period within the pacemaker, limits the pacing in this circumstance to a safe rate. As will be seen, the ventricular inhibited pacemaker is inhibited by electromagnetic interference.

2. *Ventricular Inhibited Pacemaker.* The ventricular-inhibited pacemaker senses the *R* wave of the ventricles and produces no stimulus until a preset time (e.g., 800–1000 msec) has elapsed. At the end of this time a pacemaking pulse is delivered; then the pacemaker waits for another *R* wave. Figure 8.10 illustrates schematically the manner in which this type of pacemaker operates. The first beat in Figure 8.10 was obvi-

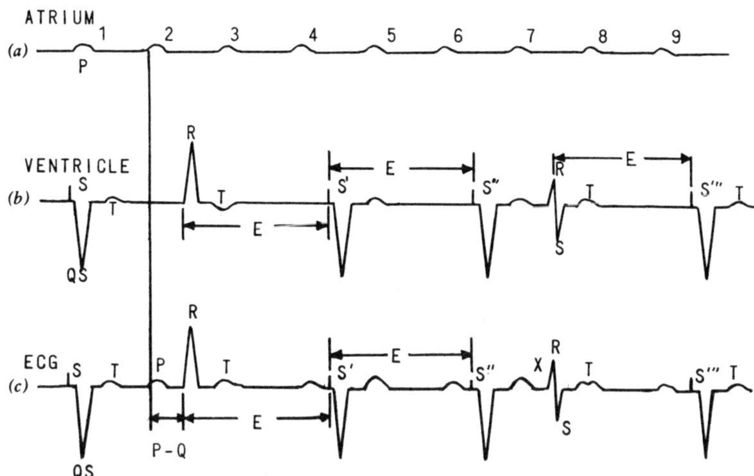

FIGURE 8.10. Diagrammatic representation of the operation of the R-wave-inhibited pacemaker. (a) illustrates atrial, (b) illustrates ventricular activity, and (c) identifies the ECG. The first P wave occurred when a stimulus (S) was delivered to the ventricles. The second P wave (P_2) was conducted and excited the ventricles and no pacemaker stimulus was delivered. A-V block then occurred for the third and fourth P waves. Meanwhile the elapsed time circuit in the pacemaker timed out and delivered a stimulus S',S'' E sec after each ventricular excitation. Later, a ventricular ectopic beat X, (R-S, T) occurred and inhibited the pacemaker for another period of E sec, after which a stimulus was delivered. (S''') because A-B block persisted.

ously initiated by the pacemaker stimulus (S). Following this beat, A-V conduction (P-Q) was restored and a normal beat (R) occurred and the pacemaker was inhibited. However, A-V block returned, and the pacemaker waited the elapsed time E sec and then delivered a pacemaking stimulus S', followed by a second stimulus S''. After the fourth ventricular beat, a ventricular ectopic beat X (R-S) occurred, and the pacemaker was inhibited, after which it waited for its preset elapsed time and then delivered a stimulus (S''') to evoke a beat.

The ventricular-inhibited pacemaker is one of the most popular pacemakers. It has a relatively long battery life and does not engage in competitive pacing. However, in a patient with a rapid ventricular rate or normal A-V conduction, it is impossible to tell if the pacemaker is functional by examining the electrocardiogram. To make the pacemaker operate, the ventricular sensing circuit is disabled, usually by an external magnet which operates a magnetic reed switch within the pacemaker.

Alternatively, in patients in whom A-V conduction has been restored, the heart rate can be reduced by eliciting the carotid–sinus reflex (i.e., by manual pressure applied to the skin over the carotid sinuses). With an adequately slow heart rate, the pacemaker will start to function.

Another interesting feature of the *R*-wave-inhibited pacemaker relates its response to electromagnetic interference. When present, such extraneous signals inhibit the pacemaker. Some pacemakers contain interference-detecting circuitry, and when interference is sensed, the pacemaker reverts to a slow fixed-rate mode.

ATRIAL TACHYARRHYTHMIAS

Owing to disease or ischemia, it is not uncommon for the atria to develop a rapid rhythm; such a condition is called a supraventricular tachycardia. When the atria beat rapidly or fibrillate, the A-V node is bombarded with impulses which it (if normal) transmits to the ventricles. The limiting ventricular rate (in beats per second) is the reciprocal of the A-V nodal refractory period (in seconds). The net result is a very rapid ventricular rate in which cardiac output is low owing to the limited time for ventricular filling. In such a case, it is useful to block transmission across the A-V node by making a lesion there, after which a pacemaker can be installed to pace the ventricles.

There are several methods of blocking the transmission of excitation from the A-V node to the ventricles. Surgical transection of the His bundle is accomplished easily. Likewise, cryogenic surgery or infiltration of the His bundle with a denaturizing solution accomplishes the same end. Finally, creation of a thermal lesion by a catheter electrode is a very convenient method, which was described by Gonzalez *et al.* (1981). The method first employs a passage of a catheter electrode via the venous system and recording the His bundle electrogram (HBE). When the catheter-borne electrode is in the correct place, as judged by the HBE, a strong shock is delivered to the catheter electrode and a large indifferent electrode on the back. Single or multiple 35-J shocks are delivered from a defibrillator to create total A-V block. In our own dog studies, slightly stronger (200-J) shocks were required to create permanent A-V block.

Clinical use of blockade of A-V nodal propagation with the implantation of a ventricular pacemaker is just beginning. It is very likely that this technique will become the therapy of choice for supraventricular tachycardias in the future.

PACEMAKER CONSIDERATIONS

It should be apparent that there are numerous possibilities for electrically pacing the heart. Moreover, there is reason to consider complex pacemakers, because in many situations the myocardium may change after pacemaker implantation. S-A node arrest, atrial fibrillation, restoration of A-V conduction, and the establishment of a stable ventricular rhythm can occur, all of which change the requirements for pacemaking. New pacemaker designs incorporating microprocessors are evolving in response to the clinical requirements. The newest type of pacemaker senses both the atrial and ventricular activity and delivers stimuli appropriately to each chamber. It may be that a universal pacemaker will be developed which is responsive to the changing needs for pacemaking. The possibility of using some physiological event that is altered by exercise to control pacing rate is being studied by many investigators. When this becomes feasible, the exercise restriction can be substantially reduced for all pacemaker patients.

PACEMAKERS AND CARDIAC OUTPUT

The subject of cardiac output in exercising subjects with fixed-rate pacemakers received considerable attention in the early days of cardiac pacing. Benchemol *et al.* (1964, 1965) measured cardiac output in eight exercising (20 kg-m/min) subjects with fixed-rate pacers. They found that cardiac output increased negligibly in two, moderately in five, and almost 50% in one. The increase in cardiac output was, of course, due to the increase in stroke volume, owing to the inotropic effect of the sympathetic nervous system on the ventricles.

The amount of exercise tolerance in a subject with a fixed-rate pacemaker is limited by the increase in cardiac output, which may be typically 10–30%. It is for this reason that there is considerable interest in creating a ventricular pacemaker that increases the pacing rate in response to exercise and is immune from atrial dysrhythmias. The only exercise-responsive pacemaker available at present is the atrial-sensed, ventricular-stimulated pacemaker (VAT). However, a variety of exercise-related physiological events is being examined for their suitability to control pacing rate. The following paragraphs present a short review of this interesting subject. Table 8.1 presents a summary of the techniques used or proposed.

TABLE 8.1. Control Methods for Exercise-Responsive Pacemakers

Sensed Quantity	Sensing Method	Principal Investigator, and Year; U.S. Patent No.
Atrial excitation (*P* Wave)	Apply delay and stimulate a ventricle	Karlof (1975) Kappenberger (1981) Krause (1982)
Respiration rate	Impedance pneumograph	Krasner (1966, 1971) 3,593,718
Respiration rate	Diaphragm motion (by piezoelectric detector)	Ionescu (1980)
pH	R-A venous blood In/In–AgCl electrodes	Cammilli 1979, 1980, 1981)
pH	In pacemaker pocket	Contini (1981)
Venous-O_2 saturation	Catheter oximeter	Wirtzfield (1980) 4,202,339
Arterial-O_2 saturation	Electrodes on Hering's nerve	Bozal-Gonzalez (1980)
Ventricular cycle	Stimulus–*T*-wave duration	Rickards (1981) 4,228,803
Core temperature	Temperature-sensitive capacitor in pacer	Fischell (1975) 3,867,950
Venous blood temperature	Thermistor R-A, R-V, P-A	Griffin (1981)
Right-ventricular blood temperature	Thermistor	Jolgren (1983)

EXERCISE-RESPONSIVE PACING

The commercial availability of the atrial-sensed, ventricular pacemaker has made it possible to identify both the indications for its use and its value in those cases. Karlof (1975) had the opportunity to compare atrially triggered and the conventional fixed-rate (VVI) pacemaker in 12 patients. At rest with the atrially triggered unit, the cardiac output was 10% higher, and during exercise it was 20% higher than with the VVI pacer. Similarly, Kappenberger et al. (1981) found that in exercising patients the atrial triggered (VAT) pacer provided 20% more cardiac output than the VVI pacer. In another recent study, Krause et al. (1982) compared the atrial-triggered pacer with the VVI pacer in 13 patients and found that the former provided 32% more cardiac output during bicycle-ergometer tests.

It is clear, that for those patients with A-V block and a normally functional sinus node, the atrial-triggered ventricular pacer is ideal.

Although an atrially triggered ventricular pacemaker is exercise responsive, a *P* wave is not always available in patients with myocardial disease. Atrial flutter, fibrillation, and sick-sinus syndrome, prevent use of the atrially triggered ventricular pacer in a number of pacemaker candidates.

Since respiratory rate increases with exercise, this physiological event has been suggested as a controller for pacing rate. Krasner (1966, 1971) proposed detecting respiration with an impedance pneumograph and Ionescu (1980) used a piezoelectric element applied to the diaphragm to detect its motion. The method involved increasing the pacing rate only when the respiratory rate increased, that is, periods of apnea did not exert control.

The pH decrease in right ventricular blood during exercise was also proposed as a pacing-rate controller by Cammilli (1979, 1980, 1981). Contini (1981) examined the pH in the tissue fluid in the pacemaker pouch and found that it tracked (but lagged) the exercise-induced decrease in venous blood pH. Cammilli has evaluated the performance of a pH-controlled pacemaker for several years, the main difficulty being with the performance and longevity of the pH-sensitive electrode system.

The decrease in venous-blood oxygen saturation that accompanies exercise has been proposed by Wirtzfield (1980) as a controller for pacing rate. A two-channel fiberoptic catheter oximeter was proposed as the detecting method.

Bozal-Gonzalez (1980) proposed to detect the decrease in oxygen saturation during exercise by measuring the action potential firing rate in Hering's nerve, which comes from the carotid body. He also proposed to use the rate of the action potentials in the synthetic nerves to the heart to control the pacing rate.

An interesting method of using the duration of the ventricular cycle to identify exercise was proposed by Rickards (1981). Working with his colleague Akhas (1981), he found that in exercising pacemaker patients, the interval between the pacing (exciting) stimulus and the end of the *T* wave (the *E-T* interval) shortened with exercise. In pacer patients with total A-V block they showed that the *E-T* interval decreased with increasing atrial rate during exercise.

It is not surprising that the rise in body temperature that accompanies exercise has been proposed for controlling the rate of a pacemaker. Fischell (1975) advocated locating a temperature sensor within the pacemaker and using the increase in temperature to increase pacing rate. The temperature rise in the pacemaker lags the rise in blood temperature.

The increase in venous blood temperature during exercising human subjects was documented by Bazett (1951) who recorded the inferior vena cava blood and rectal temperatures during exercise on a bicycle ergometer. Typically the venous blood temperature increased 1.5°C with exercise. Recently, Griffin (1981) and Jolgren (1983) also measured venous blood temperature during exercise in animals. Jolgren has used this event as a rate controller for a ventricular pacemaker.

IDENTIFICATION OF PACEMAKERS

There are two methods for identifying cardiac pacemakers. One method employs three letters to describe the functional characteristics (e.g., stimulation and/or sensing); the other method employs radioopaque symbols to identify the type and manufacturer of a pacemaker after the device has been implanted in a patient.

Three-letter Code

A three-letter code has been adopted by the Inter-Society Commission for Heart Disease Resources. The report of the deliberations of this group was edited by Personnet et al. (1974). The code adopted is shown in Table 8.2. The first letter identifies the chamber that is paced, that is, atrium (A) or ventricle (V) or doubly (D). The second letter identifies the chamber sensed (A, V, D), and the third letter specifies the mode of operation, I being used to identify inhibited and T designating triggered. The letter O is used to identify that a particular descriptor is inapplicable. For example, the original (asynchronous), fixed-rate ventricular pacemaker would be designated (VOO). The popular ventricular-demand pacemaker is identified by the letters VVT or VVI to specify whether the pacemaker is triggered or inhibited by ventricular activity. Table 8.3 presents a summary of the various pacemaker types.

TABLE 8.2. Three-Letter Identification Code[a]

1st Letter	2nd Letter	3rd Letter
Chamber Paced	Chamber Sensed	Mode of Response
V—Ventricle A—Atrium D—Double Chamber		I—Inhibited T—Triggered O—Not Applicable

[a] From Parsonnet, V., et al. (1974).

TABLE 8.3. Suggested Nomenclature Code for Implantable Cardiac Pacemakers[a]

Chamber Paced	Chamber Sensed	Mode of Response	Generic Description	Previously Used Designation
V	O	O	Ventricular pacing; no sensing function	Asynchronous; fixed rate; set rate
A	O	O	Atrial pacing; no sensing function	Atrial fixed rate; atrial asynchronous
D	O	O	Atrioventricular pacing; no sensing function	A-V sequential fixed rate (asynchronous)
V	V	I	Ventricular pacing and sensing, inhibited mode	Ventricular inhibited; *R* inhibited; *R* blocking; *R* suppressed; noncompetitive inhibited; demand; standby
V	V	T	Ventricular pacing and sensing, triggered mode	Ventricular triggered; *R* triggered; *R* wave stimulated; noncompetitive triggered; following *R*, synchronous; demand; standby
A	A	I	Atrial pacing and sensing, inhibited mode	Atrial inhibited; *P* inhibited; *P* blocking; *P* suppressed
A	A	T	Atrial pacing and sensing, triggered mode	Atrial triggered; *P* triggered; *P* stimulated; *P* synchronous
V	A	T	Ventricular pacing, atrial sensing, triggered mode	Atrial synchronous, atrial synchronized, A-V synchronous
D	V	I	Atrioventricular pacing, ventricular sensing, inhibited mode	Bifocal sequential demand, A-V sequential

[a]From Parsonnet, V., *et al.* (1974).

X-Ray Identification

At present there does not appear to be a standardized code of ratioopaque numbers and letters for identifying pacemakers, although many manufacturers include such symbols in their pacemakers. In some cases, from these symbols it is possible to identify manufacturer, year of construction, and pacemaker type. In other instances, it is possible to identify the pacemaker type by characteristics in the radiograph, for example, location and number of batteries and integrated circuits, etc. Morse and

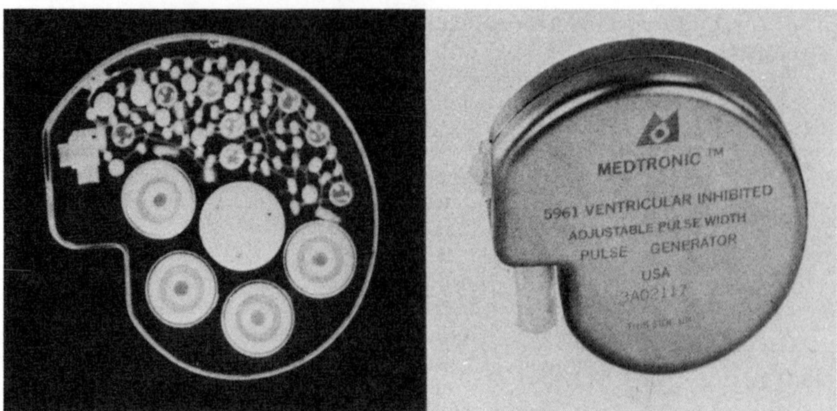

FIGURE 8.11. Pacemaker and radiograph of the same pacemaker (Medtronic 5961, VVI type).

Steiner (1978) presented a compendium of symbols and radiographs of a large number of pacemakers; Figure 8.11 is a radiograph of a typical implanted cardiac pacemaker.

ELECTRODES

Two electrodes are required to deliver the pacemaking stimuli to the ventricles and two types of stimulation, bipolar and unipolar (monopolar), are used. With bipolar stimulation, both electrodes are in contact with cardiac muscle. With unipolar stimulation, only the negative (active) electrode is in contact with myocardium; the other (indifferent or reference) electrode is some distance from the heart. The indifferent electrode is often the metallic case of the pacemaker.

A number of different types of stimulating electrode is used. Some are inserted into the myocardium and others (catheter electrodes) are placed in contact with the interior of the right ventricle by passing them down a vein. One of the first electrodes used for permanent ventricular pacemaking was the Hunter–Roth (1959) patch electrode, which is sketched in Figure 8.12*a*. This bipolar electrode consisted of a rectangular patch of silicone rubber with two 0.5-cm-long stainless-steel pins. The pins were pressed into an area of low vascularity on the surface of a ventricle, and the patch was sutured to the myocardium. Teflon-coated multistrand stainless-steel wires connected the electrode to the implanted pacemaker.

The Hunter–Roth electrode was found to have a limited life owing to

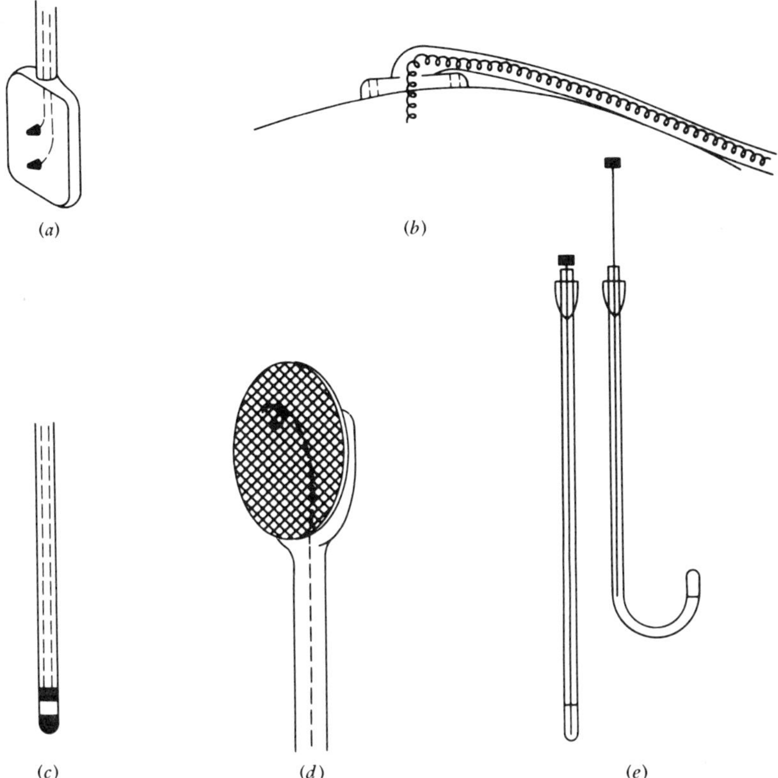

FIGURE 8.12. Pacemaker electrodes: (*a*) Hunter–Roth bipolar electrode; (*b*) Chardack coil-type electrode; (*c*) bipolar catheter electrode; (*d*) the corkscrew electrode; (*e*) the J (atrial) electrode.

the constant flexing of the wires with each heart beat. With a pacing rate of 70 per minute, the number of flexures occurring in a year is about 36.8 million, indicating that pacemaking electrodes have special requirements for mechanical durability.

A mechanically durable myocardial electrode was described by Chardack *et al.* (1961). This electrode, which could be used singly or as a pair, is illustrated in Figure 8.12*b*. The electrode consists of a long slender coil of platinum–iridium wire (0.01 in. in diameter). The electrode tip, lead wire, and terminal connected to the pacemaker consisted of a single piece of wire. A solid piece of platinum–iridium is inserted into the coil to stabilize the point where the coil takes a right-angle bend to form the electrode tip. Two-thirds of the length of the bent coil is covered with a silicone rubber sleeve to achieve a small area of contact with the myocardium. Silicone rubber is used as the insulation for the electrode cable.

The Chardack coil electrode is inserted into the myocardium via a small stab wound. The silicone rubber plate is then sutured to the heart muscle. This type of electrode functions well and is still in use. Stainless steel and other alloys have been used to fabricate this electrode. Frequently, the coils at the tips of the electrode are opened slightly to gain access to more myocardium without increasing the area of the electrode.

There are many types of unipolar and bipolar catheter electrodes available for temporary and permanent pacing. Figure 8.12*c* illustrates a typical bipolar catheter electrode, which is located at the apex of the right ventricle by advancing the catheter through a vein. Some electrodes are placed in the right ventricle with the assistance of a stylet. For permanent pacing, many catheter electrodes incorporate some type of hook, barb, or tyne which anchors the electrode to the inside wall of the right ventricle, usually at the apex.

As easily applied, sutureless corkscrew electrode was developed by Hunter *et al.* (1973). This electrode, which is sketched in Figure 8.12*d*, consists of a two-turn spiral mounted on a Dacron-mesh plate. The electrode is advanced into the myocardium by turning it three times. The rough Dacron plate stimulates the growth of fibrous tissue and soon the electrode becomes firmly attached to the myocardium.

Figure 8.12*e* illustrates the atrial J lead. It is inserted pervenously with the stylet, which is then withdrawn and the tip enters the atrial appendage.

STIMULATION THRESHOLD

With all myocardial electrodes, the threshold current required for stimulation rises gradually for about two weeks following implantation. This phenomenon is due to the growth of a fibrous tissue capsule around the electrode. This inexcitable tissue capsule lowers the current density presented to the myocardial cells. To accommodate this natural event, the stimulus strength at the time of implantation, is set to about twice the threshold as measured at implantation. Some types of implanted pacemakers can be adjusted for higher output after implantation by placing a magnetic pulser on the skin over the pacemaker. With some pacemakers, the pacing rate and duration of the pulse can be adjusted in a similar manner.

In the early days of cardiac pacemaking, little attention was paid to the importance of electrode area. The phenomenon of threshold increase was slow to be correlated with the reduced current density due to fibrous tissue growth. However, it was soon realized that it is current density that stimulates irritable tissue, and pacemaking electrodes began to appear with reduced area. Reducing the area permits attainment of the desired current density with less current. Since all of the current in the stimulus must come from the pacemaker battery, the use of smaller-area electrodes increases the life of the pacemaker battery. Furman et al. (1971) were the first to recognize this fact and develop small-area electrodes. Theoretical considerations relative to the practical minimum area for cardiac pacemaking electrodes were presented by Irnich (1975). He recommended that a practical minimum electrode area 1.13 mm^2.

ENERGY SOURCES

Irrespective of the type of pacemaker, that is, external or implanted, the pulse generator within it requires a source of electrical energy. With external pacemakers, power-line or battery operation is possible. With implanted pacemakers, some internal source of electrical energy is required. To date, chemical batteries are by far the most popular; however, nuclear-powered cells are used occasionally. Although chemical and nuclear-powered cells are the preferred power sources, many other ingenious methods have been used to produce electrical energy. For example, biogalvanic cells, which use the body fluids as electrolytes, have been created. Piezoelectric generators, which use the force developed by muscular contraction to produce a voltage, have also been reported but are not now in use. Implanted passive receivers, which recover the stimulus from modulated radiofrequency energy passing through the skin, are in limited use. Radiofrequency energy transmitted through the skin has been used to charge batteries within a pacemaker. Despite the attractive features of many of these ingenious methods for energizing pacemakers, they have not received widespread use. Experience has shown that patients do not wish to be hampered by carrying an external device and physicians prefer to install a completely implantable pacemaker, notwithstanding the fact that it may have a limited lifetime.

Chemical Cells

Prior to discussing chemical sources of electrical energy, several important points should be made. For example, the chemical cell is the functional unit that produces electrical energy. A battery is merely a group of cells arranged in series or parallel. In each cell there are two electrodes (anode and cathode) and an electrolyte. Electrons, the flow of which constitutes an electric current, are produced by a chemical reaction within the cell. The chemical action alters the composition of the electrodes and the electrolyte. Often gas is evolved as the cell is used.

Owing mainly to internal leakage current, a cell will discharge slowly when no current is drawn from its terminals. The term shelf life is often used to identify the self-discharging propensity of chemical cells. With the passage of time, in some cells, the open-circuit voltage decreases; in others, the open-circuit voltage is relatively constant and the internal resistance rises. In both cases, after prolonged periods of storage, the cell can no longer deliver its rated output. Although a universally agreed-upon definition for shelf life is lacking, the term means that after a period of time the cell cannot deliver its rated ampere-hours (charge). Obviously, however defined, a cell with a long shelf life may be stored for a long period "on the shelf," and when put into service, will deliver a substantial amount of its ampere-hour rating. The concept of a long shelf life for a cell is of obvious importance in pacemaker technology, since the cells are sealed in the pacemaker at the time of manufacture, and implantation may not occur for a considerable time.

Another important characteristic of the cells that are used in pacemakers relates to the by-products of the chemical reaction that produces the current. Cells that liberate substantial amounts of gas are not candidates for pacemaker construction. The gas-evolution problem may be solvable by the use of getters, which would combine chemically with the gas.

The production of reliable chemical cells places obvious requirements on the manufacturer. A premature failure of a cell in the ordinary world is merely an inconvenience. Failure of a pacemaker cell may result in a death. The need for premature replacement necessitates a surgical procedure. To produce pacemaker cells with a high reliability, manufacturers take special care in production. Quality control is maintained at every step of the manufacturing process. Samples are obtained from a production run and put on an aging test, that is, they are required to deliver the rated (or an elevated) current for a period of time, during which the terminal voltage is measured. This latter technique is called accelerated testing and extrapolation of expected lifetime is made with caution.

Mercury–Zinc Battery

Many of the implanted pacemakers now in use are energized by the mercury–zinc alkaline cell, which contains a porous zinc cathode and an anode composed of a compressed mixture of mercuric oxide, graphite, and silver oxide. The electrolyte is largely potassium hydroxide, and the chemical reaction that takes place to yield electrons is

$$Zn + HgO + H_2O \rightarrow Zn(OH)_2 + Hg$$

The open-circuit voltage is 1.35 V and typical cells provide 1 ampere-hour of charge when discharged at 40 μA. The power density is on the order of 500 mW-hr/cm^3 of cell. At present, a group of such cells can provide a useful pacemaker life of 48–60 months.

The mercury–zinc battery was in existence long before it was called into pacemaker service. Its outstanding characteristics are a long shelf life and relatively constant voltage throughout its useful life.

Lithium–Iodide Battery

Greatbatch, the pioneer developer of the implanted, battery-containing pacemaker, described the lithium–iodide cell, which has characteristics that are unusually attractive for pacemaker use. In this cell the anode is lithium and the cathode is a proprietary iodide (MI_2). Instead of a liquid electrolyte, a pasty salt of lithium is used. The chemical reaction, which releases electrons, was given by Greatbatch *et al.* (1971) as follows:

$$2Li + MI_2 \rightarrow M + 2LiI$$

In this reaction, no gas is liberated. The open-circuit voltage of the cell is 2.8 V, and present models have a rating of 1.1 ampere-hours. The power density is similar to or slightly higher than that of the mercury–zinc cell.

The lithium–iodide cell has several unique features that make it an ideal candidate for pacemakers. For example, since no gas is liberated, the cell can be completely sealed. This feature allows the whole pacemaker to be enclosed in a welded metal container, thereby rendering it fluid tight and reducing susceptibility to electromagnetic interference. Although the lithium–iodide cell has only been used for a decade, the characteristics and present experience indicate that today's units will have a lifetime of 10 years or more. In addition, although the shelf life is unknown, the extremely low self-discharge rate indicates a very long shelf life.

As a result of success with the Greatbatch lithium–iodide cell, many companies have developed similar lithium cells and pacemaker manufacturers are incorporating these cells into pacemakers. Initial highly successful clinical trials indicate that the lithium–iodide cell may very well displace the mercury–zinc cell for cardiac pacemaking.

Nuclear-Power Cells

Two methods are employed to obtain electrical energy from radioactive isotopes. One method employs plutonium 238 (^{238}Pu), which emits alpha particles (helium nuclei) and the other employs promethium 147 (^{147}Pm), which emits beta particles (electrons). With plutonium, heat is produced, which is converted to electrical energy; the basic reaction can be called thermoelectric. With promethium, a voltage is produced by a silicon cell, not unlike a solar cell. The promethium cell is often called a betavoltaic cell.

Plutonium Thermoelectric Cell. The element ^{238}Pu emits alpha particles as it decays. The alpha particles strike the wall of the plutonium container as shown in Figure 8.13*a*. Absorption of the alpha particles raises the wall's temperature to about 110°C. Applied to the wall is a series of thermocouples, the opposite ends of which are in contact with the case of the pacemaker that is maintained very nearly at body temperature as shown in Figure 8.13*a*. Thus, the two thermojunctions are at different temperatures and, via the Seebeck effect, produce a small voltage. To obtain a larger voltage, a series configuration of about 30 thermocouples is used. To obtain the maximum voltage, bismuth and tellurium are used to form the couples.

In summary, the energy exchange process starts with the ejection of alpha particles from the ^{238}Pu, the production of heat which gives rise to a temperature difference that is then converted to a voltage by a thermopile. A thermopile is the name given to a group of thermocouples connected in series.

Although there is more than adequate current developed by the thermopile, the output is too low ($\sim$ 1 V) to energize the pacemaker circuitry. In order to raise the voltage, a DC-to-DC converter is used. This device is merely an oscillator which is driven by the low-voltage thermopile. A transformer is used to step up the alternating voltage to the desired level, and it is then rectified and filtered to obtain a constant voltage of sufficient magnitude (e.g., 10–20 V) to energize the pacemaker circuit.

The amount of plutonium used in a pacemaker is small, amounting to about 0.25 g, being present in the oxide form. The half-life of ^{238}Pu is 86.4 yr; therefore, the life expectancy of such a pacemaker is long. To date only a few thousand "atomic-powered" pacemakers have been produced and not all have been implanted, although clinical trials are underway.

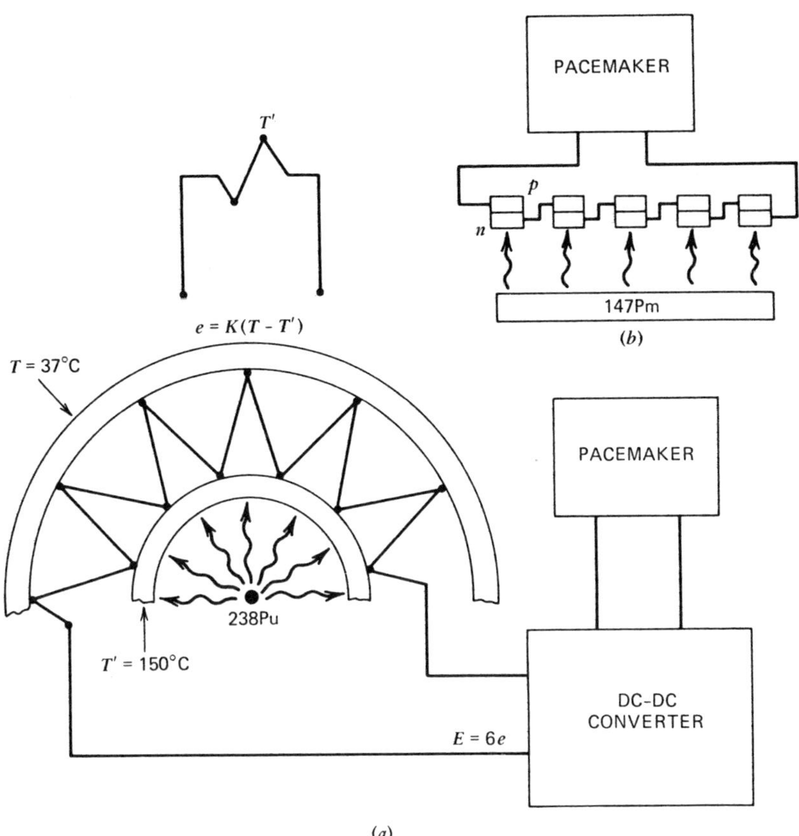

FIGURE 8.13. Nuclear-power cells. (*a*) 238 Pu energy source which emits alpha particles that strike its container and raise its temperature. The outer container is at body temperature; this temperature difference is detected by a series of thermocouples. The voltage produced thereby is used to drive a DC–DC converter to obtain a higher voltage, which energizes the pacemaker. (*b*) The betavoltaic cell consists of 147 Pm which emits beta particles (electrons). The electrons strike a series of *n-p* junctions, and a voltage is produced. The *n-p* junctions are connected in series to obtain a voltage, which energizes the pacemaker.

One of the reasons for slow progress relates to the very strict federal controls. In a preliminary clinical report, Smyth et al. (1977) provided many very interesting facts on this topic. For example, they stated that the International Nuclear Energy Agency and the Atomic Energy Commission have issued guidelines which require that radioactive release must not occur under conditions of cremation, fire, crush, impact, and corrosion. Cremation testing is performed at 1300°C, followed by a water quench. Smyth et al. stated that the amount of radiation absorbed by the pacemaker patient amounts to about 350 mrem/yr, which compares with a dental X-ray exposure of 200–1000 mrem, or equal to the exposure of an average airline pilot or stewardess, amounting to about 400 mrem/yr.

The Betavoltaic Cell. In the betavoltaic cell, promethium 147 (^{147}Pm), which emits beta particles (electrons), is employed. The beta particles are absorbed by a silicon *p-n* junction semiconductor detector, as shown in Figure 8.13*b*. The *n* and *p* materials become the negative and positive terminals and therefore constitute a voltage source. In order to obtain a voltage that is adequately high to operate a pacemaker, many *p-n* junctions are arranged in series. When connected in this way, the current available is related to the total area that receives the beta particles.

It is interesting to note that in the betavoltaic cell the energy conversion is direct, without the production of heat as in the plutonium cell. Therefore, no thermal insulation is required. The voltage available from the series circuit of semiconductor detectors is adequate to power the pacemaker without a DC-to-DC converter. These characteristics reduce the overall size and the manufacturing cost, when compared to the plutonium cell.

The half-life of ^{147}Pm is 2.67 yr, which is considerably less than that of ^{238}Pu. However, at the half life, the remaining 50% of the nuclear fuel is more than adequate to continue driving the pacemaker for some time. The betavoltaic pacemakers that have been produced have a life expectancy of 7–9 yr. With minor improvements, life expectancy of 10–12 yr is projected.

Martinis et al. (1977) presented a report covering 200 clinical implantations of betavoltaic-powered pacemakers. No failure attributable to the nuclear-power source was reported.

The average radiation level on the skin over a betavoltaic-powered pacemaker was reported by Martinis et al. (1977) to be 2.5 mrad/hr (0.75–5.10 mrad). On the back, the average level was 0.1 mrad/hr (0.02–0.2 mrad). These intensities are considered to be within safe limits.

Observations on Nuclear-Power Sources. There is no doubt that nuclear-powered devices offer unique possibilities for long-term cardiac pacemaking, as well as for energizing other implanted devices. However, there are a number of very practical characteristics peculiar to radiation-emitting devices that tend to increase their cost, such as manufacturing problems, quality control, and regulation–compliance requirements. Although nuclear-powered devices are about 10% efficient, they are being given strong competition by improvements in battery technology. Short-half-life nuclear-power sources will obviously have a reduced life expectancy if placed in storage for long periods prior to implantation. On the other hand, there is a limit to the amount of battery power that can be implanted. If, for example, several watts of power are required to energize a left-ventricular assist pump, the nuclear-power plant is perhaps the only candidate for long-term use. At present, regulatory agencies are allowing the research with nuclear-powered devices to progress slowly. Whether this is wise or not, or whether the type of controls presently enforced are too strict or inappropriate, will be for the future to decide. Ultimately, however, it is very likely that this process of slow progress will identify the tasks that are ideal for nuclear-powered devices and those that lend themselves to the use of chemical cells.

CLOSED-CHEST CARDIAC PACING

It is important to recall that the first clinical applications of cardiac pacing were due to Zoll (1952) who used transchest electrodes. This lifesaving technique was used successfully for about a decade, but patient discomfort and introduction of the implanted pacemaker led to abandonment of precordial pacing. However Zoll et al. (1981) pointed out quite correctly that there are emergency situations of ventricular arrest when pacing with chest electrodes is very appropriate. Zoll reintroduced the technique with two major improvements to minimize skin sensation: (1) the use of larger electrodes and (2) the use of a longer duration pacing pulse. Zoll advocated the use of high-resistivity electrode paste with the larger electrodes and a pacing pulse up to 40 msec in duration. The use of a longer duration pacing pulse represents a compromise between ease of myocardial stimulation and minimization of sensation and superficial muscle stimulation.

The optimum location for the electrodes is not entirely settled. However, placing the cathode over the apex beat area, or the ECG–V_3 lead position, appears to be a good choice. The location for the anode is less critical; usually it is on the right chest, below the clavicle. Alternatively, it can be placed on the back. Electrodes of about 4 in. diameter, covered with a saline-soaked sponge, are satisfactory.

When pacing is achieved with a rectangular pulse of 20 msec duration, a current in the range of 50–100 mA is required for ventricular capture in the adult. The pacing rate is typically 80 per minute.

The demand feature can be incorporated into the closed-chest pacer so that VVI operation is achieved. However, *R*-wave sensing with precordial leads is more difficult, owing to the increased susceptibility to artifacts. If competitive pacing occurs, Zoll et al. (1981) reported that the threshold for ventricular fibrillation, owing to vulnerable-period stimulation, is 10 or more times the pacing threshold in normal dogs.

To date Zoll et al. (1981) have applied the technique to 18 subjects using equipment devised by Zoll. Precordial cardiac pacemakers are becoming available commercially in the United States. Typically, the pacing rate is 80 per minute, the pulse duration is 20 msec, and the maximum pacing current is 100 mA.

HISTORICAL POSTSCRIPT

There are many excellent detailed accounts on the history of cardiac pacemaking; therefore, it is not the intent to duplicate the important accounts such as those presented by Davies and Sowton (1964), Escher (1973), and Schecter (1971–72). Instead, only the highlights, as the author sees them, will be presented.

That the arrested heart could be stimulated to contract by mechanical and electrical stimuli has been known for more than a century. Demonstrations of this fact have been routine in physiology courses to illustrate this important property of cardiac muscle. What is rather surprising is the tardy adoption of this fact by clinicians, who were well aware of the presence of cardiac arrest during the induction of anesthesia and the slow ventricular rate in total A-V block (Strokes–Adams disease) which resulted in fainting spells and death in many patients. Despite the lateness in using rhythmic stimuli clinically, there were several important animal and even human studies in which rhythmic electrical stimuli were delivered directly to the arrested heart, long before the lifesaving value of this technique was realized.

Anesthesia was brought to clinical medicine in the mid-1800s. One of the undesirable side effects with many of the early anesthetics, notable chloroform, was cardiac arrest. This fact was easily demonstrated in the experimental animal and several investigators sought to restart the heart in chloroformed animals with electrical stimuli. Among the first was Steiner (1871) who produced cardiac arrest in 3 horses, 1 donkey, 10 dogs, 14 cats, and 6 rabbits with chloroform anesthesia. Interrupted galvanic (DC) stimuli were delivered via a needle electrode (1 mm diameter × 13 cm long) thrust through the chest into the heart. The other electrode was a moistened conducting sponge placed against the epigastrum on the lower chest wall.

In the meantime, clinicians dealt with the problem of cardiac arrest by thrusting a hypodermic needle through the chest wall into the heart and injecting epinephrine. Intentional cardiac pacing did not occur until 1932 when Hyman demonstrated that cardiac pacemaking was practical clinically. He stated that Gould in Australia had stimulated a baby's heart using a chest electrode and a needle electrode thrust into the heart. Pointing out that cardiac arrest was a common clinical event and that "random and badly executed procedures are used within the last minute in the hope of resuscitating the stopped heart," he offered a solution designed to combat the cardiac arrest. He called attention to the dubious value of the technique in which epinephrine was injected directly into the heart via a needle thrust into the thorax. He pointed out quite correctly (1) that it was the needle prick that evoked ventricular contractions, rather than the epinephrine, which obviously requires cardiac pumping to distribute it, and (2) the considerable danger of ventricular fibrillation from the needle stimulus and epinephrine, particularly in hypoxic hearts. Accordingly he offered two solutions: (1) inject the epinephrine into an atrium and (2) apply rhythmic electrical stimuli to the needle thrust through the thorax into an atrium. With the atrial injection of epinephrine, the risk of ventricular fibrillation is eliminated. It is unimportant if atrial fibrillation occurs because the ventricles would only be driven at a rapid rate and the epinephrine would be pumped through the circulatory system. The atrial fibrillation could be treated later with drugs. At that time there was no way of arresting ventricular fibrillation.

Hyman proceeded to make a batteryless electrical pacemaker for delivery of induction-shock stimuli (60–120 per minute) to the atria. At that time, battery life was uncertain, therefore his pacemaker was powered by a hand-wound, spring-driven generator which provided 6 min of pacemaking without rewinding. He demonstrated the success of his portable, manually energized pacemaker by pacing guinea pig, rabbit (and one) dog hearts that had been arrested by asphyxiation. He then used the pacemaker on a small number of human subjects. Unfortunately, there are no details of his clinical success, although he stated that the method of electrical cardiac pacemaking was gaining acceptance.

If it had been heeded, the paper by Callaghan and Bigelow (1951) would undoubtedly have advanced cardiac pacemaking by a decade. In 1951 these investigators described cardiac pacemaking in animals using a catheter electrode passed into the heart via the right external jugular vein. Using 24 dogs and 9 rabbits, cardiac arrest was produced by reducing body temperature or by continuous right vagal stimulation. Pacing was achieved by delivery of rhythmic electrical stimuli to their home-made #12F catheter electrode, which was advanced to the sinoatrial (S-A) node. In one case, cardiac pacing was continued for 70 minutes using 2-msec stimuli. In normothermic animals, rhythmic stimulation at a rate in excess of the S-A node firing, captured the rate and permitted pacing up to 200 beats per minute.

The report by Callaghan and Bigelow clearly demonstrated the value and practicality of cardiac pacemaking with a catheter electrode. If only they had advanced their catheter electrode into the right ventricle and paced it, clinical cardiac pacemaking may well have been advanced by a decade.

Starting in 1952 Zoll and his colleagues reported successful cardiac pacemaking in patients with cardiac arrest by using electrodes placed on the surface of the chest. The electrodes were 3 in. in diameter, were covered with a conducting paste, and were found to be effective in a variety of locations; the criterion for location was pacing with the lowest voltage applied to the electrodes. In one configuration, the negative electrode was located over the apex beat area and the other electrode was on the right chest. Another location, which appeared to produce less muscular twitching, employed the negative electrode in the V_4-V_6 site for electrocardiography; the positive electrode was in the V_2-V_4 region. With either location it was recommended that the spacing between the electrodes exceed 3 in. The stimulus used had a duration of 2 msec and an intensity ranging from 0 to 150 V. The repetition rate was controllable from 30 to 180 per minute.

Despite the considerable success in pacing numerous patients by Zoll and his colleagues, the technique of external cardiac pacemaking was not adopted by other clinicians, probably because of pain and twitching of the chest muscles. However, it is timely to revive Zoll's external cardiac pacemaking for emergency use, because following ventricular defibrillation there sometimes occurs a period of cardiac arrest or atrioventricular block, particularly if the period of circulatory arrest has been long. A pacemaker could easily be built into existing defibrillators to restart the ventricles in such cases.

Perhaps the most influential paper on clinical cardiac pacemaking was presented by Weirich et al. (1958), who called attention to the fact that temporary atrioventricular block was one of the side effects of surgical repair of ventricular septal defects. Weirich and his colleagues demonstrated that direct heart stimulation in closed-chest patients eliminated the need for myocardial stimulation with chest electrodes. In a series of experimental animals, single and double electrodes were implanted in the ventricular myocardium and brought out through the chest. Complete control of ventricular rate (above the normal rate) was obtained. On January 30, 1957, the method was applied to human subjects, and their paper reports successful ventricular pacing in 18 patients with complete A-V block. One patient was paced for 21 days before the pacemaking could be discontinued. In these patients a single myocardial electrode was implanted at the time of surgery. A chest electrode was used to complete the circuit. When pacing was to be discontinued, the myocardial electrode was withdrawn by a gentle pull. Interestingly, such electrodes were frequently installed during cardiac surgery and gained considerable popularity.

Aware of Zoll's (1952) precordial pacing and Weirich et al.'s (1958) use of myocardial electrodes, but apparently unaware of the catheter electrode used in dogs by Callaghan and Bigelow (1951), Furman and Schweibel (1959) developed a catheter electrode designed for ventricular pacing. Using dogs to perfect the catheter and the technique, they then applied this method to humans. The electrode was mounted at the tip of a #6F catheter, which was passed into the right ventricle via the median basilic vein. The indifferent electrode consisted of a silver-plated copper wire implanted subcutaneously in the right chest wall.

Furman and Schweibel's paper describes successful pacing in two patients with atrioventricular block. The first patient was paced for 2 hr and when pacing was stopped, asystole occurred and pacing had to be reinstated. They found that it was possible to wean the patient from the pacemaker by reducing the rate slowly from 60 per minute, being the rate adopted for pacing, following which, the heart resumed its normal rhythm. Then the stimulus strength was reduced and the catheter electrode was withdrawn.

Furman and Schweibel's second patient was paced for more than 13 weeks. During this period they had to develop what later became known as the standby technique, that is, the pacemaker was arranged to turn on if more than a 5-sec period of asystole was identified in the ECG being recorded on the patient monitor. Interestingly enough, the patient was ambulatory and the energy to drive the pacemaker/monitor equipment was derived from a long cord connected to the domestic power outlet. Thus, when the patient walked around the ward, he brought his life-support equipment with him on a small cart.

Furman et al. clearly demonstrated that cardiac pacemaking could be instituted on an emergency basis with very little surgery required, consisting only of insertion of the catheter electrode into the right ventricle via a vein. The threshold for pacing was low, amounting to only about 1.5 V at 0.75 mA. No muscular twitching or sensation could be perceived by the patient. If the electrode migrated into the pulmonary artery, the pacing threshold increased to 12–15 V. However, withdrawal slightly returned the catheter to the right ventricle and the original pacing threshold was restored. In the patient who had been paced for 13 weeks, no myocardial damage was observed as judged by ECG changes.

The final step in modern cardiac pacemaking was taken by Chardack and his associates (1960), who described a totally implantable pacemaker, and in the following year presented the clinical experiences accumulated

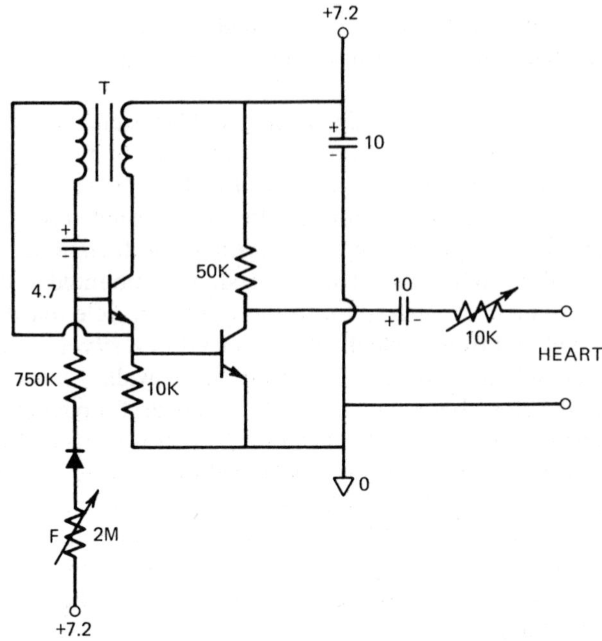

FIGURE 8.14. Circuit diagram of the Greatbatch–Chardack implantable pacemaker. [Redrawn from Chardack et al. (1964). *Ann. N.Y. Acad. Sci.* **111,** 1075–1092.]

with 15 patients. The pacemaker consisted of a transistor oscillator and amplifier energized by 10 mercury–zinc batteries. The batteries and electronic circuitry were potted in epoxy and covered by a double shell of silastic. Figure 8.14 illustrates the circuit diagram of the first implantable pacemaker. The pacemaker used the Hunter–Roth electrode (Figure 8.12*a*), which was about the size of a postage stamp with two protruding pins. The pins were advanced into the left ventricular myocardium in an area of low vascularity. Sutures held the "patch electrode" in the myocardium. The pacing rate was fixed at 60 per minute and the duration was 2 msec. The stimulus intensity was equivalent to 10 mA delivered into a 1000-ohm resistor. At a lower current stimulus (3 mA), an estimated battery life of 5 yr was postulated. In addition, battery fatigue was identifiable by a gradual increase in pacing rate. Unfortunately, the projected 5-year life was not realized.

From April 1960 to March 1961 Chardack implanted pacemakers in 15 patients. The pacemaker was located subcutaneously in the left upper quadrant of the abdomen (Figure 8.15*a*). Despite the considerable success in pacemaking, the major difficulty reported was electrode failure due to breakage. At a rate of 60 per minute, the electrodes and their cables

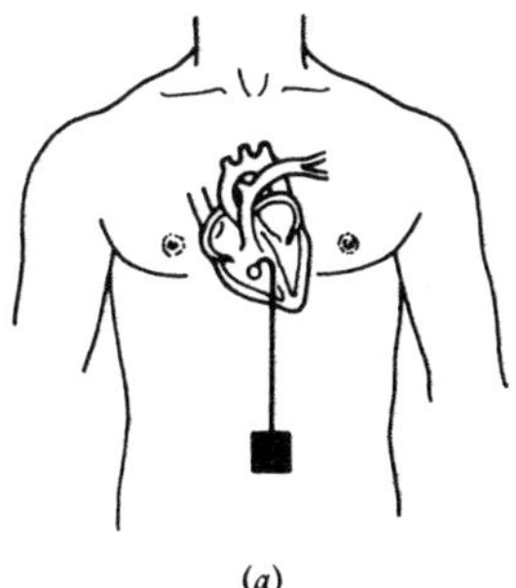

(*a*)

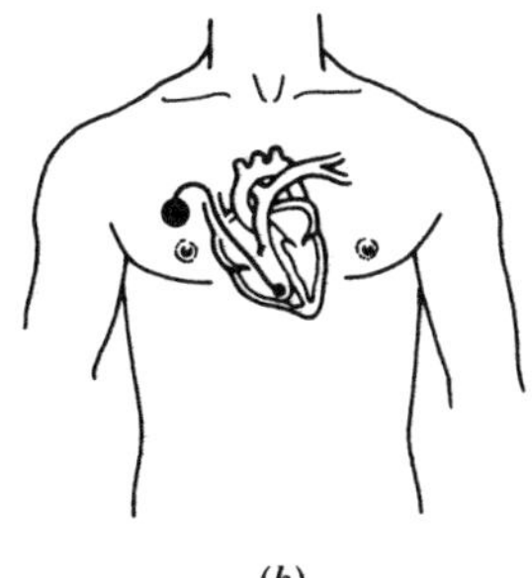

(*b*)

FIGURE 8.15. Location of pacemakers. (*a*) Abdominal site used in the early days of pacemaking. (*b*) The site most frequently used at present.

are subjected to more than 31 million flexions each year. To solve the breakage problem, Chardack et al. proposed to use monopolar electrodes made of coiled wire which extended all of the way to the pacemaker (Figure 8.12*b*).

At this point, three methods for cardiac pacemaking were available. One method, developed by Weirich, employed surgically implanted myocardial electrodes; the second, developed by Furman et al., used a catheter electrode in the right ventricle; and the third, developed by Chardack et al., employed surgical implantation of the pacemaker and its electrodes. Because of the practicality of the latter two, direct surgical implantation of myocardial electrodes became less attractive and less popular. The clinical expediency of the catheter electrode and the practical aspects of the implanted pacemaker led Parsonnet *et al.* (1962) to combine these two techniques. This contribution meant that the application of a pacemaker was reduced to a minimal surgical technique. By gaining access to a major vein in the right subclavicular region, a catheter electrode could be advanced into the right ventricle. The pacemaker could be joined to the catheter electrode and implanted in a subcutaneous pouch (Figure 8.15*b*). Both procedures could be performed in a short time without thoracic surgery and often under local anesthesia. It is obvious that this technique brought pacemaking to many more patients.

The pacemakers used up to this time were fixed-rate (asynchronous), that is, they continued to deliver stimuli irrespective of the need. In other words, if a ventricular rhythm, or a normal supraventricular rhythm developed, competitive pacing occurred. Amid the successes of these early days of ventricular pacing, there was a growing awareness that some of the sudden deaths may have been due to ventricular fibrillation caused by competitive pacing, that is, a pacemaker stimulus falling in the vulnerable period of a normally conducted or ventricular ectopic beat. In fact, there was considerable debate over this point [see reviews by Lemberg et al., (1965), and Jones and Geddes (1977)]. It was also recognized that in normal myocardium, the possibility of ventricular fibrillation was remote, but that in ischemic hearts the threshold for fibrillation was reduced markedly. In order to eliminate the danger of such competitive pacing, Lemberg et al. (1965) introduced the demand pacemaker. In this device the electrodes that are used for ventricular pacing are sampled by electronic circuitry within the pacemaker to determine if there is any electrical activity present; if so, the pacemaker was inhibited for a preset time. In other words ventricular activity inhibited the pacemaker by starting a timing circuit which established the pacemaker rate if no further ventricular activity occurred. Thus if A-V conduction returned, or if ventricular ectopic beats occurred, the pacemaker was inhibited. If no ventricular activity was present, the pacemaker operated as a fixed-rate pacemaker, being inhibited at any time by the presence of ventricular activity.

The first ventricular demand pacemaker developed by Lemberg was not an implantable unit. However, it made its point very well, for Parsonnet *et al.* (1966) reported clinical trials with the first implanted *R*-wave inhibited pacemaker. Soon commercial production began, and this type of pacemaker is one of the most popular type today since it solves the competitive pacing problem. Because only needed stimuli are delivered, battery life is prolonged.

Meanwhile, Neville et al. (1966) had developed the *R*-wave synchronous pacemaker that delivered an ineffective stimulus when an *R* wave occurred and an effective stimulus if one did not occur after a preset time. It would continue to pace if no ventricular excitation occurred within the preset time after a stimulus or an *R* wave.

Recognizing that in many clinical situations of total A-V block, the atria are still functioning, many investigators used the *P* wave to develop a stimulus that was delivered to ventricular electrodes. Folkman and Watkins (1957) developed a transistor amplifier that enlarged the atrial *P* waves and delivered them to the ventricles of dogs to evoke ventricular contractions. The unit was carried in a shoulder harness. The method was proven in dogs with surgically induced A-V block. Stephenson et al. (1959) developed a *P*-wave-triggered stimulator with a built-in delay to simulate the A-V conduction time. The unit was used in dogs with A-V block. A similar study was reported by Kahn et al. (1960). Shortly thereafter, Nathan et al. (1963) examined the use of this concept for human patients and correctly pointed out that the atrial rate (if present) is modulated by physiological needs for cardiac output. The use of a fixed-rate pacemaker in such patients obviously neglects the opportunity for deriving rate-control information for a ventricular pacemaker. Accordingly,

Nathan and his colleagues developed an implantable atrial-triggered pacemaker (which they called a *P*-wave triggered pacemaker). In their pacemaker, a single atrial lead sensed the *P* wave and a bipolar lead was used for ventricular pacing. Within the pacemaker, an 0.1 sec delay was incorporated between the sensed *P* wave and delivery of the ventricular stimulus. This delay roughly corresponds to the A-V conduction time in the normal heart. If no *P* wave occurred, or if no *P* wave was sensed, the pacemaker reverted to the fixed-rate mode of operation at a rate of 60 per minute. If an atrial tachyarrhythmia such a tachycardia, flutter, or fibrillation occurred, the ventricular pacing rate was controlled in an interesting way. For example, the ventricular rate would track the atrial rate up to 150 per minute. If the atrial rate was between 151 and 300 per minute, the ventricular rate would be one-half. If the atrial rate exceeded 300 per minute, the ventricular rate was one-third.

With the atrial-triggered pacemaker, the atrial component to ventricular filling is restored. In addition, the ventricular rate becomes responsive to the atrial rate which is normally modulated by the physiological need for cardiac output. Often, the disease process that necessitated pacemaker therapy, causes an atrial arrhythmias such as flutter, fibrillation, and asystole. The excessively high ventricular pacing rate, owing to atrial tachyarrhythmias, makes the atrial-triggered pacemakers less attractive for such patients.

Pacing of both the atria and ventricles was described by Costello et al. (1970). In this pacemaker, both atrial and ventricular electrical activity are monitored and ventricular stimulation was *R*-wave inhibited. Two sets of bipolar electrodes were used for sensing and stimulating the atria and ventricles. When the atrial rate slowed, only the atria were stimulated. When atrial slowing was associated with A-V block, or when the atrial stimuli were not effective in exciting the atria, the ventricles were stimulated after a short delay. Ventricular activity inhibited the ventricular stimulating to eliminate competitive pacing.

The dual, that is, bifocal pacemaker described by Costello et al. has been used in patients. It is, however, too early to provide evaluative comments on this new type of pacemaker.

REFERENCES

Akhas, F. and Rickards, A. F. (1981) The relationship between Q-T interval and heart rate during physiological exercise and pacing. *Jpn. Heart J.*, **22**(3), 345–351.

Bazett, H. C. (1951) Theory of reflex controls to explain regulation of body temperature at rest during exercise. *J. Appl. Physiol.*, **4**(4), 245–262.

Benchemol, A., Wu, T-Lu, and Liggett, M. S. (1965). Effect of exercise and isoproterenol on the cardiovascular dynamics in complete heart block at various heart rates. *Am. Heart J.*, **70**(3), 337–347.

Benchemol, A., Li, Y-B, and Dimond, E. G. (1964). Cardiovascular dynamics in complete heart block at various heart rates. *Circ.*, **30**, 542–553.

Bozal-Gonzalez, J. L. (1980). Cardiac pacemaker. U.S. Patent 4,201,219, May 4, 1980.

Bozal-Gonzalez, R., Scheinman, M., Margaretten, W., and Rubinstein, M. (1981). Closed-chest electrode-catheter technique for His bundle ablation in dogs. *Amer. Journ. Physiol.* H283–H286.

Callaghan, J. C. and Bigelow, W. G. (1951). An electrical artificial pacemaker for standstill of the heart. *Ann. Surg.* **134**, 8–17.

Cammilli, L. (1979). pH-triggered pacemaker. *Pace.* **2**, A6.

Cammilli, L., Green, G. D., Ricci, D., and Risani, R. (1980). pH-triggered pacemaker: Design and clinical results. *Proc. 6th World Symp. on Cardiac Pacing,* Chap. 19-8.

Cammilli, L., Alcidi, L., and Bisi, G. (1981). Results, problems and perspectives in the autoregulating pacemaker. *2nd European Symp. on Cardiac Pacing,* May-June 1981. *Pace,* **4**, A-36.

Chardack, W. M., Gage, A. A., and Greatbatch, W. (1960). A transistorized self-contained implantable pacemaker for long-term correction of complete heart block. *Surgery* **48**, 643–654.

Chardack, W. M., Gage, A. A., and Greatbatch, W. (1961). Corrections of complete heart block by a self-contained and subcutaneously implanted pacemaker. *J. Thoracic Cardiovasc. Surg.* **42**, 814–825.

Contini, C., Papeschi, G., and Ricci, D., et al. (1981). pH changes in chronic pacemaker packet: A new means of increasing rate during exercise; preliminary results. *Pace,* **2**, 366.

Costello, C., Lemberg, L., Castellanos, N., and Berkovits, B. Y. (1970). Bifocal (sequential atrioventricular) demand pacemaker for sinoatrial and atrioventricular conduction disturbances. *Am. J. Cardiol.* **25**, 87 (Abstract).

Davies, J. G. and Sowton G. E. (1964). Cardiac pacemakers. *Phys. Med. Biol.* **9**, 257–272.

Escher, D. (1973). Historical aspects of pacing. In *Cardiac Pacing* by P. Samet. Grune and Stratton, New York.

Fischell, R. R. (1975). Fixed-rate rechargeable cardiac pacemaker. U.S. Patent 3,867,950.

Folkman, M. J., and Watkins, E. (1957). An electrical conduction system for the management of experimental complete heart block. *Clin. Congr. (Amer. Coll. Surgeons)* **8**, 331–334.

Furman, S. and Hurzeler, P. (1975). Pulse duration variation and electrode size as factor in pacemaker longevity. *J. Thoracic Cardiovasc. Surg.* **69**, 382–389.

Furman, S. and Schweibel, J. B. (1959). An intracardiac pacemaker for Stokes-Adams seizures. *New Engl. J. Med.* **26**, 943–948.

Furman, S., Denize, A., Escher, D. W., and Schwedel, J. B. (1966). Energy considerations for cardiac stimulation as a function of pulse duration. *J. Surg. Res.* **6**, 441–445.

Furman, S., Parker, B., and Escher, D. (1971). Decreasing electrode size and increasing efficiency of cardiac stimulation. *J. Surg. Res.* **11**, 105–110.

Greatbatch, W., Lee, J. H. Mathias, W., Eldridge, M., Moser, J. R., and Schneider, A. A. (1971). The solid-state lithium battery: A new improved chemical power source for implantable cardiac pacemakers. *IEEE Trans. Bio-Med. Eng.* **BME-18**, 316–324.

Griffin, J. C., Tutzy, K. R., and Claude, J. P., et al. (1981). Non-electrographic indices of pacemaker rate. *Proc. AEMB,* **34,** 202.

Hickman, D. M., Geddes, L. A., Hoff, H. E., Hinds, M., Moore, A. G., Francis, C. K., and Engen, T. (1961). A portable miniature transitorized radio-frequency coupled cardiac pacemaker. *I.R.E. PGBME Trans.* **BME-8,** 258–262.

Hunter, S. W., Bolduc, L., Long, V., and Quattelbaum, F. W. (1973). A new myocardial pacemaker lead. *Chest* **63,** 430–433.

Hunter, S. W., Roth, N. A., Bernardez, D., and Noble, J. D. (1959). A bipolar myocardial electrode for complete heart block. *Lancet* **79,** 506.

Hyman, A. S. (1932). Resuscitation of the stopped heart by intracardial therapy. *Arch. Int. Med.* **50,** 289–308.

Ionsecu, V. L. (1980). An "on demand" pacemaker responsive to respiratory rate. *Pace* **3,** 375.

Irnich, W. (1975). Engineering concepts of pacemaker electrodes. In *Advances in Pacemaker Technology.* M. Schaldach and S. Furman (Eds.), Springer Verlag, New York.

Jolgren, D., Fearnot, N. E., and Geddes, L. A. (1983). A rate-responsive controlled by right ventricular blood temperature. Proc 32nd Ann. Sci. Session. *Am. Coll. Cardiol. J. Acc.,* part 1 (1), 720.

Jones, M. and Geddes, L. A. (1977). Strength-duration curves for cardiac pacemaking and ventricular fibrillation. *Cardiovascular Research Center Bulletin* **15,** 101–112.

Kahn, M., Senderoff, E., Shapiro, J. Bleifer, S. B., and Grishman, A. (1960). Bridging of interrupted A-V conduction in experimental heart block by electronic means. *Am. Heart J.* **59,** 548–559.

Kappenberger, L. *et al.* (1981). Differentiated pacemaking therapy. *Schweiz. Med. Wochenschrift* **111,** 45–48.

Karlof, I. (1975). Hemodynamic effects of atrial-triggered versus fixed rate pacing at rest and during exercise in complete heart block. *Acta. Med. Scand.* **197,** 195–206.

Krasner, J. L., Voukydis, P. C., and Nardella, P. C. (1966). A physiologically controlled cardiac pacemaker, *J.A.A.M.I.* 20.

Krasner, J. L. and Nardella, P. (1971). U.S. Patent 3,593,718.

Kruse, I., Arnman, K., Conradson, T., and Ryden, L. (1982). A comparison of the acute and long-term hemodynamic effects of ventricular inhibited and atrial synchronous-ventricular inhibited pacing. *Circulation* **65,** 846–855.

Lemberg, L., Castellanos, A., and Berkcovits, B. V. (1965). Pacemaking on demand in A-V block. *J. Am. Med. Ann.* **191,** 12–14.

Martinis, A. J., Matheson, W. E., and Schaldack, M. (1977). Current status of betavoltaic pacemaker systems. In *Cardiac Pacing* (Proc. 5th Int. Symp. Tokyo, Mar. 14–18, 1976) Y. Watanabe (Ed.), Excerpta Medica, Amsterdam, the Netherlands.

Morse, D. and Steiner, R. M. (1978). *Pacemaker Identification Handbook,* Medical Examination Publishing Co., Garden City, NY.

Nathan, D. A., Center, S., Wu, C. Y., and Keller, W. (1963). An implantable synchronous pacemaker for the long-term correction of complete heart block. *Circ.* **27,** 682.

Neville J., Millar K., Keller W., and Abildskuv J. A. (1966). An implantable demand pacemaker. *Clin. Res.* **14,** 256.

Parsonnet V., Zucker I. R., and Asa M. (1962). Preliminary investigation of a permanent implantable pacemaker utilizing an intracardiac dipolar catheter. *Clin. Res.* **10,** 391 (see also *Am. J. Cardiol.* **10,** 261).

Parsonnet V., Zucker, I. R., Gilbert L., and Myers G. H. (1966). Clinical use of an implanted standby pacemaker. *JAMA* **196,** 784.

Parsonnet, V., Furman, S., and Smyth, M. P. D. (1974). Implantable cardiac pacemakers status report and resource guideline. *Circulation* **50,** A21–A35.

Rickards, A. F. (1981). Physiologically adaptive cardiac pacemaker. U.S. Patent 4,228,803.

Rickards, A. F., Norman, J., and Thalen, A. et al. (1981). The use of stimulus-T interval to determine cardiac pacing rate. *Pace,* **4,** A68.

Rickards, A. F. and Norman, J. (1981). Relation between Q-T interval and heart rate. *Brit. Heart J.* 45:56–61.

Schecter, D. C. (1971–72). Background of clinical cardiac electrostimulation. Parts I-Vii. *New York State J. Med.* 2576–25, 81, 2794–2805, 270–284, 395–404, 605–619, 953–961, 1165–1191.

Smyth, N. P. D., Basu, A. P., Bacos, J. M. et al. (1971). Permanent transvenous synchronous cardiac pacing. *Chest* **59,** 493–497.

Smyth, N. P. D., Magovern, G. J., Cushing, W., and Kerkishian, J. M. (1977). Preliminary experience with a new radioisotope powered cardiac pacemaker. In *Cardiac Pacing* (Prac. 5th Int. Symp., Tokyo Mar. 14–18, 1976) Y. Watanabe (Ed.), Excerpta Medica, Amsterdam, the Netherlands.

Steiner, F. (1871a). Ueber die Electropunctur des Herzens als Wiederbelebungsmittel in der Chloroformsyncope. *Archiv. klin. Chir.* **12,** 748–790.

Stephenson, S. E., Edwards, W. H., Jolly, P. C., and Scott, H. W. (1959). Physiologic P-wave cardiac stimulator. *J. Thoracic Cardiovasc. Surg.* **38,** 604–609.

Weirich, W. L., Paneth, M., Gott, V. L., and Lillehei, C. W. (1958). Control of complete heart block by use of an artificial pacemaker and a myocardial electrode. *Circ. Res.* **6,** 410–415.

Wirtzfield, A. (1980). Cardiac pacemaker. U.S. Patent 4,202,339.

Zoll, P. M. (1952). Resuscitation of heart in ventricular standstill by external electric stimulation. *N. Engl. J. Med.* **247,** 768.

Zoll, P. M., Zoll, R. M., and Belgard, A. H. (1981). External non-invasive electric stimulation of the heart. *Crit. Care Med* **9,** 393.

CHAPTER 9

The Defibrillator and Defibrillation

A defibrillator is an electrical device that sends a pulse of current through the heart to arrest several types of arrhythmias. The pulse of current can be applied to electrodes directly on the heart, to electrodes on a catheter in the heart, or to electrodes placed on the thorax. Considerably more voltage, current, and energy are required in the latter case.

CARDIAC ARRHYTHMIAS

Arrhythmias can arise in the atria or ventricles and cause the affected chamber to beat rapidly or to fibrillate. A high rate of organized contraction and relaxation is called a tachycardia. Fibrillation is a disorganized contraction and relaxation of all of the individual fibers of the affected chamber. Therefore, the blood-pumping capability of a fibrillating chamber is lost.

Tachycardia can develop in the atria or ventricles. With atrial tachycardia, the rapid atrial rate drives the ventricles at a rapid rate. Ventricular filling time is compromised and cardiac output is reduced. With ventricular tachycardia, the ventricles are beating independently of the atria and the rapid rate compromises ventricular filling time, thereby reducing cardiac output. There are some types of atrial and ventricular tachycardia that are resistant to drugs and electric countershock can be used effectively.

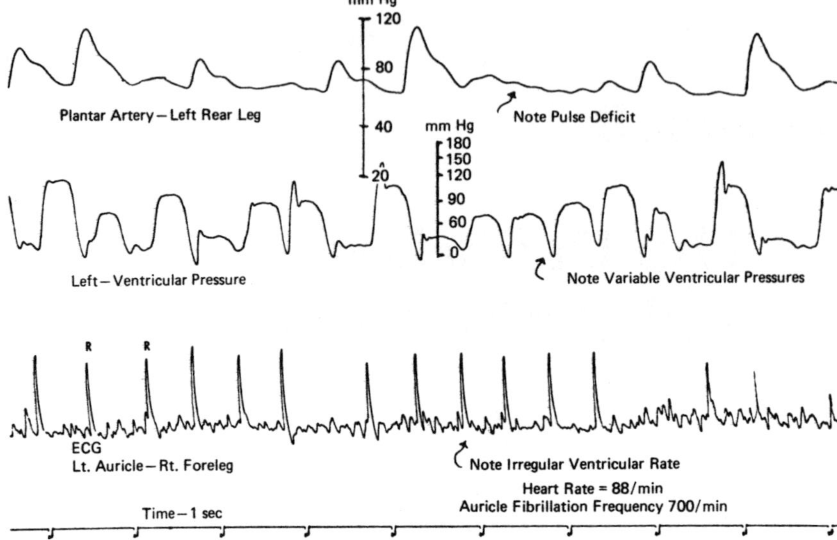

FIGURE 9.1. Atrial fibrillation in the horse. The top channel displays the pressure in the plantar artery; the middle channel shows left-ventricular pressure; and the bottom record is the semidirect electrocardiogram (ECG).

Atrial Fibrillation

Fibrillation can occur in the atria (or auricles) of the heart, and when present, all pumping action of these chambers is lost. In atrial fibrillation, the rapid asynchronous excitations bombard the atrioventricular node of the ventricules with repetitive excitation waves, resulting in a very rapid and irregular ventricular rate. So rapid is the rate that there is not always adequate time for adequate ventricular filling; therefore, the stroke volume varies widely and results in a rapid irregular pulse, both in force and in rate. Figure 9.1 illustates the ECG, arterial, and left-ventricular pressures in atrial fibrillation; note the pulse deficit in the plantar artery recording.

Atrial fibrillation is compatible with life, but owing to the rapid irregular stroke volume, cardiac output is reduced. Medication to reduce the number of impulses reaching the atrioventricular node, or defibrillation of the atria by drugs or electric shock, are the therapies available. Drug-resistant atrial tachycardia or fibrillation can be treated by creating permanent A-V block and installing a ventricular pacemaker.

When the atria are defibrillated electrically, chest electrodes are used. The technique is called "elective cardioversion," since it is possible to schedule the time for atrial defibrillation. In the early days of atrial defibrillation, an anesthetic was used to prevent the patient from feeling the considerable electric shock delivered to the thoracic electrodes. As experienced accumulated, it was found that a heavy dose of a tranquilizing drug was satisfactory. With damped sine wave current applied to thoracic electrodes, atrial defibrillation is accomplished in adults with 20–200 W-sec (J), the lower energy being used at first; often multiple shocks are administered. The energy requirements for other waveforms may be different.

Termination of atrial tachycardia is carried out in the same way as is atrial defibrillation. Likewise, the technique for terminating ventricular tachycardia is the same, except that the energy levels may differ. In all three cases, it is necessary to use synchronization so that the countershock is not delivered during the vulnerable period of the ventricles. Although unsynchronized countershock is sometimes used, the danger of ventricular fibrillation is always present in such a case.

Vulnerable Period

When applying a countershock to terminate atrial tachycardia and fibrillation (and ventricular tachycardia), it is necessary to deliver the pulse of current outside of the vulnerable period of the ventricles. The vulnerable period is that period in the ventricular cycle when a single pulse of current will precipitate ventricular fibrillation. The ventricular vulnerable period occurs during most of the *T* wave of the electrocardiogram and is illustrated in Figure 9.2 (inset). Note that a single stimulus (X), delivered during the *T* wave, caused ventricular fibrillation. In the normal heart a strong stimulus is needed to evoke fibrillation; in an ischemic heart the intensity is much less.

To eliminate vulnerable-period stimulation, many defibrillators permit delivery of the current only during, or slightly after, the *QRS* wave. Such defibrillators have a "synchronizing" circuit and require either feeding an ECG signal into the defibrillator or applying ECG electrodes to the subject and connecting them to the ECG amplifier in the defibrillator. Some defibrillators acquire the ECG through the defibrillating electrodes.

Ventricular Fibrillation

With ventricular fibrillation, all pumping action of the ventricles ceases and blood pressure falls to a near zero level immediately. Figure 9.3 illustrates the EEG, ECG, and blood pressure before, during, and after precipitating ventricular fibrillation. If circulatory support is not provided within about 3 min, irreversible changes start to occur in the brain. Note

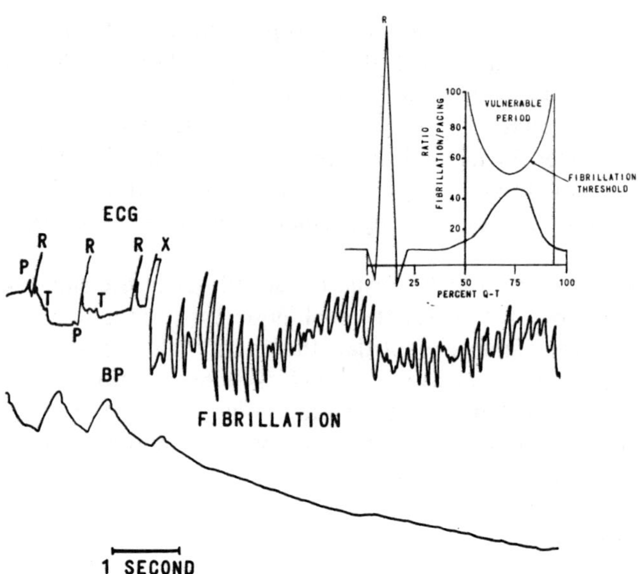

FIGURE 9.2. Location of the vulnerable period in the ventricular cycle. The stimulus strength required to evoke ventricular fibrillation is minimum near the apex of the *T* wave. An example of fibrillation by vulnerable period stimulation is shown at *X*.

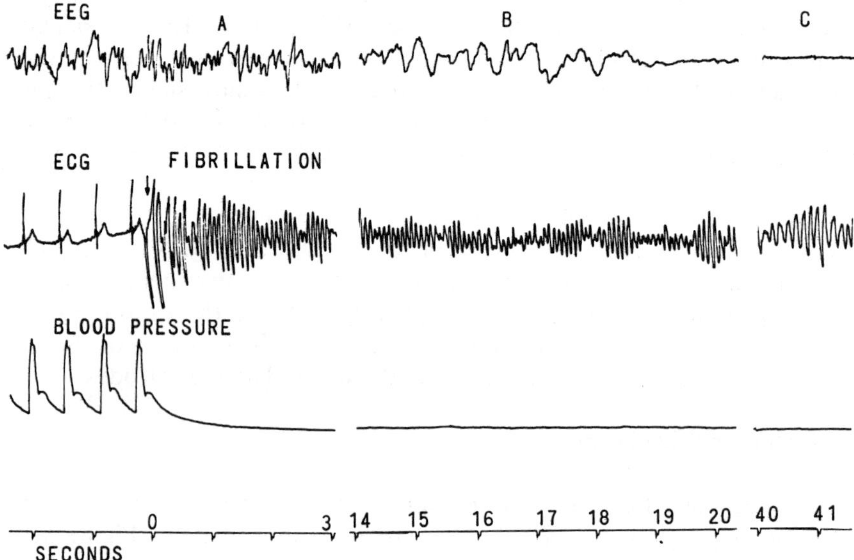

FIGURE 9.3. Electroencephalogram (EEG), electrocardiogram (ECG), and femoral artery blood pressure of a dog, prior to and after the onset of ventricular fibrillation at time 0. About 19 sec after the onset of fibrillation, the EEG became isolectric.

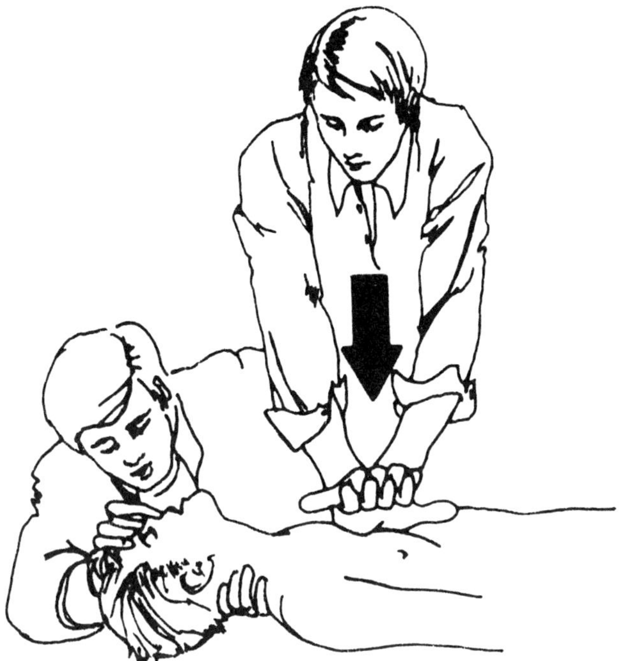

FIGURE 9.4. Cardiopulmonary resuscitation.

that in Figure 9.3, the EEG became inactive 19 sec after ventricular fibrillation started. Circulatory support can be provided by the use of cardiopulmonary resuscitation (CPR), in which the chest is rhythmically forced down toward the spinal column (to squeeze blood out of the fibrillating ventricles). Mouth-to-mouth respiration is used to oxygenate the blood that is forced through the pulmonary circulation by cardiac compression; Figure 9.4 illustrates the technique. In the open-chest subject, the ventricles can be squeezed manually; the result is shown in Figure 9.5. Note the gradual reappearance of the EEG after 18 cardiac compressions and the dramatic increase in EEG activity after 24 cardiac compressions, indicating brain pertusion with oxygenated blood. Open- or closed-chest cardiac compression can be continued for a prolonged period.

The only safe and effective method of defibrillating the ventricles consists of passing a pulse of current through them. As stated earlier, electrodes can be placed directly on the heart when the chest is open or on the chest surface in the intact subject. In either case, the goal is to achieve an adequately high current-density distribution in the ventricles to extinguish the random circulating excitatory waves that characterize fibrillation.

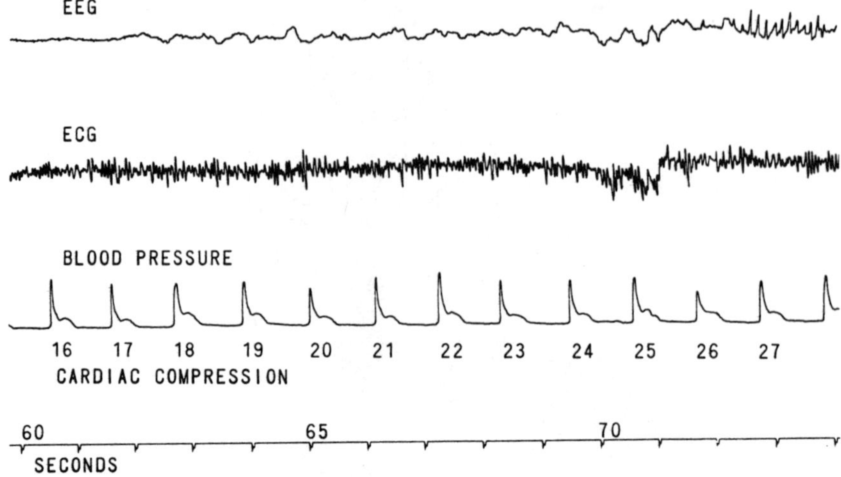

FIGURE 9.5. The EEG, ECG, and blood pressure during ventricular fibrillation while rhythmic cardiac compression was being carried out. Note that after about 18 cardiac compressions the EEG started to reappear, following 24 cardiac compressions, spindling appeared in the EEG indicating restoration of oxygenated blood flow to the cortex. During this time artificial respiration was applied.

When the appropriate output is selected from a defibrillator and the current pulse is delivered, defibrillation is instantaneous, and cardiac pumping usually resumes in a few seconds. If not, CPR is reestablished until forceful ventricular contractions return. Figure 9.6 illustrates defibrillation of the animal subject just discussed, using 5 W-sec of damped sine wave current applied to electrodes directly on the ventricles.

The electrical output required to achieve ventricular defibrillation depends on heart size and body size, electrode location, and the type of current waveform. These factors will be discussed in this chapter. For the moment, it is merely necessary to state that the output available from a defibrillator is described in energy units, watt-seconds or joules. It is important to note that the energy requirements for defibrillation are slightly different for the different current waveforms and clinicians are just beginning to adopt the dose concept; that is, for a given waveform, a specified number of joules per gram of heart or kilogram of body weight is required.

ELECTRODE PLACEMENT

Termination of atrial and ventricular tachycardia and fibrillation is achieved with electrodes placed on the anterior chest wall (Figure 9.7) or

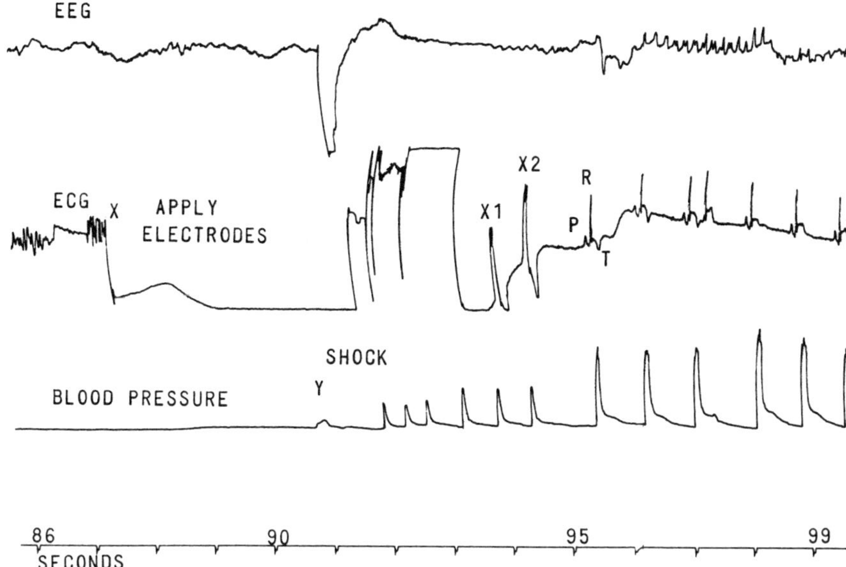

FIGURE 9.6. The EEG, ECG, and blood pressure following rhythmic cardiac compression and while the defibrillating electrodes were placed around the heart (*X*). At *Y*, the defibrillating shock was delivered. In about 1 sec the ventricles started to beat and 2 sec later the ECG amplifier became unblocked revealing two ectopic beats (X_1, X_2), followed by a normal sinus rhythm (*P*, *QRS*, *T*).

with one electrode on the chest and one on the back (Figure 9.8). The latter placement is favored for terminating atrial fibrillation. The equivalent electrical circuit will be discussed subsequently.

CURRENT WAVEFORMS

A variety of current waveforms has been used for ventricular defibrillation; the first was 60-Hz alternating current, derived from the power line. The duration of application was about 0.1 sec. This waveform is shown in Figure 9.9*a*. The simple capacitor-discharge current pulse (Figure 9.9*b*) was used to defibrillate animal and a few human hearts. the slightly underdamped (Figure 9.9*c*) and critically or overdamped (Figure 9.9*d*) sine wave displaced the 60-Hz defibrillators for human application. More recently, the truncated exponential or trapezoidal waveform (Figures 9.9*e* and 9.9*f*) is provided by some defibrillators. When the capacitance is large and the discharge time constant is long, an almost square wave of current is obtained, as shown in Figure 9.9*e*. In some defibrillators, the capacitance is less and there is a considerable decrease in the current during the pulse, that is, there is a tilt on the top of the

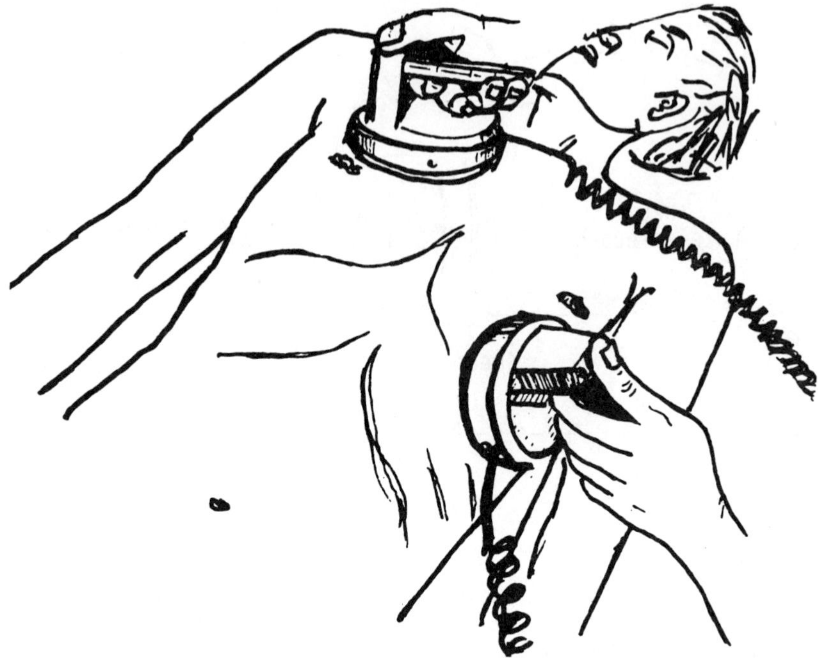

FIGURE 9.7. Location of electrodes on the chest for precordial defibrillation. One electrode is placed on the left chest over the region of the apex beat. The other electrode is on the right chest, to the right of the sternum and just below the clavicle.

wave. Figure 9.9*f* illustrates a high-tilt trapezoidal wave. Tilt is defined as the percentage decrease in the current during the pulse. In Figures 9.9*e* and 9.9*f* the tilt is 100 $(I_i - I_f)/I_i$, where I_i and I_f are the initial and final currents. The capabilities of these waveforms to achieve defibrillation will be presented following a discussion of the principles of defibrillation.

THE FIVE PRINCIPLES OF DEFIBRILLATION

There are five important aspects of defibrillation that can be drawn together in quantitative terms; the author has designated them the principles of defibrillation. Since they apply to fibrillating myocardium, they apply equally well to atrial and ventricular defibrillation. However, only their importance to ventricular defibrillation will be discussed here. The five principles are embodied in the strength-duration curve, the distribution of thresholds, the average current in a pulse of defibrillating current, the dose concept, and myocardial depression due to overdose defibrillating current. These five principles will now be discussed; supporting data will be presented throughout this chapter.

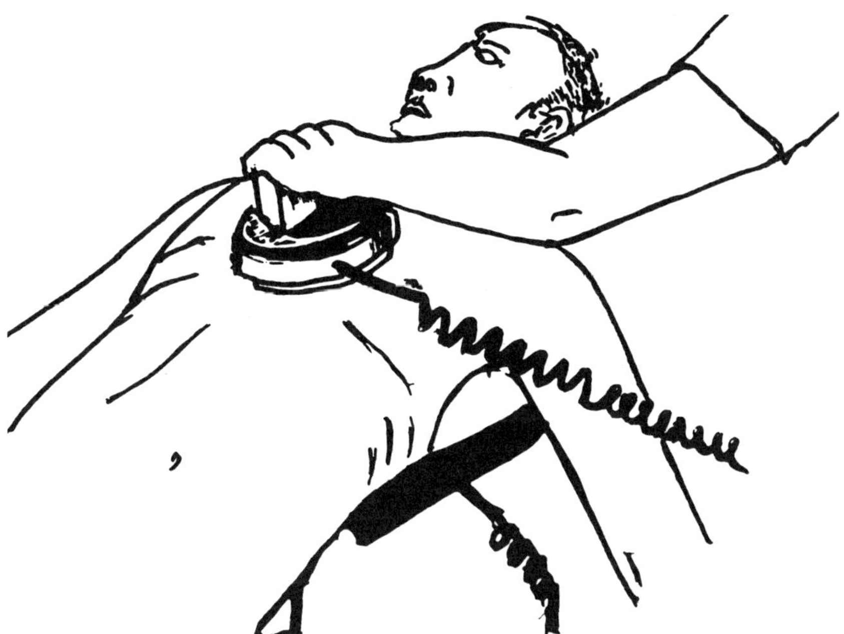

FIGURE 9.8. Location of electrodes for chest-to-back defibrillation. One electrode is over the area of the apex beat; the other, often a much larger electrode, is centered over the lower border of the left scapula. Sometimes this electrode is placed between the scapulae.

The Strength–Duration Curve

The first principle of defibrillation relates to the intensity and duration of the pulse of current required to achieve defibrillation in a given heart. Just as for tissue stimulation, for any defibrillating current waveform there is an inverse Lapicque-type relationship between the lowest (threshold) current intensity and duration of the current pulse to achieve defibrillation. A plot of this relationship is known as the strength-duration curve. That the strength-duration relationship applies to defibrillating current was reported by Geddes et al. (1970).

To achieve defibrillation, an adequate current density must be established in the ventricles for an adequate time, brief as it may be. With a specified duration of current pulse, the lowest current that achieves defibrillation is known as the threshold. The strength-duration curve is often expressed empirically as

$$I = \frac{k}{d} + b$$

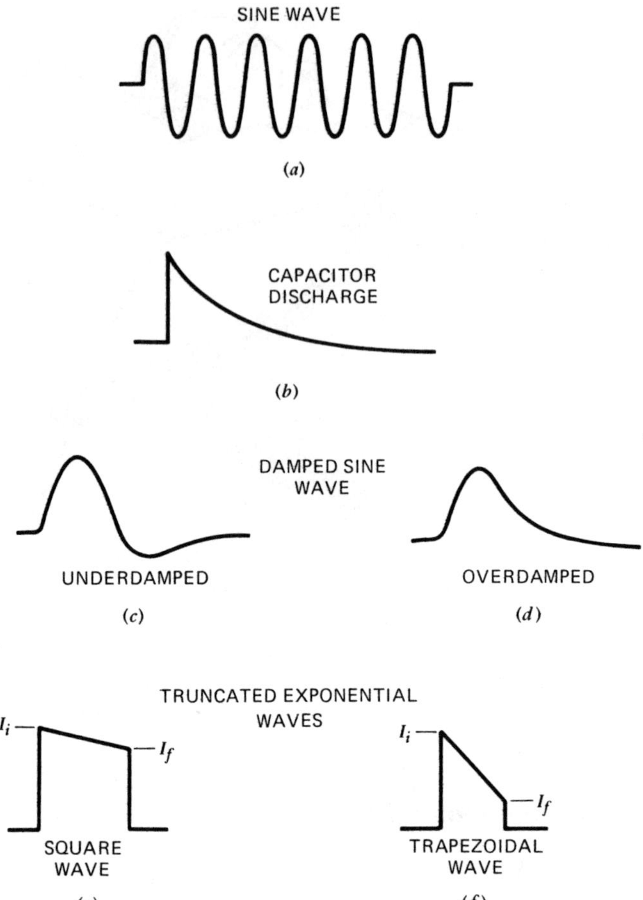

FIGURE 9.9. Current waveforms used for ventricular defibrillation (*a*) sine wave, (*b*) capacitor discharge, (*c, d*) damped sine waves, and (*e, f*) trapezoidal waves.

where I is the threshold defibrillating current, d is the duration of the current pulse, b is the defibrillation threshold for an infinitely long duration pulse (i.e., the rheobase), and k is a constant. Figure 9.10 is a plot of this expression.

The charge (Q) delivered is the average current (I_{av}) during the pulse multiplied by the duration; therefore $Q = I_{av}d$. The charge-duration curve is also shown in Figure 9.10.

Because energy is used to describe shock strength, the energy-duration relationship is also shown in Figure 9.10. The duration for minimum energy corresponds to the duration of a current that is twice the rheobasic value. For a pulse the energy (U) is the integral of the square of the

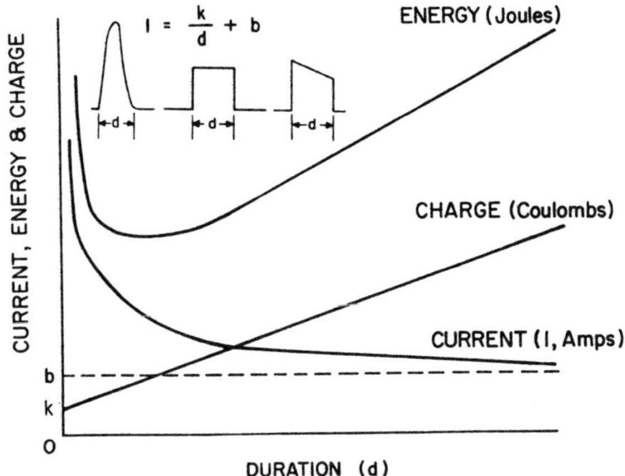

FIGURE 9.10. Strength-duration curve for current, energy, and charge.

current (I) multiplied by the resistance (R) through which it flows and the duration (d) of the pulse of current. Mathematically

$$U = \int_0^d I^2 R \, dt$$

In the following paragraphs, strength-duration curves will be presented for threshold current and energy for the various waveforms used for defibrillation.

In summary, the first principle of defibrillation states that there is an inverse relationship between pulse duration and the threshold current required for defibrillation.

Threshold Distribution

The threshold distribution principle recognizes that although the threshold current required to defibrillate a given heart is well defined, the threshold for another heart (of the same size and species) will not be exactly the same. A plot of number of hearts versus threshold current (per gram of heart) will exhibit a typical distribution curve. The consequences of this fact is that by increasing the shock strength (mA/g or A/kg), an increasing percentage of hearts can be defibrillated.

Average Current Principle

The average current principle permits comparing the efficacy of one waveform with that of another. Bourland et al. (1978) noted that with four trapezoidal waves of different tilts, a plot of the charge delivered (area under a current pulse) versus duration produced four straight lines that were virtually superimposed. The consequence of this charge-duration relationship is that, given a duration, the average current for each of the four waveforms is the same. Another consequence of the finding is that the strength-duration curves for average current is the same for these four waveforms. Bourland et al. (1978) showed that the strength-duration curves for average current with the damped sine wave and high and low tilt trapezoidal waves were virtually superimposed.

Stated more simply, the average current principle predicts that given a duration of current pulse, the threshold average current required for defibrillation with different waveforms, will be the same. In the following paragraphs the evidence to support this statement will be offered. To date, the principle has been verified for damped sine and low and high-tilt trapezoidal waves.

Dose Concept

The fourth principle of defibrillation is the dose concept which states that the shock strength required to defibrillate with a given current waveform increases with heart size. Shock strength can be measured in terms of current or delivered energy. MacKay and Leeds (1953) proposed the use of energy to describe the shock strength required for defibrillation. Energy is still used to describe shock strength, and this fact causes some difficulty because delivered energy is always less than stored energy in the defibrillator and the energy delivered is seldom known.

To illustrate the dose concept, it is necessary to choose a current waveform and determine the threshold current required to defibrillate hearts of widely differing weights. When this is done, it is found that the current intensity (and delivered energy) required to defibrillate increase with increasing heart weight. The same type of relationship is revealed if thoracic electrodes are used to defibrillate animals of increasing body weight. In the following paragraphs, evidence will be given to support the dose concept.

Myocardial Depression

The fifth principle of defibrillation states that the amount of loss of postdefibrillation contractile force (myocardial depression) is related to the shock overdose ratio. The overdose ratio is the ratio of shock strength used to the threshold shock strength required for defibrillation. It will be shown that, despite differences in threshold among the various current

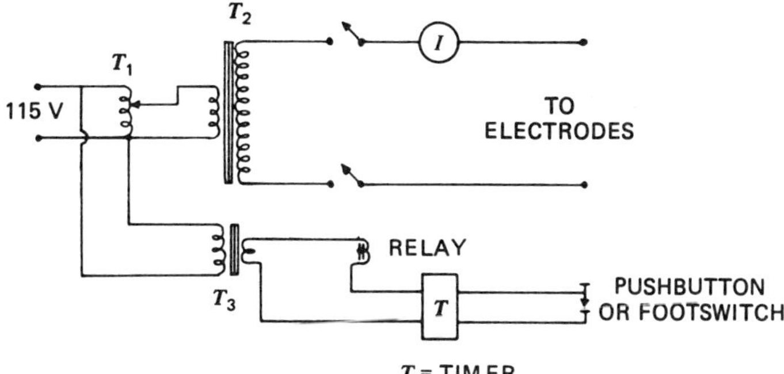

FIGURE 9.11. Circuit diagrams of a typical 60-Hz defibrillator. T_1 is a variable transformer which controls the output voltage presented to the electrodes. T_2 is a step-up transformer. T_3 is a step-down transformer used to energize the relay which controls delivery of the output. When a pushbutton or footswitch is operated, the timer circuit (T) closes the output relay for a fraction of a second.

waveforms, the myocardial depression is quite similar for the same overdose ratio (among the waveforms studied to date).

60-Hz ALTERNATING CURRENT

Sinusoidal alternating current (60 Hz) from the domestic power line (Figure 9.9*a*) was the first waveform used for routine defibrillation. As early as 1933, Hooker *et al.* found that 60-Hz current could defibrillate dog hearts; but it was not until 1947 when Beck *et al.* used it to defibrillate the human heart with directly applied electrodes. The voltage used was 110 (rms), which was applied for about one-half second. It was not until 1956 that the first human transchest defibrillation was performed by Zoll *et al.*, who used up to 750 V (rms) applied to thoracic electrodes; the current level was about 15 A (rms), which flowed for about one fifth of a second.

A typical 60-Hz defibrillator is shown in Figure 9.11. In a given subject, the amount of 60-Hz current required to achieve defibrillation is inversely related to the duration of its application; Figure 9.12*a* illustrates this point derived from a study carried out by Gullett *et al.* (1968) with electrodes applied directly to dog hearts. These data show that there is little decrease in current required when the duration is beyond about 0.15 sec. In typical 60-Hz defibrillators, the duration of current flow is 0.1–0.2 sec, that is, 6–12 sinusoids are delivered. Figure 9.12*b* shows that the energy required increases with the duration of current flow.

As stated previously, when the 60-Hz defibrillator was used with chest electrodes, the voltage applied varied between 500 and 750 V rms. For a

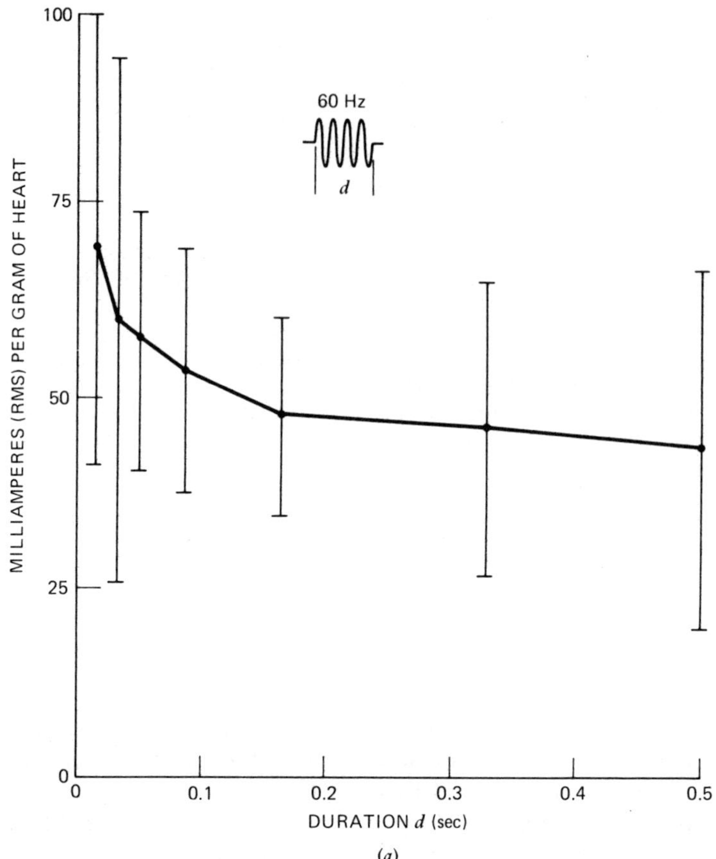

(*a*)

FIGURE 9.12. Strength-duration curve for (*a*) 60-Hz alternating current and (*b*) energy applied to transventricular electrodes on dog hearts. [Redrawn from Gullett et al. (1968).]

variety of reasons, which includes the high current drawn from the domestic power line, the large physical size of such defibrillators, the inability to use synchronization, and the strong tetanic contractions in the subject, the use of 60-Hz current soon gave way to the damped sine wave, which is now in widespread use.

CAPACITOR DISCHARGE

For a short time, the simple capacitor-discharge (Figure 9.9*b*) defibrillator was used in animal and human studies. It did not gain popularity and was displaced by the damped-sine-wave defibrillator, probably because the

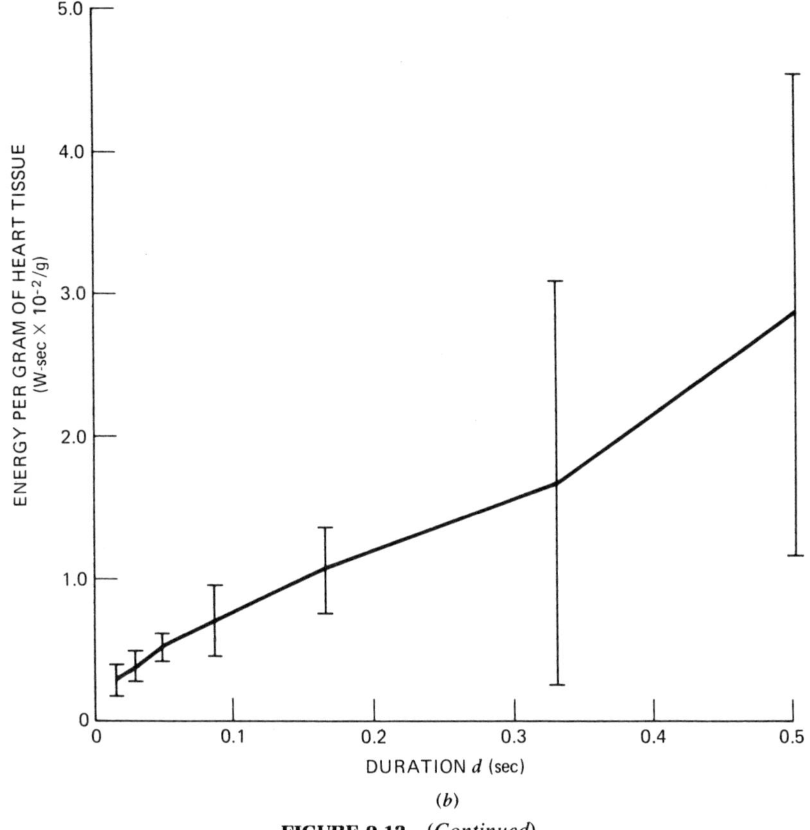

(*b*)

FIGURE 9.12 (*Continued*)

addition of the inductor permitted defibrillation with less peak current. Moreover, Tacker *et al.* (1968) showed that the A-V block, often seen with the capacitor-discharge waveform, was reduced by the addition of an inductor. Typical strength-duration curves were presented by Geddes *et al.* (1970).

DAMPED-SINE-WAVE DEFIBRILLATION

The damped-sine-wave defibrillator (Figure 9.13) consists of a capacitor (*C*) which is discharged through an inductor (*L*) in series with the electrodes on the heart or thorax. The damped sine waveform often carries the name Gurvich, Lown, or Edmark, because of its use by these pioneering investigators. Gurvich and Yuniev (1947) first used it on animals; Lown (1964) and Edmark et al. (1966) applied it to humans. Although the

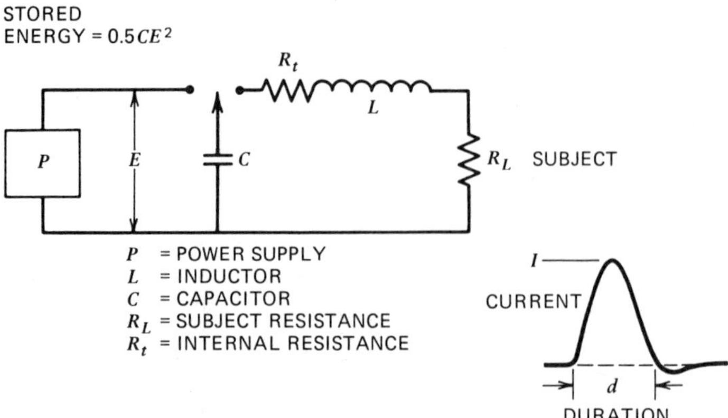

FIGURE 9.13. Essential features of the damped-sine-wave defibrillator, consisting of a capacitor C which is charged from a direct current supply (P) to a voltage E. By connecting the capacitor to the subject via an inductor (L), current flows through the subject (R_L). The energy in joules or watt-seconds stored in the capacitor is $0.5CE^2$, where C is the capacitance in farads and E is the voltage on the capacitor. The energy delivered to the subject is always less than the stored energy, owing mainly to resistive losses in the inductor (L). R_t is the internal resistance of the defibrillator.

waveform used by each of these investigators is a damped sine wave, the sizes of the capacitors and inductors used were different, resulting in slightly different waveforms and durations. The damped sine wave used by Lown is typically 5 msec in duration and slightly underdamped, that is, the current flow reverses direction slightly, as shown in Figure 9.9*c*. The damped sine wave used by Edmark [and now advocated by Pantridge *et al.* (1975)] is longer in duration (about 10 msec), and is critically or overdamped, as shown in Figure 9.9*d*, that is, the current flows in the same direction throughout the duration of the current pulse. Whether the waveform is underdamped, critically damped, or overdamped depends on the value of the inductor, capacitor, and resistance of the electrode–subject circuit.

The importance of pulse duration is demonstrated by strength-duration curves, which have been obtained on animals with electrodes applied directly to the heart; Figure 9.14*a* presents such a curve for dogs, normalized to heart weight. It is clear that the duration for minimum current is in the range of 5–10 msec.

The applicability of the strength-duration principle to a wide variety of hearts from several species is shown in Figure 9.14*b*. In this illustration the defibrillation threshold is expressed in milliamperes (peak) per gram of heart. If a single species is chosen, for example, the dog, it will be seen that for the 8-msec duration, there is a range of thresholds, offering evi-

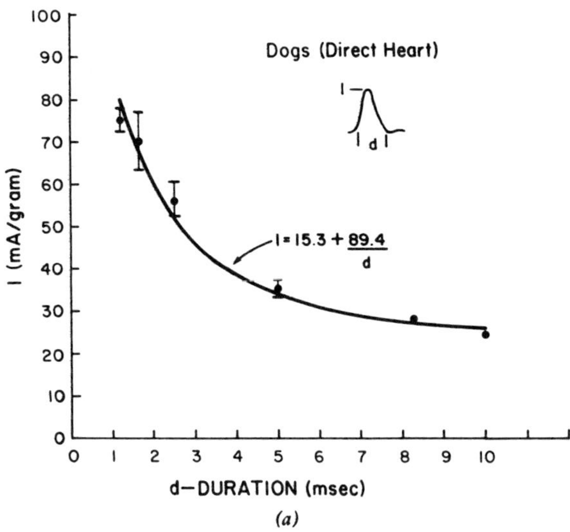

(a)

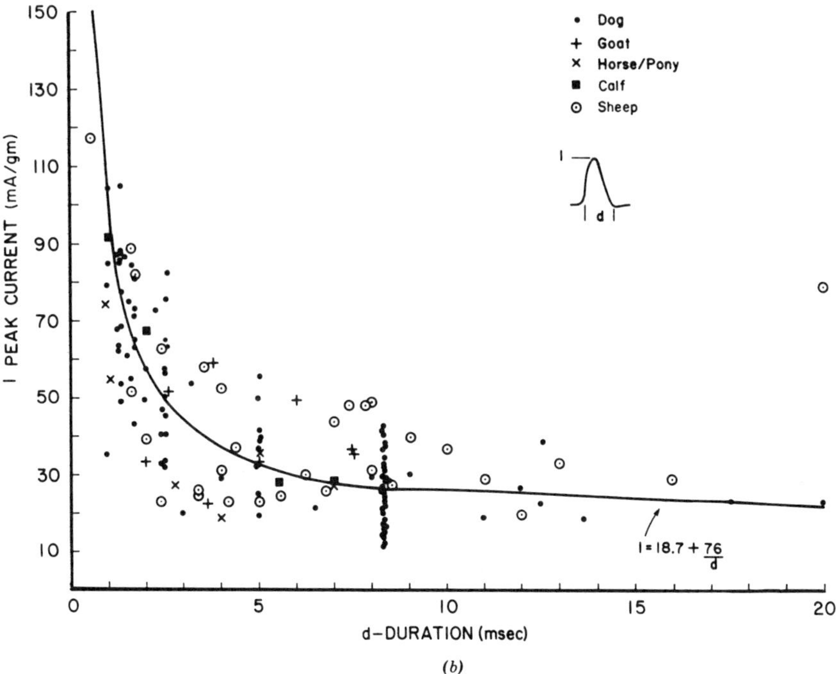

(b)

FIGURE 9.14. Strength-duration curve for direct-heart defibrillation with damped sine wave current applied (*a*) to dogs and (*b*) to five species.

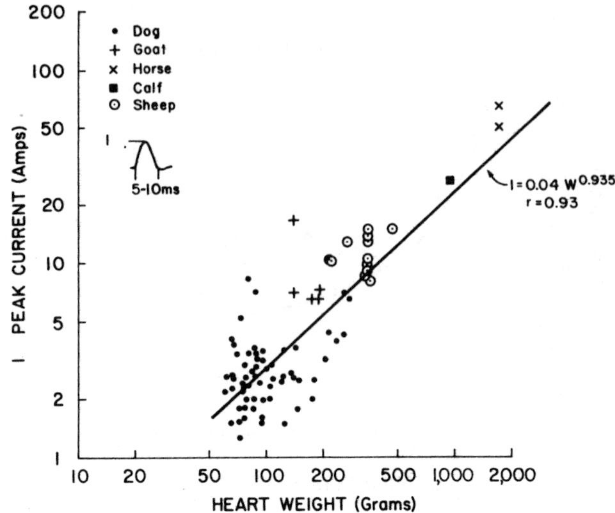

FIGURE 9.15. Threshold peak current versus heart weight for defibrillation with 5–10 msec damped sinusoidal current applied to transventricular electrodes. [Redrawn from Geddes et al. (1974).]

dence of the principle of distribution of thresholds. Figures 9.20, 9.21, and 9.22 offer additional evidence for this principle.

It was stated previously that the output of present-day defibrillators is described in energy units, either stored or delivered into a 50-ohm resistive load (which simulates the human thorax). It is current flow that effects defibrillation and in the case of the damped-sine-wave defibrillator, the current intensity is related to the setting of the energy control on the defibrillator.

Direct-Heart Defibrillation with 5–10 msec Pulses

Animal Subjects. The threshold peak current and energy required to defibrillate small and large animal hearts with 5–10 msec damped sinusoidal current is shown in Figures 9.15 and 9.16. Both illustrations show that more peak current and energy are required as heart weight is increased; this is the dose concept.

Human Subjects. Tacker *et al.* (1975) determined the energy required to defibrillate human hearts with directly applied electrodes. The subjects were on cardiopulmonary bypass and the measurements were made with body temperatures ranging from 26°C to 36°C. Figure 9.17*a* presents the data obtained in Tacker's study which reveals that hearts weighting 400 g were defibrillated with 5 J; hearts weighing 500 g required

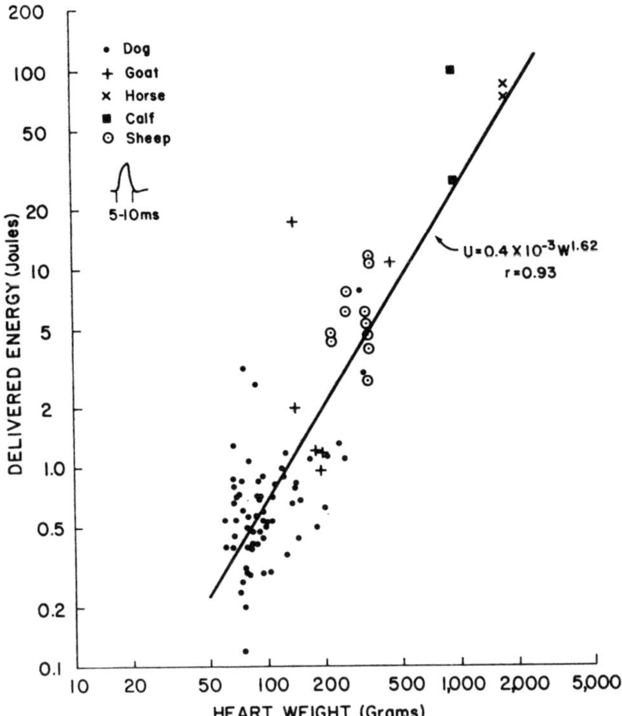

FIGURE 9.16. Threshold delivered energy versus heart weight for defibrillation with 5–10 msec damped sinusoidal current applied to transventricular electrodes. [Redrawn from Geddes et al. (1974).]

10 J. On only one occasion, a 550-g heart required 20 J. Tacker therefore recommended that 5 J should be used as the initial energy setting for direct-heart defibrillation of adult hearts with damped sine waves.

Kerber *et al.* (1980) also carried out a study to determine the threshold current and energy required to defibrillate the adult human heart. Using damped sinusoidal current applied to 202 human hearts, they found that the peak current required ranged from 8 to 34 A, with the mean and standard deviation being 12 ± 5 A. The transventricular impedance was 23 ± 9 ohms and the delivered energy required varied between 5 and 20 J. The percent successful defibrillation varied with shock strength and whether one or two shocks were delivered. Figure 9.17*b* presents a summary of their experience.

An analysis of Tacker's and Kerber's data reveals that a typical 350-g human heart requires about 10 A (peak) for defibrillation. A typical value for the impedance of the electrode–heart circuit is about 25–35 ohms. It is interesting to note that the peak current and energy required for a 350-g

(a)

(b)

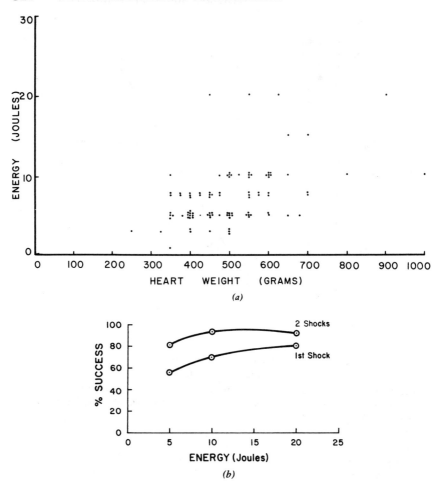

FIGURE 9.17. (*a*) Threshold damped sinusoidal energy required to defibrillate the human heart [data from Tacker, and Geddes (1980)]. (*b*) Percent successful defibrillation of the adult human heart with damped sinusoidal current using one and two shocks of different delivered energy [data from Kerber et al. (1980)].

animal heart, using 5–10 msec damped sinusoidal current, are 10 A and 5 J, respectively (Figures 9.15 and 9.16), indicating a considerable similarity for direct-heart defibrillation.

Closed-Chest Defibrillation

The current required for ventricular defibrillation with thoracic electrodes depends on a variety of factors that include subject size, electrode size

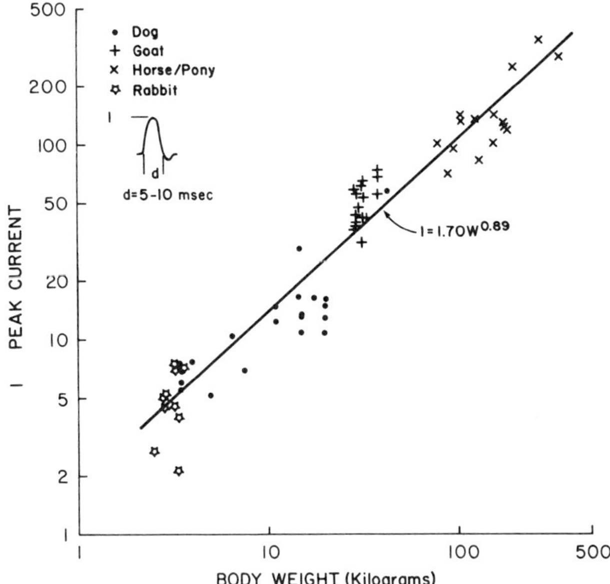

FIGURE 9.18. Threshold peak current required for defibrillating animals of different body weights using 5–10 msec damped sine wave current. [Redrawn from Geddes et al. (1974).]

and placement, and the presence of myocardial disease and/or drugs. The two most important factors are subject size and electrode location. At present it is recommended that one electrode is placed over the apex-beat area and the other is either on the right chest below the clavicle or on the back, below the left scapula. Figure 9.7 shows the precordial placement and Figure 9.8 shows the chest-to-back placement. Frequently, the electrode placed on the back is larger (e.g., 15 cm) than the chest electrodes (9 cm). The posterior electrode is sometimes located between the scapulae. One manufacturer provides a very large electrode that is slipped under the subject's back. As yet there is no strong evidence to indicate whether the precordial or chest-to-back placement is optimal for ventricular defibrillation, although the chest-to-back placement is preferred for atrial defibrillation (Lown, 1964).

Animal Subjects. In studies on a large number of animals ranging from 5 to 750 lb, the author (Geddes *et al.*, 1974) reported the relationship between threshold current and body weight for a first-shock successful defibrillation; Figure 9.18 presents this relationship for 5–10 msec damped sinusoidal current.

Figure 9.19 illustrates the threshold energy versus body weight rela-

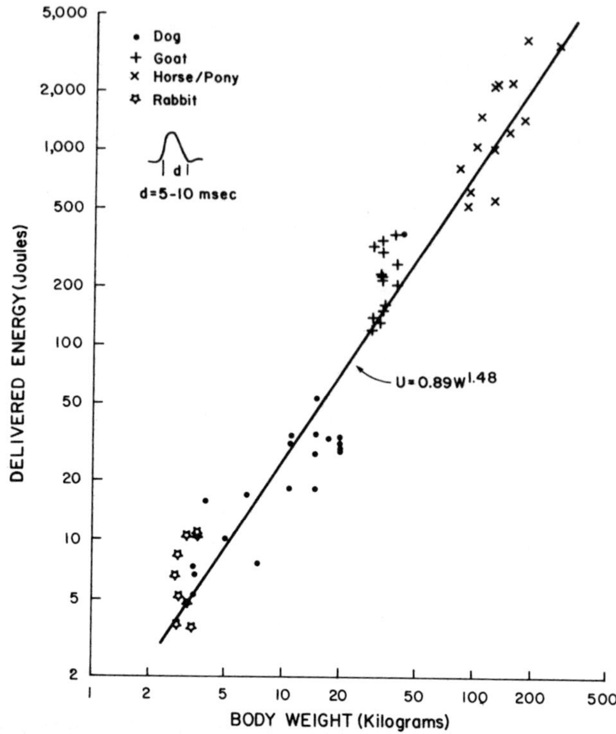

FIGURE 9.19. Threshold energy required for defibrillating animals of different body weights using 5–10 msec damped sine wave current. [Redrawn from Geddes et al. (1974).]

tionship for the same population of animals using 5–10 msec damped sine wave current.

Figures 9.15, 9.16, 9.18, and 9.19 clearly indicate the dose concept, that is, more energy and current are required as heart and body weight are increased. However, at any body weight, it is clear that some animals require less and others require more energy and current for defibrillation. For example, some dogs require 0.9 J/kg, while others require about 3.6 J/kg. This is evidence of the threshold-distribution principle. Figure 9.20 presents the energy and current dose distribution for dogs. In Figure 9.20 if any dose is selected, all of the animals to the left of this dose will be defibrillated; those to the right will not because the energy and current are too low. Therefore, by counting the number of subjects to the left of a selected dose, a plot can be composed to show the percentage of animals successfully defibrillated versus the dose; Figure 9.21 presents such a relationship for energy and peak current. It is for this reason that it has been customary to discuss percent successful defibrillation when identifying a particular energy and body or heart weight.

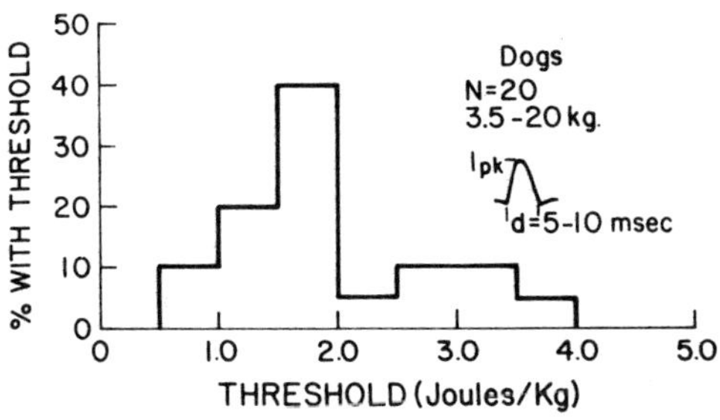

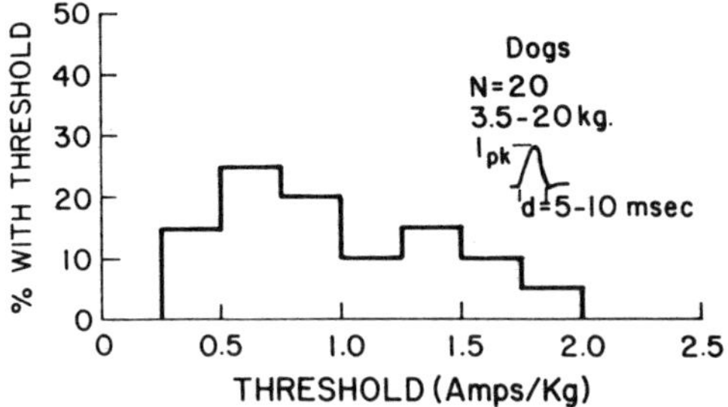

FIGURE 9.20. Energy and current per kilogram required to defibrillate dogs with 5–10 msec damped sine wave current with precordial electrodes.

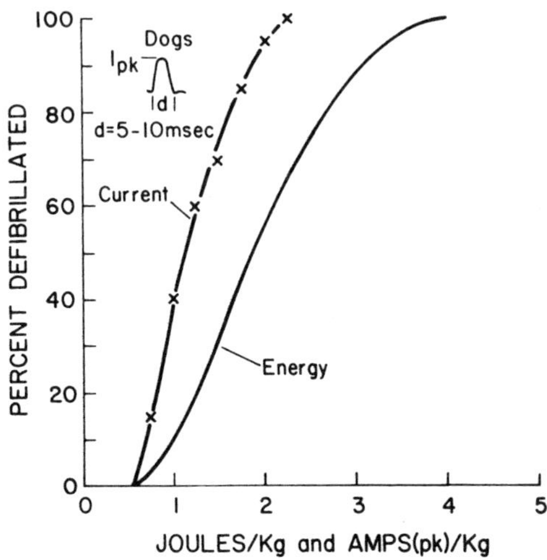

FIGURE 9.21. Percent of dogs defibrillated with increasing energy and current per kilogram.

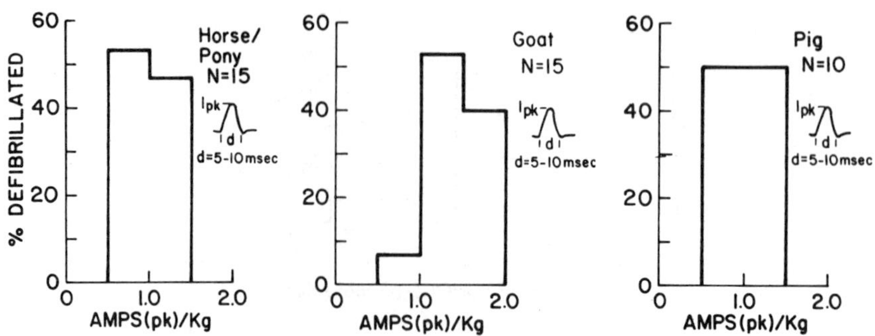

FIGURE 9.22. Range of peak current per kilogram required to defibrillate the horse/pony, goat, and pig.

To demonstrate the threshold distribution for peak current among different species, Figure 9.22 is presented. This illustration shows that the defibrillation threshold ranges from 0.5 to about 2 A/kg using 5–10 msec damped sine wave current.

Human Subjects. For defibrillation of the ventricles of children with transchest electrodes, Gutgesell et al. (1976) recommended a dose of 2 J/kg be used for subjects ranging in weight from 2.5 to 50 kg. Figure 9.23 presents Gutgesell *et al.'s* data.

At present, there appears to be little controversy over the energy dose for defibrillating children. However, there is some disagreement on the energy levels required for human adults, particularly those who weigh 100 kg or more. The controversy relates, in part, to the technique used and, in part to the definition for successful defibrillation, and also in part, to the type of patient (e.g., in-hospital or out-of-hospital). Moreover, two techniques are employed; with one, multiple low-energy shocks (often interspersed with cardiopulmonary resuscitation) are delivered and with the other, a single higher energy first shock is employed. The controversy is by no means settled and is unlikely to be for some time.

Presently available damped-sine-wave defibrillators store 400 J of energy and deliver about 350 into a 50-ohm resistor. A few manufacturers provide experimental defibrillators with higher stored energy levels. However, the most important point relative to using such devices for transchest defibrillation is to adopt a dose concept, that is, the strength of the shock required is related to the size of the subject's heart. The practice of turning the output control to a maximum and delivering full output to all adult subjects is very ill advised and can be dangerous. As stated earlier, the output used should be selected on the basis of subject size. The low-energy, multiple-shock advocates recommend starting with an

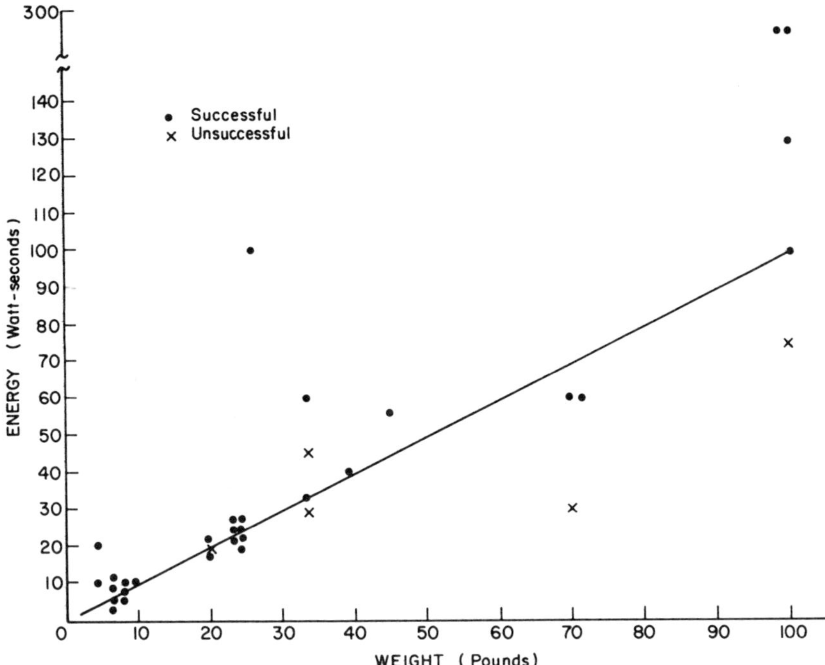

FIGURE 9.23. Energy–body weight relationship for defibrillating children with damped sine wave current. [Redrawn from Gutgesell et al. (1976).]

energy dose of about 2 J/kg of body weight for adult human subjects using damped-sine-wave current. Those who advocate the use of a single shock believe that the starting dose required is about 4 J/kg of body weight for adult subjects.

It is a common experience that very large subjects are difficult to defibrillate. Two published studies which report percent success in achieving defibrillation versus body weight were reported by Tacker et al. (1974) and Pantridge et al. (1975). The defibrillators used by both groups were capable of storing 400 J and delivering about 320 or slightly more. Figure 9.24 presents the percent success data reported by these two groups.

Adgey *et al.* (1978) carried out studies in which single and multiple 100- and 200-J shocks were used to defibrillate human subjects, ranging in weight from 30 to 100 kg. Figure 9.25 presents the percent success versus body weight histograms for the 100- and 200-J shocks. By dividing the energy by the body weight and calculating the percent success, a percent success versus energy dose curve can be composed as shown in Figure 9.26. This illustration clearly shows an increasing percent success with an

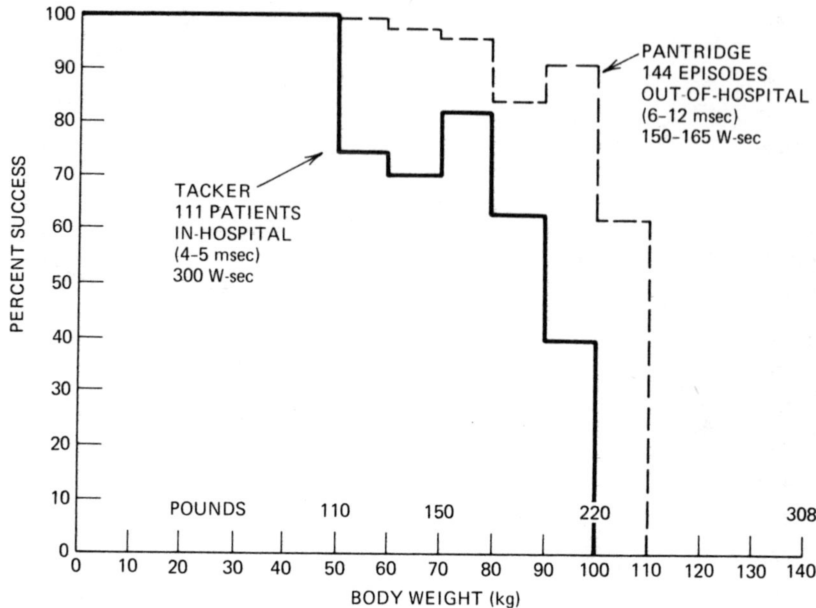

FIGURE 9.24. Percent successful defibrillation versus body weight for damped sine wave defibrillators with 400 J of stored energy. [Redrawn from Tacker et al. (1974) and Pantridge et al. (1975).]

increasing energy dose. Almost 100% successful defibrillation was achieved with about 4 J/kg.

TRAPEZOIDAL-WAVE DEFIBRILLATION

Schuder *et al.* (1964, 1966) showed that the square (Figure 9.9*e*) and trapezoidal waves (Figure 9.9*f*) were effective in defibrillating the ventricles of dogs using thoracic electrodes. Based on this demonstration, defibrillators delivering these waveforms became available commercially. The circuitry used to produce both the low- and high-tilt waveforms is the same and is shown in Figure 9.27. The energy is stored in a capacitor *C*. When the pulse of current is to be delivered, a silicon-controlled rectifier (SCR1) is triggered to become conducting and current flows from the capacitor into the subject. As the capacitor discharges, the current decreases exponentially. Current flow through the subject is arrested by triggering SCR2, which short circuits the capacitor. Thus the current waveform is a truncated exponential, which is sometimes designated a

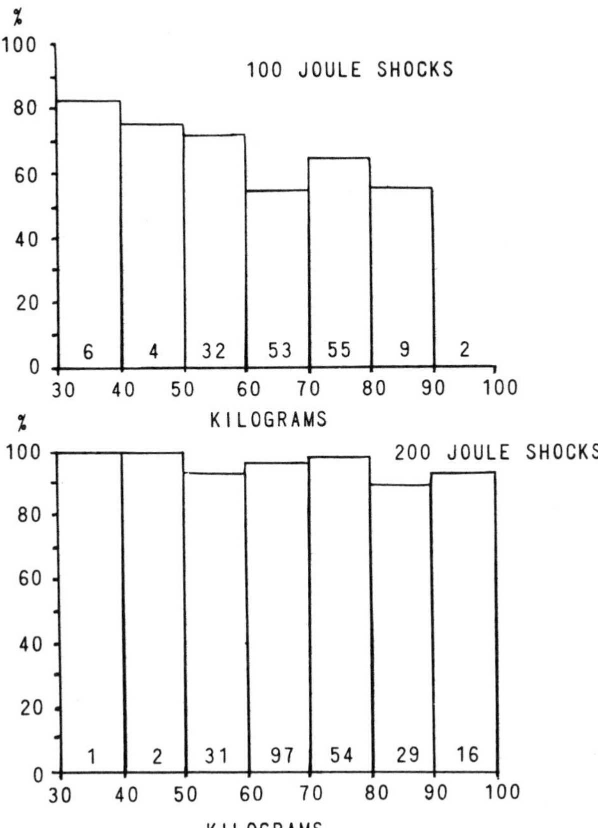

FIGURE 9.25. Percent successful defibrillation of human subjects with damped-sine-wave current. (*a*) The percent success with single and multiple 100-J shocks. (*b*) The percent success with 200-*J* shocks. [Composed from data presented by Adgey et al. (1978).]

trapezoidal wave. If the decrease in current during the pulse is small, the wave is called a square wave or low-tilt trapezoid. If the decrease in current is considerable (e.g., more than 50%), the waveform is called a high-tilt trapezoid. The fractional decrease in current is called the tilt, being defined as $(I_i - I_f)/I_i$, where I_i and I_f are the initial and final currents. The percent tilt is merely 100 times the tilt. Whether the tilt is high or low depends on the size of the capacitor (C), the resistance of the electrode–subject circuit (R_L), and the duration (d) of the pulse of current. The average current for a truncated exponential (trapezoidal) wave depends on the initial current (I_i) and the tilt (T). The average current is $I_iT/\log_e [1/(1 - T)]$.

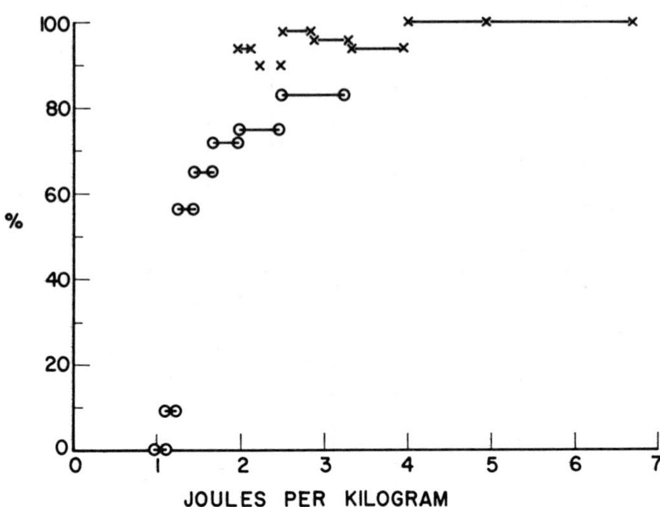

FIGURE 9.26. Percent successful defibrillation for human subjects using different energy doses of damped-sine-wave current. [Composed from data presented by Adgey et al. (1978).]

Direct-Heart Defibrillation

Animal Subjects. The importance of pulse duration in achieving defibrillation with a square wave was demonstrated by Koning et al. (1975) who determined the threshold current necessary to defibrillate dog hearts. Figure 9.28 presents the results of his study, which indicates that

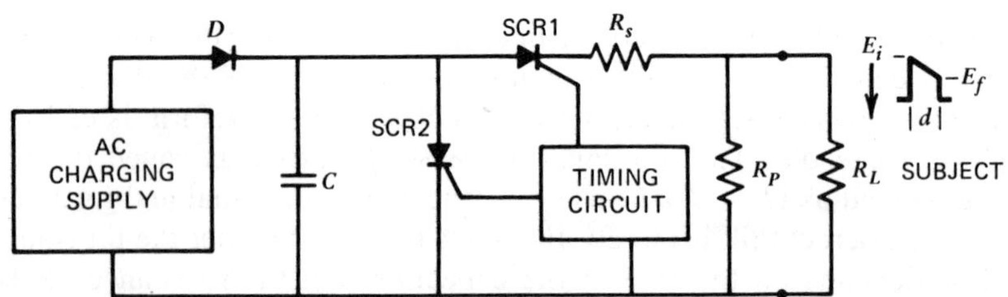

FIGURE 9.27. The circuit employed in the square and trapezoidal waveform defibrillators. The capacitor C is charged by an AC power supply via diode D. When current is to be delivered, SCR1 is turned on and current flows from the capacitor through the subject. The timing circuit terminates the current flow through the subject by turning on SCR2 which short circuits the capacitor. The duration of the pulse of current is determined by the timing circuit.

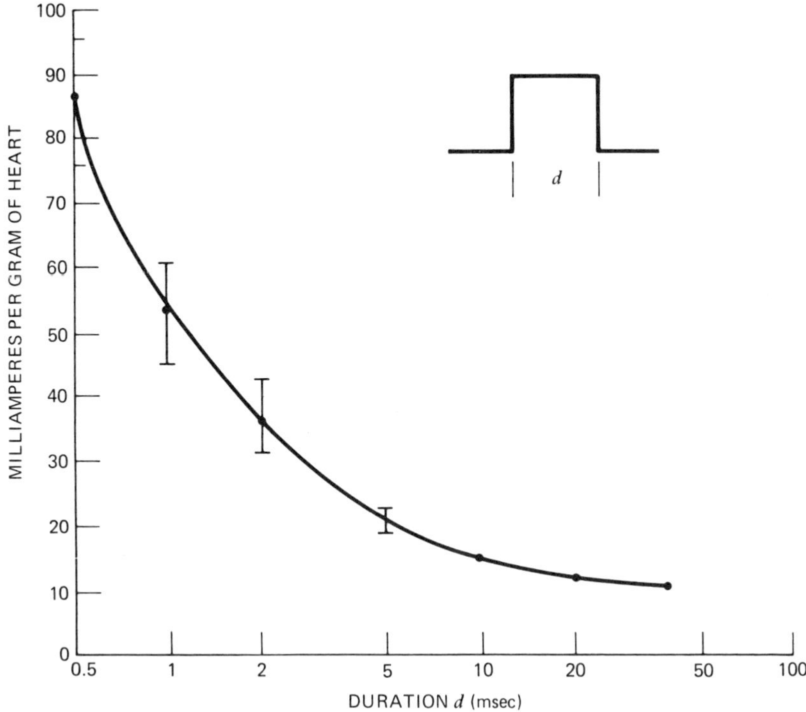

FIGURE 9.28. Threshold square-wave peak current required to defibrillate dog hearts with directly applied electrodes. [Redrawn from Koning et al. (1975).]

the current/gram of heart increases as the duration decreases, thereby offering additional proof of the strength-duration principle.

When the current is allowed to fall during the pulse, the peak current required is increased. To date there are no studies with transventricular electrodes that demonstrate this point. However, information comes from a dog study by Wessale et al. (1980) in which defibrillation was achieved with one electrode in the right ventricle and the other (100-mm distant) in the superior vena cava. The data in Figure 9.29 were scaled from this study to provide equivalent transventricular values and indicate that with increasing tilt, the peak current required increases for all durations that were measured. These extrapolated data allow comparison with the damped-sine wave data in Figure 9.14.

At present, there are no data on the energy required for ventricular defibrillation with trapezoidal waves applied to electrodes on the hearts of animal subjects of different sizes. Interpolation of animal data indicates that the energy levels for the low-tilt trapezoid will be less than those

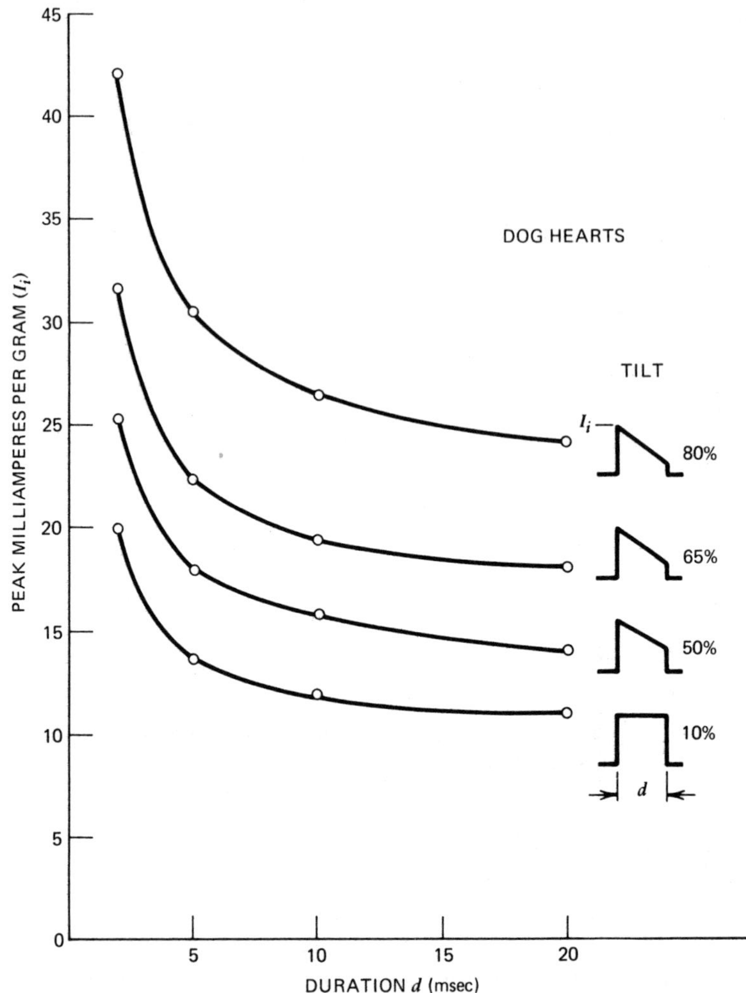

FIGURE 9.29. Calculated threshold peak current per gram of heart required for defibrillation using trapezoidal waves applied transventricular electrodes. [Redrawn from data provided by Wessale et al. (1980) and Koning et al. (1975).]

required with the damped sine wave. With the high-tilt trapezoidal wave (~ 80%), the energy levels are similar to those required with the damped sine wave. This statement can be made because of the equivalence of current comparisons shown in Figures 9.14, 9.28, and 9.29.

Human Subjects. To date there have no published data on the energy and current levels required to defibrillate the human heart with transventricular electrodes using trapezoidal waves. However, the interpolation just presented can be applied, that is, in comparison to the damped sine wave, less energy will be required with the low-tilt trapezoid. The high-tilt trapezoid (~ 80%) should require about the same energy as with the damped sine wave.

Closed-Chest Defibrillations

Animal Subjects. Defibrillation has been accomplished with low- and high-tilt trapezoidal waves applied to small and large animals. A most interesting study was reported by Gold et al. (1979) who examined the increased energy and current required to defibrillate calves as they increased their weight from 50 to 150 kg. A 4-msec square wave was used, and the current and electrode diameter were scaled on the basis of body weight. Figures 9.30*a* and 9.30*b* present the results of this study, and illustrate that for 91–96% success and 49–66% success, the energy required increased with increasing body weight. For the higher percent success (91–96%) the energy dose is about 3 J/kg. Similarly, the peak current (Figure 9.30*b*) required increased with increasing body weight for both the higher and the lower percent success. For the higher-percent success (91–96%), the current dose is about 0.6 A/kg. These two illustrations clearly demonstrate the validity of the dose concept in the same species.

Geddes et al. (1980) reported a similar relationship of increased energy and current with increasing body weight in animals ranging from 6.4 to 101 kg when defibrillated with trapezoidal waves 10 msec in duration with 10%, 50%, 70%, and 90% tilt. The energy dose for the lighter animals (2 J/kg) was less than was required for the heavier animals (4.5 J/kg). Interestingly enough, the dose expressed as average current per kilogram was the same for all animals and for all tilts, for example, 0.4–0.48 A/kg for the 10-msec pulse.

Comparison of Damped-Sine and Trapezoidal Waves

Animal Studies. Animal studies permit determination of the relative efficacies of the damped sine and trapezoidal waveforms, such a comparison that cannot be performed readily in man. As stated previously, it is current flow through the ventricles that achieves defibrillation. Accordingly, it is reasonable to compare these two waveforms on the basis of current. Bourland et al. (1978) measured the peak threshold current required for defibrillation with damped sine waves and trapezoidal waves of the same duration having 90% tilt. Figure 9.31 presents the results of this

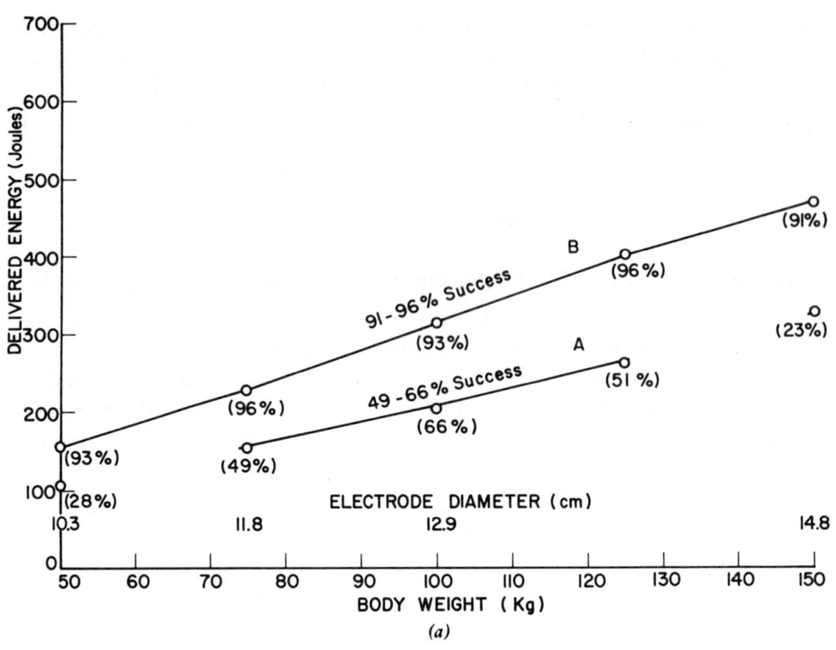

(a)

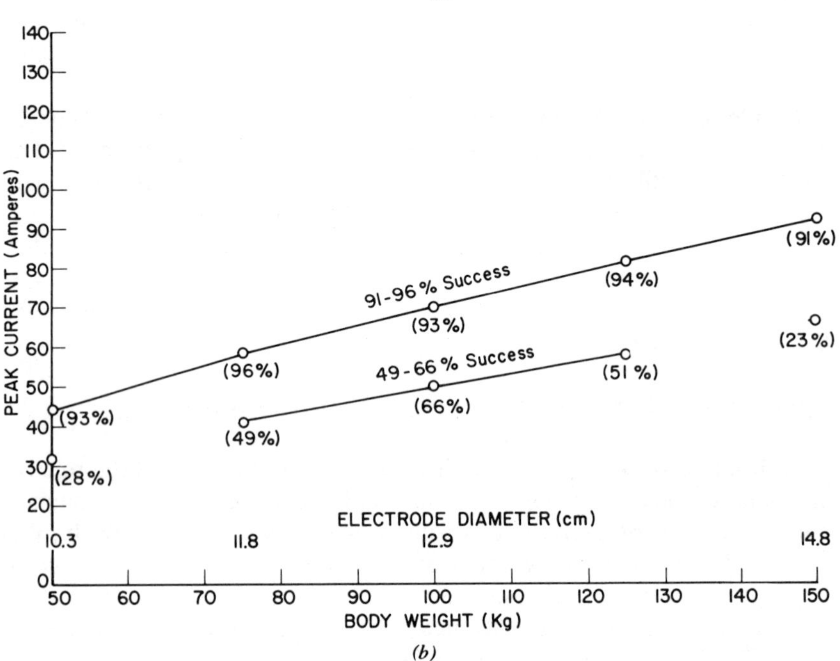

(b)

FIGURE 9.30

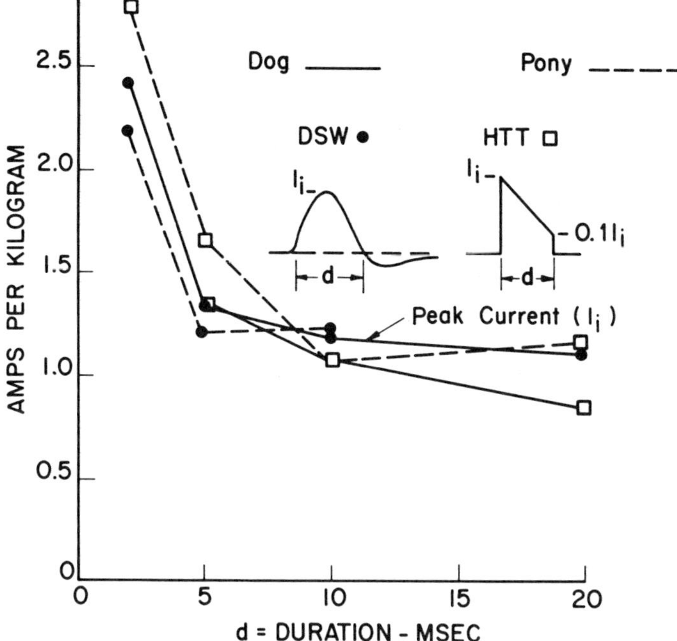

FIGURE 9.31. Comparative efficacy of damped sine wave and high-tilt (90%) trapezoidal waves in achieving ventricular defibrillation with transchest electrodes. [Redrawn from Bourland et al. (1978).]

study, which used dogs and ponies. It is apparent that the threshold peak currents required for defibrillation are essentially the same for these two waveforms. Because of this, the energy levels would be expected to be similar, although not identical.

Average Current Principle. A better method of comparing waveform efficacy was suggested by Bourland *et al.* (1978). They noted that when the average currents were compared among waveforms of the same duration, there was a striking similarity. Bourland tested the validity of this observation by measuring the threshold peak current required for defibrillation with a critically damped sine wave and trapezoidal waves

---

FIGURE 9.30. (*a*) Energy and (*b*) current required for defibrillating calves as they grew from 50 to 100 kg using a 4-msec rectangular wave. The electrode diameter (*d*) in cm was scaled according to $d = 10.1\,(W/50)^{1/3}$, where *W* is the animals weight (kg). The peak current (*I*) was scaled according to $I = I_0\,(W/50)^{2/3}$, where I_0 was 32 or 44 A when the animals entered the study at 50 kg. The line representing the higher percent success results from the higher starting current. [Composed from data reported by Gold et al. (1979).]

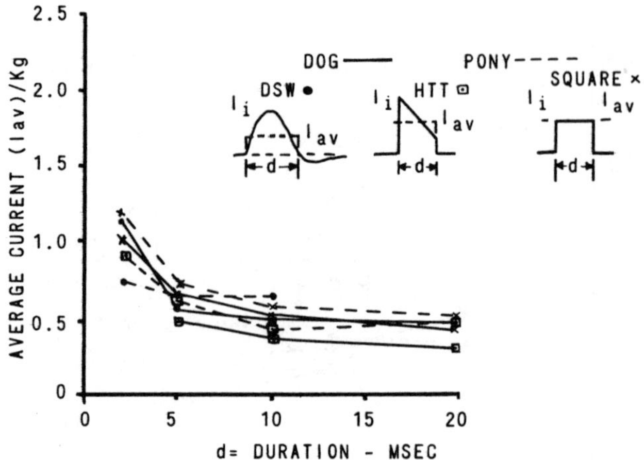

FIGURE 9.32. Strength-duration curves showing the average current required for defibrillation with the damped sine wave and low- and high-tilt trapezoidal waves. [Redrawn from Bourland et al. (1978).]

with 90% and less than 10% tilt, using dogs and ponies. For each waveform the average current was determined from the delivered charge. Figure 9.32 presents the resulting strength-duration curves for average current versus duration. To this illustration has been added the average current data for the damped sine wave. It is interesting to note that despite the wide differences in waveform, the threshold average currents are similar for the range of durations studied.

Human Subjects. At present, there is one square, or low-tilt, trapezoidal waveform defibrillator available commercially. In this device the energy available (250 J) is controlled by varying the duration of the current pulse from a few to about 30 msec. The output voltage is 1200 V and therefore it is capable of delivering 24 A into a 50-ohm resistor. With this defibrillator, Anderson and Suelzer (1956) presented efficacy data relating percent success with body weight; precordial electrodes were used. Figure 9.33 presents the data. It is important to note that the electrodes provided with this 250-J defibrillator are larger than those used with many other defibrillators. In some applications with this defibrillator, a large electrode is placed under the subject and the other electrode is placed on the chest.

At present there is available a defibrillator which produces a 10-msec constant-duration pulse with about 80% tilt. The output is adjustable from 0 to 400 J by varying the output voltage. The device is capable of delivering about 50 A (peak) into a 50-ohm resistor. With this unit, clinical

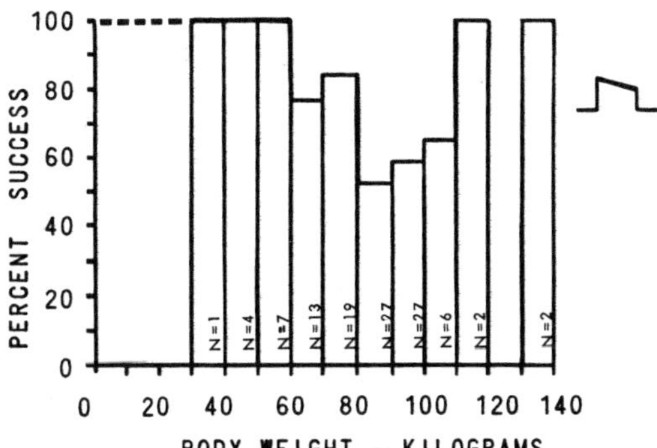

FIGURE 9.33. Percent success versus body weight for a low-tilt trapezoidal waveform defibrillator in which the energy output (max = 250 J) is regulated by varying the duration of the pulse. [Redrawn from Anderson and Suelzer (1976).]

experience indicates that the efficacy is virtually the same as with a 400-J damped-sine-wave defibrillator (Tacker et al., 1976). This evidence is consistent with data obtained by Bourland et al. (1978), in which the threshold current for defibrillation was determined using the damped sine and high-tilt trapezoidal waveforms in the same animal.

MYOCARDIAL DAMAGE

There is no doubt that the use of energy and current levels that are much in excess of the threshold required for defibrillation will depress contractility and even damage myocardial cells. It is therefore especially important to avoid the practice. However, it is of equal importance to know if there is a safety margin, that is, the level between the threshold for defibrillation and the threshold for myocardial damage. Unfortunately, it is difficult to obtain such information because human hearts that are defibrillated usually have underlying cardiac disease, and it would be difficult to quantify defibrillator-induced damage from that due to the disease. Nonetheless, animal studies provide some information on the safety margin for defibrillating current waveforms.

At present myocardial damage is a term that is used loosely. For example, some ascribe postdefibrillation changes in the ECG to myocardial damage; others require that there be histologic evidence of alteration in myocardial cells. Some accept an elevation in serum enzymes (of cardiac origin); others require that there be scintigraphic evidence of myocardial cell injury. Although all four indicators can identify myocardial damage, they do not always predict the amount of physiologic impairment.

Animal studies with damped-sine-wave current provide useful information. For example, the data reported by Peleska (1965) reveal that the threshold for arrhythmias was about 1.8 times the threshold energy for defibrillation. Lown (1967) reported a somewhat higher value. Tacker et al. (1978) reported no damage to the myocardium with a threshold defibrillating shock. Van Vleet et al. (1978) reported mild cellular damage with a single shock of nine times threshold energy. Ehsani et al. (1976) reported ECG changes and gross and microscopic cardiac damage with 10 shocks of 3–4 times threshold. Di Cola et al. (1976) reported data which showed that about 0.15% of the heart was damaged following a single shock of about three times threshold energy. Dahl et al. (1974) showed that the overdose damage was less with larger electrodes and when the time between multiple shocks was increased. Finally, Babbs et al. (1976, 1978) reported that a single shock of 15 times threshold energy produced myocardial damage in 50% of the animals studied.

From all of these studies, it appears that threshold shocks do not damage the normal animal heart. Shocks with three times threshold energy can produce cellular damage in the myocardium. Whether these data apply to the human heart is not known.

Despite these well-conducted and informative studies on myocardial response due to overdose defibrillator shocks, they do not provide direct evidence on the functional degree of myocardial impairment. In addition, none of these studies have directed themselves toward comparison of the postdefibrillation pumping capability differences due to the different current waveforms. In order to obtain this type of information, Niebauer et al. (1982) conducted studies with a metabolically supported working dog heart suspended in an isoresistive and isotonic volume conductor. In the volume conductor were placed two large area defibrillating electrodes (1,2) as shown in Figure 9.34. Because of the resistivity matching, the current density distribution was virtually uniform. A support dog provided oxygenated blood delivered retrograde into the aortic stump. After passing through the coronary arteries, the blood from the right ventricle was returned to the support dog. The left ventricle contracted isovolumically and the pressure therein was recorded as a measure of the ventricular force. The left ventricular diastolic loading could be selected as desired.

The method for determining myocardial depression consisted of fibrillating the ventricles and determining the threshold current for defibrillation. Then with the heart fibrillating, shocks above threshold strength were delivered and the percent myocardial depression was calculated. Percent myocardial depression was defined as the difference between the peak preshock systolic pressure minus the immediate peak postshock systolic pressure, divided by the peak preshock systolic pres-

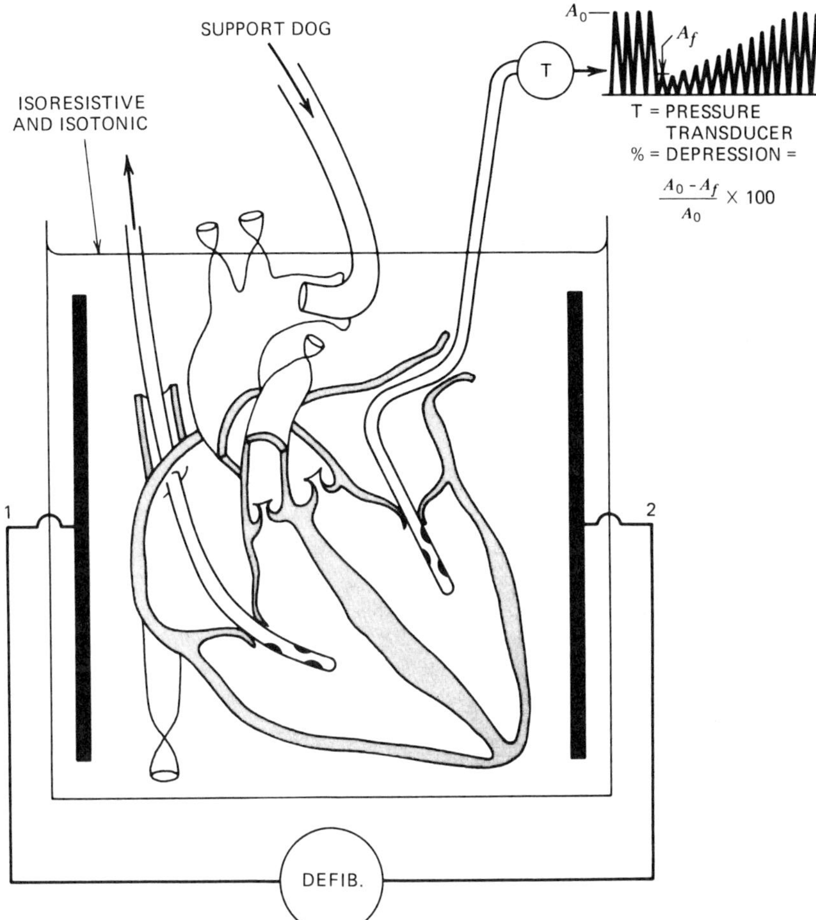

FIGURE 9.34. Isolated heart preparation used for myocardial depression studies. [Courtesy M. Niebauer (1982).]

sure; multiplying this quotient by 100 provided percent myocardial depression. Figure 9.34 (inset) illustrates this definition.

Niebauer determined the percent myocardial depression versus the overdose ratio for several different waveforms. Overdose ratio is the ratio of the shock strength to threshold strength for defibrillation. Figure 9.35 presents the results of Niebauer's study and indicates that the amount of myocardial depression increases with the overdose ratio for all waveforms tested; it also indicates that there is little difference between the various waveforms (except for the 2-msec square wave). It is important to

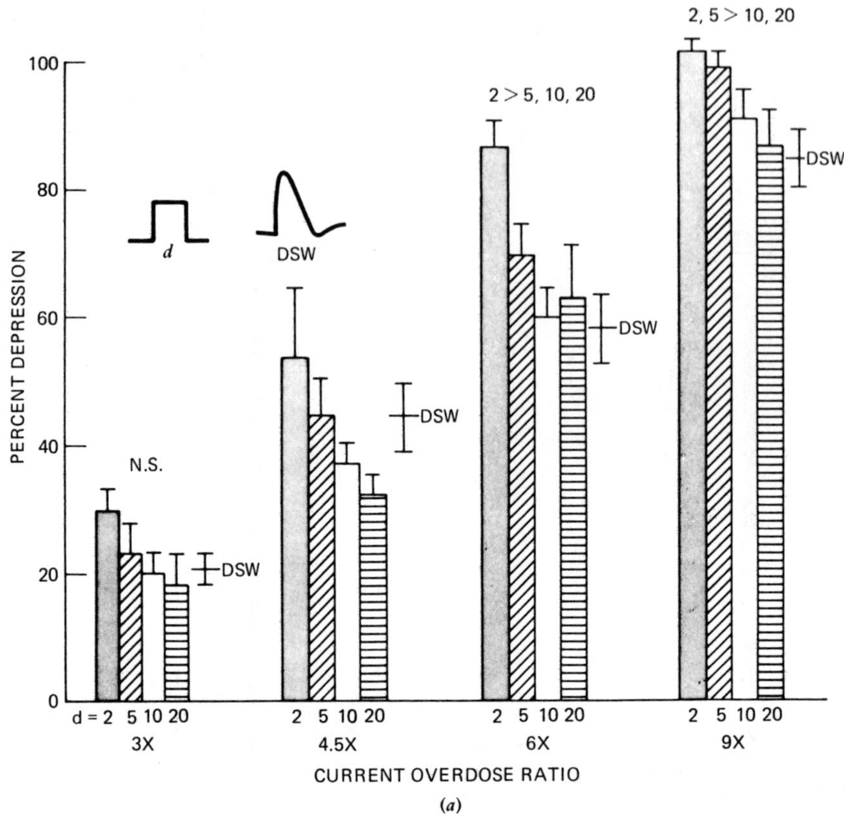

(*a*)

FIGURE 9.35. (*a*) Percent myocardial depression for different current overdose ratios. A illustrates the percent myocardial depression with square waves of 2-, 5-, 10-, and 20-msec duration and damped sine waves of 4–6 msec in duration. (*b*) The percent myocardial depression with trapezoidal waves (10 msec in duration) having < 10%, 45%, 65%, and 80% tilt. [Courtesy M. Niebauer (1982).]

recall that the threshold peak current for defibrillation is different for the different waveforms, but the effect of overdose is remarkably similar in producing myocardial depression. Niebauer found that myocardial depression is minimal with a threshold defibrillating shock. Therefore, the price of overdose shock is temporary myocardial depression.

SUMMARY

At this time, the output of all defibrillators is described in terms of energy. This practice originated with the studies by MacKay and Leeds (1953) in

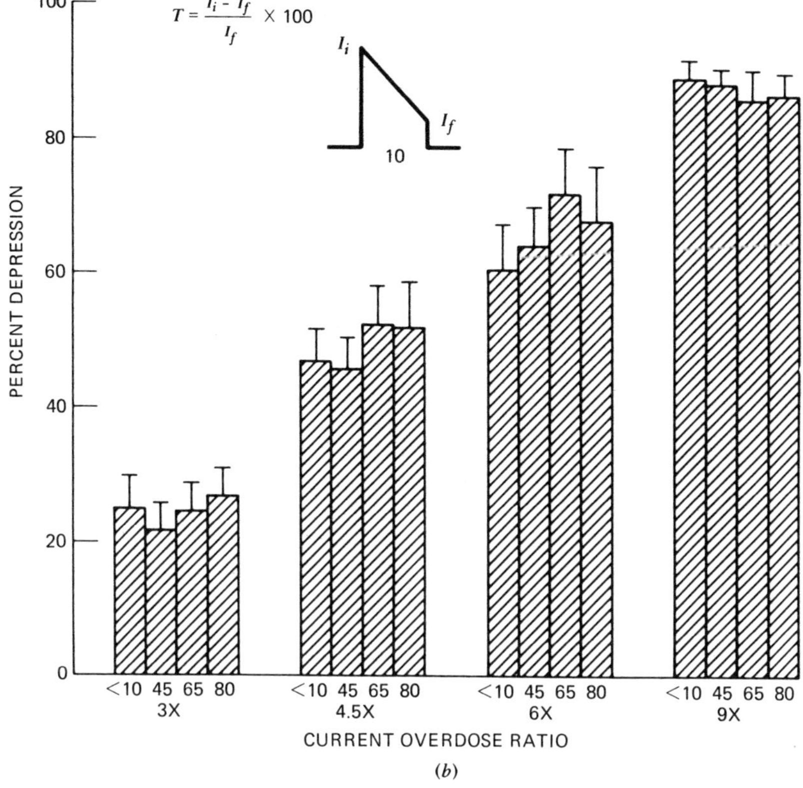

(*b*)

FIGURE 9.35 (*Continued*)

which it was postulated that the energy delivered is the best electrical descriptor of what is required for ventricular defibrillation. It is well known, and clearly stated by MacKay and Leeds, that it is the current that flows through the ventricles that achieves defibrillation. Thus there is a need to establish an adequate current density in a critical mass of the ventricles for an adequate time, short as the latter may be. For this reason, there is a relationship between current intensity and duration of current flow, and heart and body weight. With most defibrillators there is a direct relationship between delivered current and the energy setting. Therefore, for each current waveform there is a relationship between body and heart weight and the energy required for defibrillation.

Of all of the factors discussed in this chapter, the dose concept is the most important. Failure to deliver an adequate energy and current results in failure to defibrillate. The use of an excessive shock strength will defibrillate but impairs the ability of the myocardium to contract, and very high current and energy will damage heart cells. There are only limited

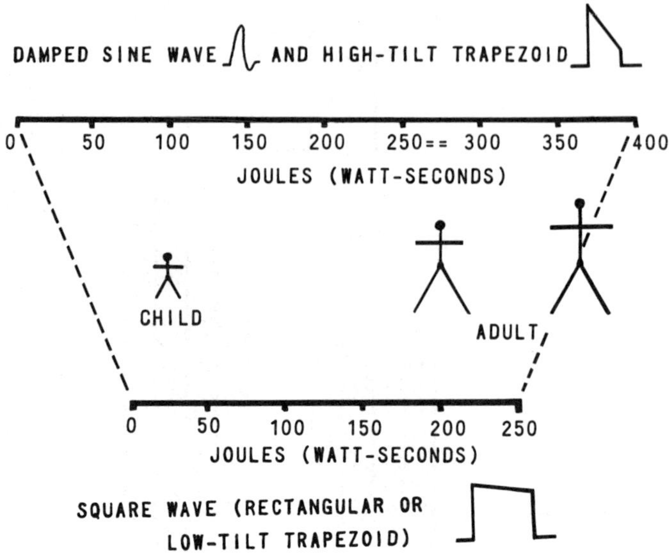

FIGURE 9.36. The dose concept for ventricular defibrillation.

human data to indicate the margin of safety, that is, the ratio of energy for myocardial damage to the threshold for defibrillation. However, it has been shown that for both the damped sine wave and trapezoidal wave, myocardial damage is not seen until nearly twice-threshold energy is delivered to normal dog hearts.

The dose concept is slowly evolving and is illustrated in Figure 9.36 for transchest (and chest-to-back) electrodes. Of some importance in using the dose concept is the technique of defibrillation. At present, two techniques are used; with one, defibrillation is achieved by delivering multiple low-energy shocks and with the other, a single, slightly higher energy shock achieves defibrillation. There are no data available to indicate which of the two techniques is optimum.

EQUIVALENT CIRCUIT FOR SUBJECT

At this point it is useful to examine the equivalent circuit for thoracic and direct-heart electrodes. Figure 9.37 presents a typical model. The electrode–subject interface consists of resistance and capacitance, the impedance of which is quite low and inversely dependent on current density and electrode area. The intervening tissue also contains resistive and capaci-

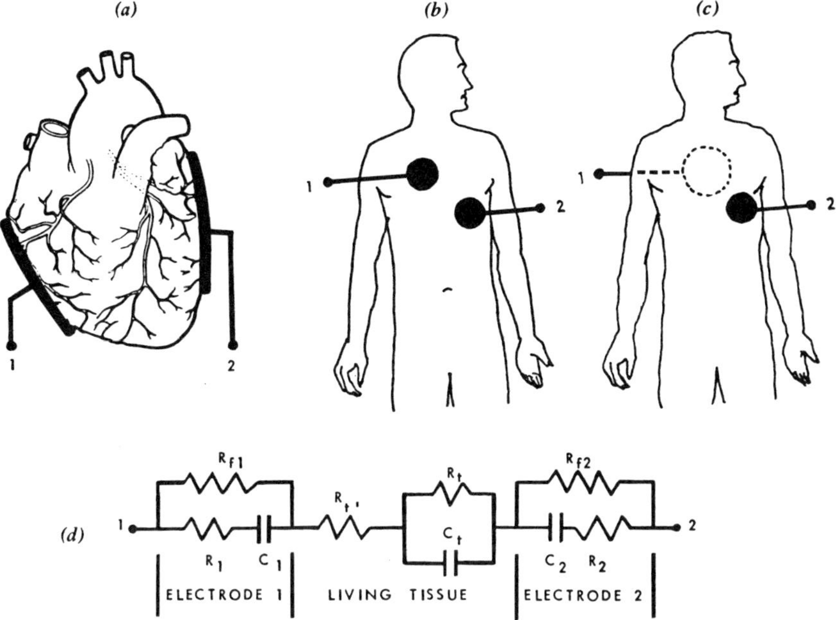

FIGURE 9.37. Typical electrode application (a, b, c) and an equivalent circuit (*d*). R_{f1}, R_1 E_1, and $R_{f2}R_2E_2$ represent the electrode–electrolyte interface impedance; R_tC_t represent the impedance of the intervening tissues.

tive components. For the high current pulses used in defibrillation, the circuit is mainly resistive.

If the impedance to low intensity sinusoidal current is measured, the reactive components of the circuit can be identified. Figure 9.38 presents the typical impedance–frequency characteristic for 3.5-in. defibrillating electrodes applied to the thorax of human subjects. Note that a direct-current ohmmeter will not measure a resistance equivalent to that offered to defibrillating current. However, the impedance measured in the 25–75 kHz region provides a fair equivalent impedance (Geddes et al., 1976).

It was stated previously that single and multiple shocks are used for defibrillation. It is important to recognize that with the same defibrillator setting, the peak current increases slightly with successive shocks owing to a decrease in thoracic impedance. Geddes *et al.* (1975) and Dahl *et al.* (1976) made this observation in dogs and Chambers *et al.* (1978) confirmed it in humans. Figure 9.39 presents data on the decrease in thoracic impedance with successive shocks.

Because the current used for human defibrillation is relatively un-

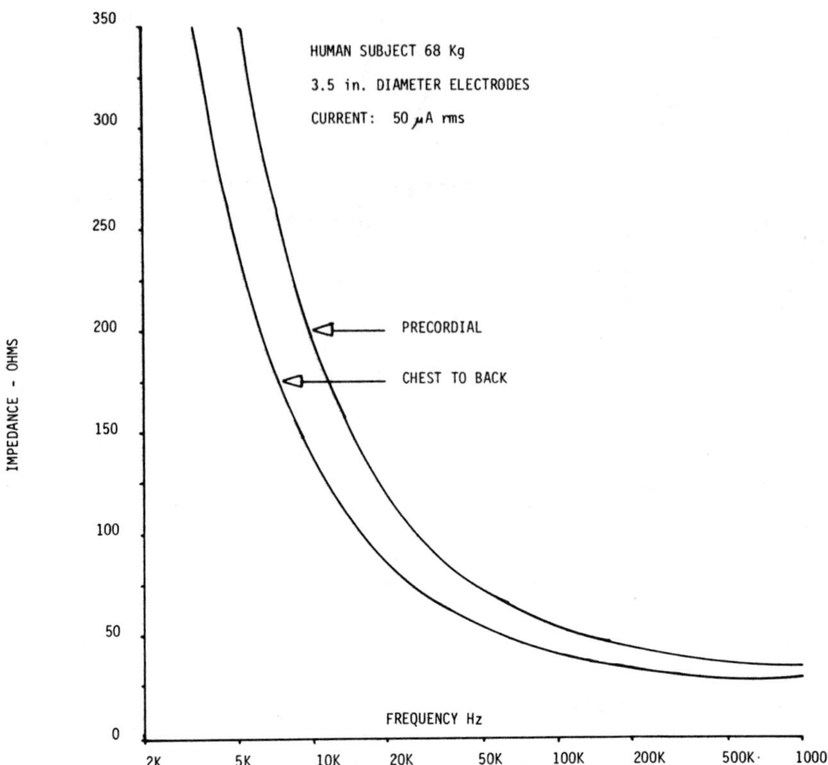

FIGURE 9.38. Sinusoidal impedance–frequency curves for 3.5-in. defibrillating electrodes applied to the thorax of an adult human subject.

known, the thoracic impedance is relatively unknown. To obtain information on this important point, Machin (1978) measured the currents and voltages used in human defibrillation and calculated the impedance. Figure 9.40 presents his data, which show that although the nominal thoracic impedance is about 50 ohms; values ranging from 25 to 125 ohms are encountered.

TESTING DEFIBRILLATORS

There are several different types of testers for evaluating the output of a defibrillator. All contain a 50-ohm load resistor. Some are simple devices that contain a neon lamp which flashes when current above a certain level has been delivered. Other types contain electronic circuitry that computes the energy delivered to the 50-ohm resistor, $\int i^2 R dt$, where i is the

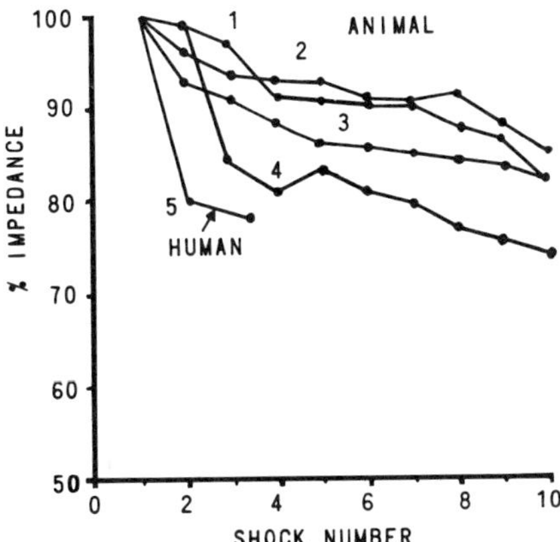

FIGURE 9.39. The decrease in thoracic impedance with successive shocks. Curve 1 represents 300-J shocks delivered to 61–64-kg sheep; 2 represents 800-J shocks delivered to 73–77-kg pigs; 3 represents 1000-J shocks delivered to 70–120-kg pigs; 4 represents 1200-V shocks delivered to human subjects. [Data redrawn from Geddes et al. (1975) and Chambers et al. (1978).]

current, $R = 50$ ohms, and t is time. The latter type of instrument is very convenient for testing all types of defibrillators.

Damped-Sine-Wave Defibrillator

Babbs and Whistler (1978) developed a simple method of determining the magnitude of the internal resistance, capacitance, and inductance, without gaining access to the internal circuitry. The method consists of discharging the defibrillator into at least two resistors which cause the waveform to be underdamped. The voltage waveform is recorded on a

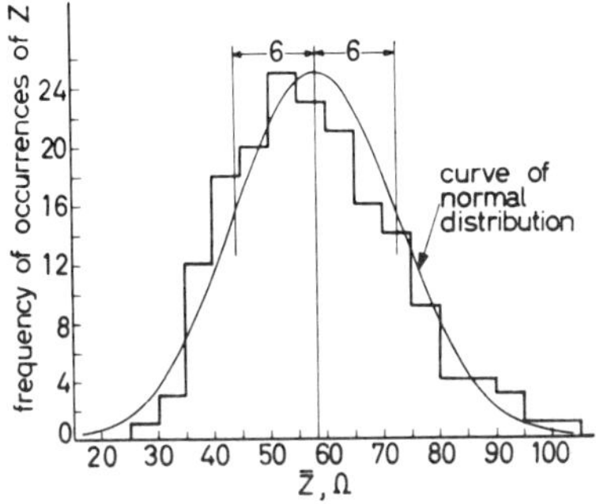

FIGURE 9.40. Human thoracic impedance offered to damped sine wave defibrillating current. [From Machin (1978).]

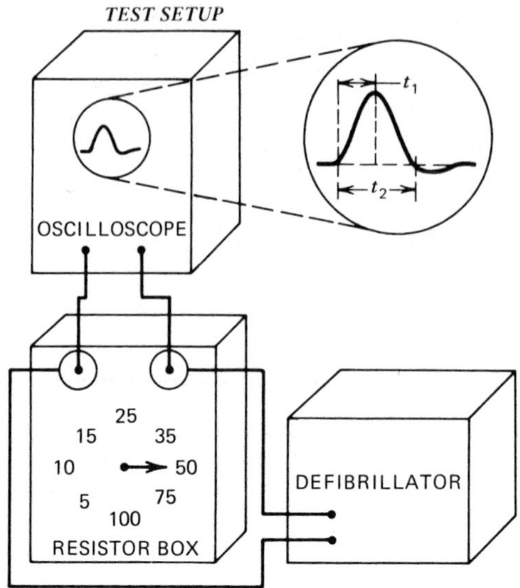

FIGURE 9.41. Arrangement of apparatus for determining the internal resistance, inductance, and capacitance of a damped-sine-wave defibrillator. [Redrawn from Babbs and Whistler (1978).]

storage oscilloscope and the time to peak (t_1) and the time to the first baseline crossing (t_2) are measured. Figure 9.41 illustrates the arrangement of equipment and the manner of measuring these two times.

Using t_1 and t_2, values for $\hat{a}$ and $\hat{c}$, are calculated as follows:

$$\hat{a} = \frac{\pi}{t_2 \tan(\pi t_1/t_2)}$$

$$\hat{c} = \frac{2\hat{a}}{\hat{a}^2 + (\pi/t_2)^2}$$

These values are plotted for the various values of resistance used to test the defibrillator. Figure 9.42 presents a plot of $\hat{a}$ and $\hat{c}$ for 10 and 50 ohms. By measuring the slopes and intercepts, the internal resistance (R_t), inductance (L), and capacitance (C) can be calculated as follows.

From the plot of $\hat{a}$ versus R:

$$R_t = \frac{\text{Intercept}}{\text{Slope}}$$

$$L = \frac{1}{2(\text{Slope})}$$

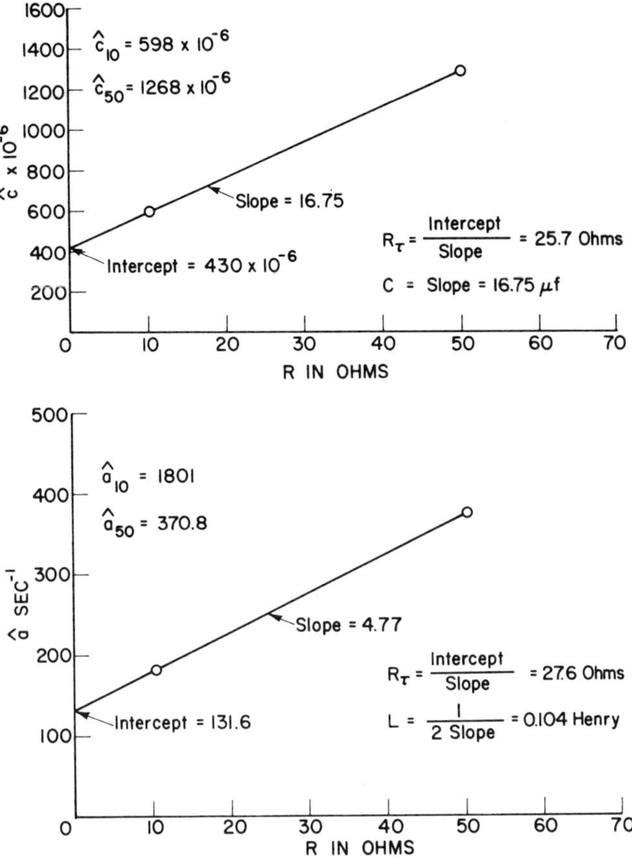

FIGURE 9.42. Plots of $\hat{a}$ and $\hat{c}$ versus R used to calculate R_t, L, and C for a damped-sine-wave defibrillator.

From the plot of $\hat{c}$ versus R

$$R_t = \frac{\text{Intercept}}{\text{Slope}}$$

$$C = \text{Slope}$$

Note that the internal resistance (R_t) can be obtained from either plot. By knowing R_t, the percent delivered energy into any load (R) can be calculated as follows:

$$\text{Percent Delivered} = \frac{100\,R}{R + R_t}$$

Trapezoidal-Wave Defibrillator

Babbs et al. (1980) described a method for determining the internal constants of the trapezoidal-wave defibrillator. The circuit diagram of such a unit, shown in Figure 9.27, reveals that there are three important components: the energy-storage capacitor (C), the internal series resistance (R_s), and parallel resistance (R_p). The method reported by Babbs et al. permits calculation of the values of all three components by measuring the output voltage waveform when the defibrillator is discharged into three or more load resistors.

Briefly, the use of Babbs' method involves measuring the initial (E_i) and final (E_f) voltages and duration (d) when the defibrillator is discharged into each load resistor (R_L). From these data the time constant (τ) is calculated as follows:

$$\tau = \frac{d}{\log_e (E_i/E_f)}$$

The open-circuit time constant (τ_∞) is calculated by making $R_L = \infty$. A plot of $\tau/(\tau_\infty - \tau)$ versus R_L provides a straight line. From the slope and intercept, it is possible to calculate R_s and R_p as follows:

$$R_s = \frac{\text{Intercept}\,(1 + \text{Intercept})}{\text{Slope}}$$

$$R_p = \frac{1 + \text{Intercept}}{\text{Slope}}$$

To determine the internal capacitance (C), the value of the equivalent internal resistance (R_{eq}) is calculated as follows:

$$R_{eq} = R_s + \frac{R_p R_L}{R_p + R_L}$$

Tabular data for R_{eq} and τ permit plotting a graph of τ versus R_{eq}. The slope of this line is C.

Figure 9.43*a* is a plot of $\tau/(\tau_\infty - \tau)$ versus R_L for an experimental trapezoidal-wave defibrillator. From the slope and intercept, R_s and R_p were calculated to be 3.40 and 486 ohms, respectively. Figure 9.43*b* is a plot of τ versus R_{eq}, the slope of which provides a value of 194 μF for the internal capacitance. The component value for C was 200 μF and R_p was 500 ohms.

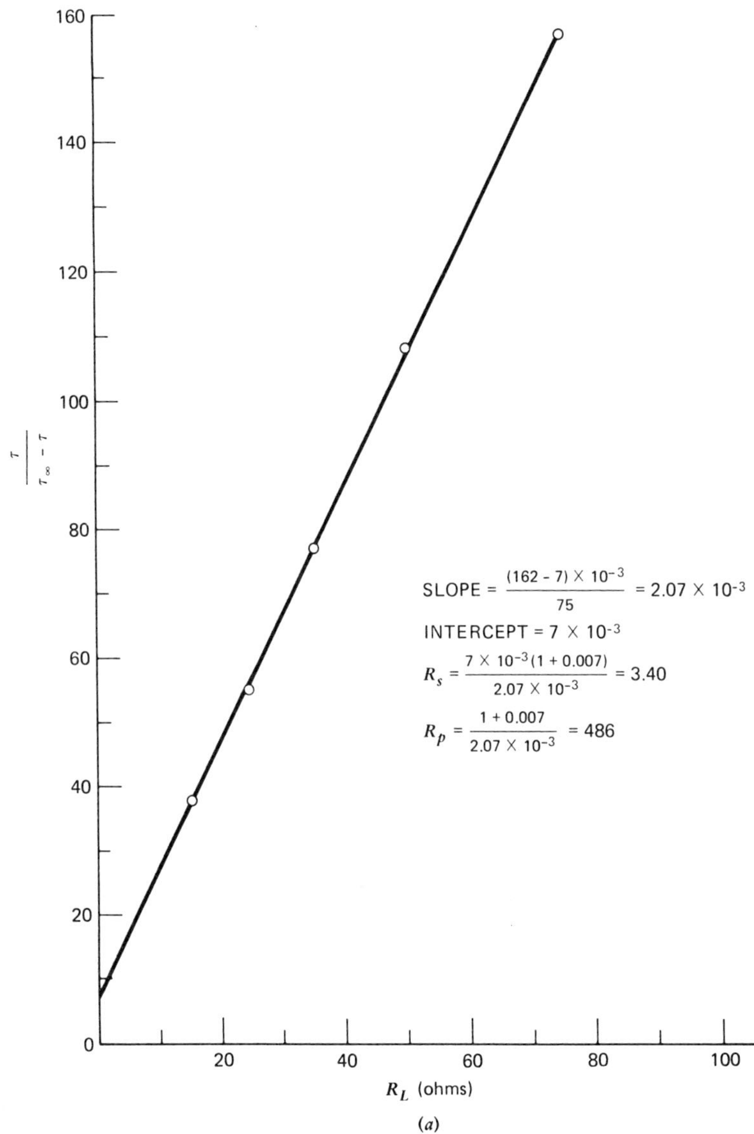

(*a*)

FIGURE 9.43. (*a*) Plot of $\tau/(\tau_\infty - \tau)$ versus load resistance R_L and calculation of R_s and R_p from slope and intercept. (*b*) Plot of τ versus R_{eq} and calculation of C.

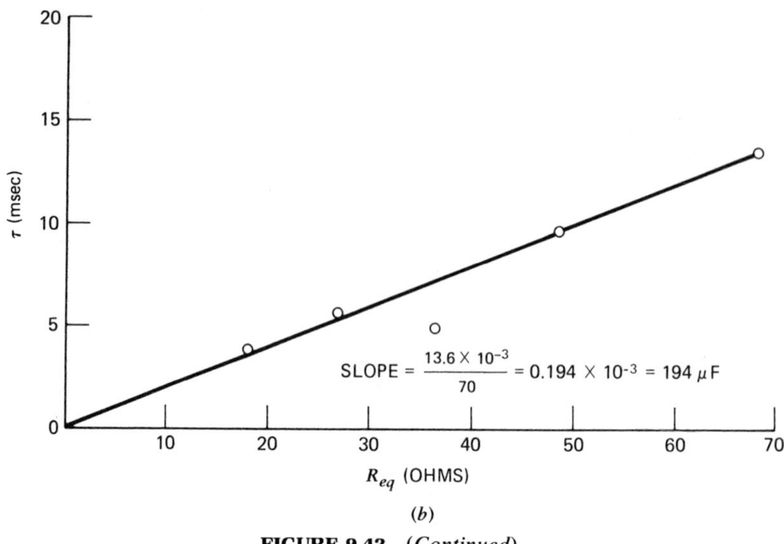

(*b*)

FIGURE 9.43 (*Continued*)

AUTOMATIC IMPLANTED DEFIBRILLATOR

It is becoming possible to identify a substantial number of patients in whom ventricular fibrillation is likely to occur. As was pointed out earlier, and elegantly demonstrated by Figure 9.3, the enemy is time, because hypoxic changes start to take place within a fraction of a minute and irreversible cellular changes start to occur in a few minutes. For patients at risk, survival depends on the immediate availability of emergency medical aid—or an automatic implanted defibrillator capable of sensing the presence of ventricular fibrillation and delivering a countershock to the heart—all within a minute or so.

The idea of developing an automatic implantable defibrillator occurred simultaneously and independently to Schuder et al. (1970) and Mirowski et al. (1970). Both team leaders have continued research in this important area, despite considerable opposition and even hostility. The end result has been the creation and implantation into humans, of an automatic defibrillator. At this time (June 1983), there are about 200 patients with implanted defibrillators. Many teams are developing automatic implantable defibrillators, but the pioneering work was conducted by Schuder and Mirowski. The following paragraphs recount the major milestones, as well as describing the important considerations for automatic ventricular defibrillation.

To identify ventricular fibrillation unambiguously, it is necessary to detect replacement of the *QRS-T* waves in the ECG by fibrillation waves and to identify the loss of cardiac output by the absence of pulsatile arterial pressure and its fall to a near-zero value. Detection of the ECG changes is relatively straightforward, but detection of circulatory collapse with an implanted device is much more difficult. Solving these two problems, or circumventing one or the other, has occupied the energies of many investigators—including the author.

Sensing

Several methods have been used for sensing fibrillation. The first automatic defibrillator developed by Schuder et al. (1970) used the absence of *R* waves in the ECG for 5 sec to trigger delivery of the shock to subcutaneous electrodes in the dog thorax. Mirowski et al. (1970) first used a right-ventricular pressure transducer, then in 1972 substituted a rugged conducting elastomer strain gauge in the right ventricle as a sensor of rhythmic pumping. The absence of ECG-*R* waves and rhythmic contractions triggered the defibrillator. Subsequently, Mirowski et al. (1975) abandoned the use of mechanical pumping for sensing and developed an ECG-processing system that identified fibrillation by the absence of isoelectric intervals in the ECG. This method is now used in the Mirowski defibrillator, which has been implanted in human subjects.

Bourland et al. (1977) developed a system that uses both the ECG changes and loss of right-ventricular pumping to identify ventricular fibrillation. A bipolar catheter is used in the right ventricle to continuously record the ECG and measure the impedance changes therein.

During diastole, the interelectrode impedance is low and during systole it is high. A logic circuit monitors the ECG, and on the basis of frequency, tentatively identifies fibrillation; the absence of rhythmic impedance changes confirms it.

As it stands now, it is not known whether the processed ECG is reliable enough to identify ventricular fibrillation. If it turns out to be so, the circuitry for the implant is somewhat simplified.

Energy-Storage and Defibrillating Electrodes

With all defibrillators, the energy-storage device is a capacitor that is charged when fibrillation is identified. The capacitor is then discharged through the electrodes, and the discharge is arrested in about 5–10 msec. Therefore, the current waveform is a truncated exponential, usually with a high tilt.

The type and location of the defibrillating electrodes merits careful consideration because their location and size importantly affect the energy and current required for defibrillation.

The most popular electrode system for defibrillation is catheter based. A catheter with an electrode at its tip is passed into the right ventricle; another electrode on the catheter (about 10 cm distant) in the superior vena cava completes the defibrillating electrode pair. The current and energy required with this type of transvenous electrode system were investigated by Schuder et al. (1971, 1972, 1973), Mirowski et al. (1971, 1973), Ewy and Horan (1976), Rubin et al. (1976, 1978), and Wessale et al. (1980). From these studies it soon became apparent that the current required for defibrillation was somewhat high, making it necessary to use a fairly large capacitor in the implanted defibrillator. However, the attractive feature of the transvenous catheter is that the ECG can be detected and the defibrillating shock can be delivered to electrodes on the catheter. More importantly, however, insertion of the catheter and implantation of the defibrillator does not require a thoracotomy.

Mirowski et al. (1977) developed a conical electrode for insertion at the cardiac apex extrapericardially. The other electrode was in the superior vena cava. With this electrode arrangement, the defibrillating current flows in the base–apex direction of the heart, and less current and energy are needed for defibrillation. Thus the size of the implanted defibrillator can be smaller than if catheter-defibrillating electrodes are used; but the price paid is a thoracotomy.

The Mirowski automatic defibrillator was initially implanted in three human subjects. A report (1980) states that the unit functioned satisfactorily in two of the three patients. To date (June 1983) the device has been implanted in about 200 patients. It is far too early to describe the clinical course of these patients for whom there was no other therapy, except perhaps a heart transplant. However, the experience is most encouraging.

HISTORICAL POSTSCRIPT

The story of ventricular defibrillation starts with the first observation of fibrillation by Ericksen (1842), who was investigating the effect of arresting blood flow in the coronary arteries. In a series of studies using artificially respired dogs and rabbits, he ligated the coronary arteries near their origin and watched the heart and counted its rate thereafter.

In his first dog experiment he wrote that "at twelve minutes after the ligature of the vessels . . . the heart was beating from 36 to 40 per minute. At seventeen minutes it has fallen to 28 to 30. At twenty-one minutes, the action of the ventricles had ceased, with the exception of a slight tremulous motion. The auricles acted and continued to do so for some time longer; the precise period, however, was not noted, as it was unimportant to the result of the experiment."

The term "tremulous motion" was obviously ventricular fibrillation. This and other terms were used repeatedly in the later literature, becoming known as ventricular fibrillation only much later.

The first study of ventricular fibrillation are usually credited to Hoffa and Ludwig (1850) who were able to record the consequences of electrically induced ventricular fibrillation in the dog and rabbit hearts. They noted a cessation of pumping and loss of pressure; they were surprised to note that with the passage of time, the ventricles became engorged.

Electrical ventricular defibrillation was performed in animals as early as 1899 by Prevost and Battelli in Switzerland. They used both capacitor-discharge and sinusoidal alternating current applied directly to animal hearts. Much later Hooker et al. (1933) found that 1 A (rms) of 60-Hz current, applied for 0.1 sec, defibrillated canine hearts with directly applied electrodes. With transchest electrodes, 6–7 A were required. Defibrillation of animals weighing up to 79 kg was accomplished by Ferris et al. (1936), who used up to 27 A (rms) applied to electrodes on various parts of the body. It was, however, the extensive studies by Kouwenhoven that demonstrated the practicality of electrical ventricular defibrillation—and resuscitation through closed-chest cardiac compression [see Kouwenhoven by Geddes (1976)].

The first human heart to be defibrillated successfuly was reported by Beck in 1947, who applied 110-V (rms), 60-Hz current to electrodes directly on the heart. In 1956 Zoll et al. defibrillated human subjects with transchest electrodes. Sinusoidal current was used with voltages ranging from 300 to 750 (rms), applied to thoracic electrodes. The 60-Hz defibrillators were very large, heavy, and drew high currents from the power line. They were abandoned when it was demonstrated that a damped sine wave was as effective. Such defibrillators were much smaller and could be operated from any conventional power outlet. Gurvich and Yuniev in Russia (1947) were the first to employ the capacitor-discharge and the damped sine wave to defibrillate animal hearts. In the United States MacKay and Leeds (1953) pointed out in animal studies that the amount of energy required was less when a capacitor discharge was prolonged by the addition of an inductor; the resulting waveform is a damped sine wave. The damped sine wave entered clinical medicine with the studies by Lown et al. (1964) and Edmark et al. (1963, 1966). Square and trapezoidal-wave defibrillators were first described by Schuder et al. (1964, 1966). Their clinical use followed rapidly because of the light weight and simplicity of such defibrillators.

Automatic Defibrillation

As shown in Figure 9.3, during ventricular fibrillation and with the passage of time, the effect of hypoxia is clearly visible within one-half minute. Therefore, it is logical to inquire if an automatic defibrillator could be created for patients with a high risk of fibrillation. Implementation of this concept has only become feasible within the last decade or so owing mainly to advances in pacemaker technology which have demonstrated that a sophisticated, implanted electronic device is practical and long lived.

The idea of creating an automatic defibrillator appears to have occurred to several investigators at the same time. Satinsky and Braslow (1970) described the use of a 70-J defibrillator which was triggered by the absence of *R* waves in the ECG to deliver a shock to transchest electrodes every 5 sec. This device obviously could not distinguish between asystole and fibrillation, but it could act as a low-rate external pacemaker or defibrillator.

Research was started toward the development of implantable defibrillators in 1970 by Schuder and Mirowski et al. Schuder's first automatic defibrillator employed the absence of *R* waves in the ECG, detected by intrathoracic electrodes, to trigger discharge of a capacitor connected to two 7.5-cm diameter subcutaneous electrodes in the dog chest. Schuder et al. (1971) then employed a catheter with one electrode in the right ventricle and the other in the superior vena cava. Studies were then carried out using a right-ventricular catheter electrode paired with chest electrodes for defibrillation. These electrode-placement studies, along with an investigation of various trapezoidal current waveforms, were designed to identify the conditions for minimum energy and current, thereby providing design information to create the smallest implantable unit.

The first studies by Mirowski et al. (1970) employed a pressure transducer in the right ventricle to detect the absence of rhythmic pressure changes to identify ventricular fibrillation. One defibrillating electrode was in the right ventricle and the other was on the anterior chest. Mirowski et al. (1972) replaced the pressure transducer with an elastic resistor on the right-ventricular catheter, which also carried the electrodes for detecting the ECG. Mirowski et al. (1973) then carried out catheter-defibrillation studies in a human during surgery using a 4-msec trapezoidal wave with about 50% tilt. Defibrillation was achieved using a superior vena cava to right-ventricular apex electrode, as well as with the right-ventricular electrode paired with saline-soaked pad on the superior vena cava.

Mirowski pointed out that although defibrillation was effective with a right-ventricular electrode, there were practical difficulties relating to electrode fixation. Accordingly, with Heilman (1978) he developed an extrapericardial apex electrode which was applied with a thoracotomy. Meanwhile, Mirowski (1975) previously developed an algorithm for detecting ventricular fibrillation using the absence of isoelectric periods in the ECG.

After numerous dog studies, Mirowski's automatic implanted defibrillator (AID) was implanted in three human subjects. The first report (Mirowski et al., 1980) indicated that the AID functioned satisfactorily in the three patients.

In closing, it should be noted that many other investigators followed the path started by Schuder and Mirowski. At present, many of the pacemaker manufacturers are contemplating the development of automatic implanted defibrillators. There is the suggestion that a pacemaker will be included in future units to initiate pacing if pumping does not resume after defibrillation.

REFERENCES

Adgey, A. A. J., Campbell, N. P. S., Webb, S. W., Kennedy, A. L., and Pantridge, J. F. (1978). Transthoracic ventricular defibrillation in the adult. *Med. Instr.* **12,** 17–19.

Anderson, G. and Suelzer, J. (1976). The efficacy of trapezoidal wave forms for ventricular defibrillation. *Chest* **70,** 298–300.

Babbs, C. F. and Tacker, W. A. (1978). Fundamental aspects of electrical ventricular defibrillation. *J. Cardiovasc. Technol.* **20,** 88–98.

Babbs, C. F. and Whistler, S. J. (1978). Evaluation of the operating internal resistance, inductance and capacitance of intact damped sine wave defibrillation. *Med. Instr.* **12,** 34–37.

Babbs, C. F., Whistler, S. J., and Geddes, L. A. (1980). Evaluation of the operating internal resistance and capacitance of intact trapezoidal waveform defibrillator. *Med. Instr.* **14,** 67–69.

Beck, C. S., Prilchard, W. H., and Feil, H. J. (1947). Ventricular fibrillation of long duration abolished by electric shock. *J. Amer. Med. Assoc.* **135,** 985–986.

Bourland, J. D., Geddes, L. A., Terry, R. S., Hinds, M., and Jones, J. T. (1977). Automatic detection of ventricular fibrillation for an implantable defibrillator. *Frontiers in Medical Signal Processing Midcon.* **5/2,** 1–5.

Bourland, J. D., Tacker, W. A., and Geddes, L. A. (1978). Strength-duration curves for trapezoidal waveforms of various tilts for transchest defibrillation in animals. Proc. 2nd Purdue Defibrillation Conf. *Med. Instr.* **12,** 38–41.

Bourland, J. D., Tacker, W. A., and Geddes, L. A. (1978). Comparative efficacy of damped sine wave and square wave current for transthoracic ventricular defibrillation in animals. Proc. 2nd Purdue Cardiac Defibrillation Conference 1977. *Med. Instr.* **12,** 42–45.

Bourland, J. D., Terry, R. S., and Geddes, L. A. (1978). Automatic detector of ventricular fibrillation using the ECG and intraventricular electrical impedance changes. *Med. Instr.* **12,** 52.

Chambers, W., Miles, R., and Strathicher, R. (1978). Human chest resistance during successful countershocks. *Med. Instr.* **12,** 53.

Dahl, C. F., Ewy, G. A., Warner, E. D., and Thomas, E. (1974). Myocardial necrosis from direct current countershock. *Circulation* **30,** 956–961.

Dahl, D. F., Ewy, G. A., Ewy, M. D., and Thomas E. (1976). Transthoracic impedance to direct current discharge: effect of repeated countershocks. *Med. Instr.* **10,** 151–154.

DiCola, V. C., Freedman, C. J., Downing, S. E., and Zaret, B. L. (1976). Myocardial uptake of technetium 99m stannous pyrophosphate following direct current transthoracic shock. *Circulation* **54,** 980–986.

Edmark, K. W., Thomas, G. I., and Jones, T. W. (1966). DC pulse defibrillation. *J. Thoracic Cardiovasc. Surg.* **51,** 326–333.

Edmark, K. W. (1963). Simultaneous voltage and current waveforms generated during internal and external direct-current pulse defibrillation. *Surg. Forum* **14,** 262–264.

Ehsani, A., Ewy, G. A., and Sobel, B. E. (1976). Effects of electrical countershock on serum creative phosphokinase isoenzyme activity. *Amer. J. Cardiol.* **37,** 12–18.

Ericksen, J. C. (1842). Influences of the coronary circulation on the action of the heart. *London Med. Gazette.* **2,** 561–564.

Ewy, G. A. and Horan, W. (1976). Electrode catheter defibrillation. *Med. Instr.* **10,** 155.

Ferris, L. P., King, B. G., Spence, P. W., and Williams, H. B. (1936). Effect of electric shock on the heart. *Elect. Eng.* **55,** 498–515.

Geddes, L. A., Tacker, W. A., McFarlane, J., and Bourland, J. (1970). Strength-duration curves for ventricular defibrillation in dogs. *Circ. Res.* **27,** 551–560.

Geddes, L. A., Tacker, W. A., Rosborough, J., Moore, A. G., Cabler, P., Bailey, M., McCrady, J. D., and Witzel, D. (1974). The electrical dose for ventricular defibrillation with electrodes applied directly to the heart. *J. Thoracic Cardiovasc. Surg.* **68,** 593–602.

Geddes, L. A., Tacker, W. A., Rosborough, J., Moore, A. G. and Cabler, P. S. (1974). Electrical dose for ventricular defibrillation of large and small animals using precordial electrodes. *J. Clin. Invest.* **53,** 310–319.

Geddes, L. A., Tacker, W. A., Cabler, P., Chapman, R., Rivera, R., and Kidder, H. (1975). The decrease in transthoracic impedance during successive ventricular defibrillation trials. *Med. Instr.* **9,** 179–180.

Geddes, L. A., Tacker, W. A., Schoenlein, W., Minton, M., Grubbs, S., and Wilcox, P. (1976). The prediction of the impedance of the thorax to defibrillating current. *Med. Instr.* **10,** 159–162.

Geddes, L. A., Bourland, J. D., and Tacker, W. A. (1980). Energy and current requirements for ventricular defibrillation in dogs and ponies using trapezoidal waves. *Am. J. Physiol.* **238,** H231–236.

Gold, J. H., Schuder, J. C., Stoeckle, H., Granberg, T. A., Hamdani, S. Z., and Rychlewski, J. M. (1975). Transthoracic ventricular defibrillation in the 100kg calf with unidirectional rectangular pulses. *Circulation* **56,** 745–750.

Gold, J. H., Schuder, J. C. Stoeckle, H. Granberg, T. A., Dettmer, J. C., and Schmidt, D. C. (1979). Scaling current and energy with body weight: requirements for the transthoracic ventricular defibrillation of calves as they grow from 50 to 150 kg. *Circulation* **60,** 187–195.

Gullett, J., Havens, W. W., Tacker, W. A., Geddes, L. A., and Hoff, H. E. (1968). Optimum duration of 60-Hz current for direct ventricular defibrillation. *Cardiovasc. Res. Ctr. Bull.* **6,** 117–123.

Gurvich, N. L. and Yuniev, G. S. (1947). Restoration of heart rhythm during fibrillation by a condenser discharger. *Am. Rev. Sov. Med.* **4,** 252–256.

Gutgesell, H. P., Tacker, W. A., Geddes, L. A., Davis, J. S., Lee, Y. T. and McNamara, D. G. (1976). Energy dose for ventricular defibrillation of children. *Pediatrics* **58,** 898–901.

Heilman, M. M., Langer, A. A., Mirowski, M.M., and Reilly, D. M. (1971). Implantable electrodes for accomplishing ventricular fibrillation and pacing, method of electrode implantation and utilization. U.S. Patent 4,030,509.

Hooker, D. R., Kouwenhoven, W. B., and Langworthy, O. R. (1933). The effect of alternating currents or the heart. *Am. J. Physiol.* **102,** 444–454.

Hoffa, M. and Ludwig, C. (1850). Einige neue Versuche über Herzbewegung. *Z. rat. Med.* **9,** 107–144.

Kerber, R. E., Carter, J., Klein, S., Grayzel, J and Kennedy, J. (1980). Open chest defibrillation during cardiac surgery: energy and current requirements. *Am. J. Cardiol.* **46,** 393–398.

Kouwenhoven, W. B., by Geddes, L. A. (1976). *Med. Instr.* **10,** 141–143.

Koning, G., Schneider, H., Hollen, A. J., and Reneman, R. S. (1975). Amplitude duration relation for direct ventricular defibrillation with rectangular current pulses. *Med. Biol. Engng.* (May) 388–395.

Lown, B. (1964). Cardioversion of arrhythmias. *Modern Concepts of Cardiovasc. Dis.* **33,** 863–868.

Lown, B. (1967). Electrical reversion of cardiac arrhythmias. *Brit. Heart J.* **29,** 469–487.

Machin, J. W. (1978). Thoracic impedance of human subjects. *Med. Biol. Eng. Comput.* **16,** 169–178.

MacKay, R. S. and Leeds, S. (1953). Physiologic effects of condenser discharge with application to tissue stimulation and ventricular defibrillation. *J. Appl. Physiol.* **6,** 67–75.

Mirowski, M. (1975). Implanted defibrillators. *Proc. Cardiac Defibrillation Conference,* Engineering Experiment Station Document 00147, Purdue University, W. Lafayette, IN.

Mirowski, M., Mower, M. M., Staeven, W. S., Tabatzink, B. and Mendeloff, A. (1970). Standby automatic defibrillator. *Arch. Int. Med.* **126,** 158–161.

Mirowski, M., Mower, M. M., Staewen, W. S., Denniston, R. H., Tabalznik, B., and Mendeloff, A. I. (1971). Ventricular defibrillation through a single intravascular catheter electrode system. *Clin. Res.* **19,** 328.

Mirowski, M., Mower, M., Staewen, W. S., Tabatznik, B., and Mendeloff, A. I. (1970). Standby automatic defibrillator. *Arch. Int. Med.* **126,** 158–161.

Mirowski, M., Mower, M. M., Staewen, W. W., Denniston, R. H. and Mendeloff, A. I. (1972). Development of the transvenous automatic defibrillator. *Arch. Int. Med.* **129,** 773–779.

Mirowski, M., Mower, M. M., Gott, V. L., and Brawley, R. K. (1973). Feasibility and effectiveness of low-energy catheter defibrillation in man. *Circulation* **42,** 79–85.

Mirowski, M., Mower, M. M., Langer, A. Heilman, M. S., and Schrellman, J. (1978). A chronically implanted system for automatic defibrillation in acute conscious dogs. *Circulation* **58,** 90–94.

Mirowski, M., Rein, P. R., Mower, M. M., Watkins, L., Gott, V. L. Schquble, J., Langer, J. A., Heilman, M. S., Kolenik, S. A., Fisch, X., and Weisfeldt, M. (1980). Termination of malignant ventricular arrhythmias with an implanted automatic defibrillator in human beings. *N. Engl. J. Med.* **303,** 322–324.

Niebauer, M. (1982). Efficacy and Safety of Defibrillation Waveforms Using an Isolated Canine Heart Model. Ph.D. Thesis, Purdue Univ. May 1982.

Pantridge, J. F., Adgey, A. A. J., Webb, S. W., and Anderson, J. (1975). Electrical requirements for ventricular defibrillation. *Brit. Med. Journ.* **2,** 313–315.

Pantridge, J. F., Adgey, A. A. J., Geddes, J. J., and Webb, S. W. (1975). *The Acute Coronary Attack.* Grune and Stratton, New York.

Peleska, B. (1965). Cardiac arrhythmias following condenser discharges led through an inductor. *Circ. Res.* **16,** 11–18.

Prevost, J. L. and Battelli, F. (1899). Some effects of electric discharge on the hearts of mammals. *Comptes Rendus Acad. Sci.* **129,** 1267–1268.

Prevost, J. L. and Battelli, F. (1899). Death due to electric currents. *Comptes Rendus Acad. Sci.* **128,** 668–670.

Rubin, L., Hudson, P., Duller J., Alexander, L., and Parsonnet, V. (1976). Automatic defibrillator and pacing with a transvenous electrode. *Proc. 4th New. Engl. Biomed. Eng. Conf.* **4,** 427–430.

Rubin, L., Hudson, P., Duller, J., and Parsonnet, V. (1978). An evaluation of ventricular defibrillation with left intracavity electrodes. *Med. Instr.* **12,** 55.

Satinsky, V. F. and Braslow, N. M. (1970). An automatic portable resuscitation unit to prevent electrical failure of the heart. *Proc. 23rd Ann. Conf. Eng. Med. Biol.* 10–16.

Schuder, J. C., Stoeckle H., West, J., and Dolan, A. M. (1964). Thoracic ventricular defibrillation with square-wave stimulus. *Circ. Res.* **15,** 258–264.

Schuder, J. C., Rahmoeller, G. A., and Stocckle, H. (1966). Transchest ventricular defibrillation with triangular and trapezoidal waveforms. *Circ. Res.* **19,** 689–694.

Schuder, J. C., Stoeckle, H., Gold, J. H., West, J. A., and Keskar, P. Y. (1970). Experimental ventricular defibrillation with a completely implanted defibrillator. *Trans. ASAIO* **16,** 207–212.

Schuder, J. C., Stoeckle, H., West, J. A., Keskar, P. Y., and Gold, J. H. (1971). Ventricular defibrillation with catheter having distal electrode in the right ventricle and proximal electrodes in the superior vena cava. *Circulation* **44,** 11.

Schuder, J. C., Stoeckle, H., West, J., Keskar, P. Y., and Gold, J. H. (1971). Ventricular defibrillation using bipolar catheter and truncated exponential stimuli. *Proc. 24th Annual Conf. Eng. Med. Biol.* 35.

Schuder, J. C., Stoeckle, H., West, J. Keskar, P. Y., Gold, J., and Denniston, R. H. (1973). Ventricular defibrillation in the dog with a bielectrode intravascular catheter. *Arch. Int. Med.* **132,** 280–290.

Tacker, W. A., Geddes, L. A., and Hoff, H. E. (1968). Defibrillation without A-V block using capacitor-discharge with added inductance. *Circ. Res.* **22,** 633–638.

Tacker, W. A., Galioto, F., Guiliani, E., Geddes, L. A., and McNamara, D. (1974). Energy dosage for human trans-chest electric ventricular defibrillation. *New Engl. J. Med.* **290,** 214–215.

Tacker, W. A., Rubio, P. A., Reyes, L. H., Korompai, F. L. and Guinn, G. A. (1975). Low energy electrical defibrillation of human hearts during cardiac surgery. *J. Thoracic Cardiovasc. Surg.* **68,** 603–605.

Tacker, W. A. and Geddes, L. A. (1980). *Electrical defibrillation*. CRC Press, Boca Raton, FL. 192 pp.

Tacker, W. A., Geddes, L. A., Van Vleet, J. F., and Davis, J. S. (1976). Cardiac damage produced by high-current defibrillation shocks. *Med. Inst.* **10, 52.**

Tacker, W. A., Cole, J. S., and Geddes, L. A. (1976). Clinical efficacy of a truncated exponential decay defibrillator. *J. Electrocardiol.* **9,** 273–274.

Tacker, W. A., Davis, J. S., Lie, S. T., Talies, J. L., and Geddes, L. A. (1978). Cardiac damage produced by transchest damped sine wave current. *Med. Instr.* **12,** 27–29.

VanVleet, J., Tacker, W. A., and Geddes, L. A. (1978). Acute cardiac damage in dogs given multiple transthoracic shocks with a trapezoidal wave defibrillator. Proc. 2nd Purdue Cardiac Defibrillation Conf. *Med. Instr.* **12,** 55–56.

VanVleet, J. F., Tacker, W. A., Geddes, L. A., and Farrans, V. J. (1978). Sequential cardiac morphologic alterations induced in dogs by single transthoracic damped sinusoidal waveform defibrillator shocks. *Am. J. Vet. Res.* **39,** 271–278.

Wessale, J. L., Bourland, J. D., Tacker, W. A., and Geddes, L. A. (1980). Bipolar catheter defibrillation in dogs. *J. Electrocardiol.* **13,** 359–366.

Zoll, P. M., Linenthal, A. J., Gibson, W., Paul, M. H., and Norman, L. R. (1956). Termination of ventricular fibrillation in man by externally applied electric countershock. *New Engl. J. Med.* **254,** 727–732.

CHAPTER 10

Electrical Hazards

In the environment of a patient experiencing medical treatment there can be identified three types of electrical hazard. One relates to sparks produced by static electricity or environmental instruments; a second results indirectly from the domestic power line which is used to energize diagnostic, monitoring, therapeutic, and assistive devices. The third type of hazard results from radiofrequency electrosurgical current which is used to cut and coagulate living tissue. These three types of hazard are variably present and depend on the particular circumstances, that is, whether the patient is in the operating room, coronary/intensive care unit, ward, or specialized diagnostic area. This chapter will discuss the electrical hazards in a medical environment. Parker (1967), van der Mosel (1970), Feldtman and Derrick (1973), and Stanley (1974) have written extensively on this subject. It should be recognized that such an environment has other hazards, such as infection and radiation of a variety of types; these, however, will not be discussed.

ELECTRIC SPARK HAZARD

Static electricity, one of the many causes of electric sparks, is the electricity of friction which was first described by Thales (640–546 BC). He found that when amber was rubbed with fur it attracted very light particles of plant and paper. Incidentally, the Greek word for amber is elektron, hence the origin of the word "electricity" that described the "amber effect." It was later found that the phenomenon of electrification could be produced when different insulating materials are rubbed together, the most familiar of these occurring when the hair is combed or when walking over a carpet on a dry day. Contact between the subject and a nearby metal object results in a spark which discharges the static charges separated by the energy of friction. Equally good static-electricity generators are clothes made of synthetic fibers. The potentials developed are in the tens of thousands of volts and the spark discharge can be centimeters in length. Such a discharge can provide the subject with a strong shock and a considerable surprise.

Because a single static-electricity discharge is accompanied by a spark, it can ignite a mixture of explosive gases. A single spark can also stimulate sensory receptors, nerve, and muscle. In the latter case, if the discharge is applied directly to an exposed motor nerve or skeletal muscle, it can evoke a twitch in the muscle, as was elegantly shown by Galvani in 1794. If such a discharge is applied to heart muscle it can evoke an extrasystole. This subject will be discussed subsequently. However, the most important hazard of a static discharge is associated with anesthetic procedures. Similarly, electric sparks from a variety of instruments can ignite mixtures of flammable gases and cause an explosion.

EXPLOSION HAZARD

When flammable gases are used with oxygen for anesthesia, the stage is set for an explosion. A single spark occurring in the environment can provide the necessary ignition, just like the spark in a spark plug ignites the gasoline–air mixture in the cylinder of an automobile engine.

Electric sparks, capable of igniting mixtures of flammable gases, can be produced by static electricity, switches, motor commutators, and the active electrode of an electrosurgical instrument. Although it is often possible to enclose switches and motor commutators, it is not possible to secure protection from the tiny electric arc that accomplishes cutting and coagulation when an electrosurgical instrument is used. Most of the older electrosurgical instruments contain spark-gap generators to provide the electrosurgical current. Proper ventilation of the environment and avoidance of leaks in the anesthetic equipment is the only means of protection against ignition of flammable gases by spark-gap generators. Walter (1966, 1967) and Bruner (1967) have discussed this subject extensively.

Explosions by the ignition of anesthetic mixtures attributable to the presence of an environmental spark have been reported. However, not all gases used for anesthesia are explosive. Moreover, it is possible to use anesthetic agents that are injected intravenously, although they are much less controllable than gaseous anesthetics.

Anesthesia is a state in which the response to noxious stimuli is suppressed reversibly. Without anesthesia, very few surgical procedures could be performed. Anesthesia can be created by substances which reach the brain via ingestion, injection (subcutaneous, intramuscular, intraperitoneal, or intravenous), or inhalation. Of the three routes of administration, inhalation is the most controllable with regard to depth and duration of anesthesia. Restoration of consciousness merely requires cessation of delivery of a volatile anesthetic presented to the airway and continued breathing. Because there are a variety of requirements relating to patient safety and controllability, many different anesthetics are used, each of which has its desirable characteristics and side effects. It is the duty of the anesthesiologist to select the anesthetic regimen that is most suitable for the patient.

In the early days of anesthesia, many of the anesthetics were flammable. With the passage of time new gaseous anesthetic agents have been found which, when combined with oxygen, are not flammable. However, some of the older flammable anesthetics have properties which require their use. Table 10.1 presents a listing of many of the popular anesthetics and their flammability characteristics which indicate the propensity for ignition and explosion. Laurence and Bostress (1959) presented combustibility data on the older anesthetic mixtures.

When explosive anesthetic gases are used, special precautions must be taken to ensure that an explosion will not occur. There are numerous codes and recommendations designed to create a safe environment when flammable anesthetic gases are used; a listing of many of these appears among the references at the end of this chapter.

Perhaps the best way of informing the reader about the hazard of explosion in anesthesia is to define the extent of the hazardous area surrounding a patient anesthetized with a flammable anesthetic. The National Fire Protection Association (NFPA) Technical Committe Report recommends an environmental temperature of 70 ± 5°F (21 ± 2.8°C) and a relative humidity of not less than 50%. The floor should be made of conducting material; the resistance of the floor should be less than 1 megohm when measured between two electrodes placed 3 ft apart at any two points on the floor. Each electrode shall weigh 5 lb and shall have a round, flat circular contact area 2.5 in. in diameter which shall comprise a surface of aluminum or tin foil 0.0005–0.001 in. thick backed by a layer of rubber, 0.25 in. thick (of a hardness ASTM D-2240-68). The ohmmeter shall have a normal open-circuit output of 500 V DC and a short-circuit current of 5 mA with an effective resistance of 100,000 ohms ± 10%. The

TABLE 10.1. Characteristics of Anesthetic Gases[a]

Substance	Boiling Point (°C)	Relative Density (air = 1)	Flammability Limits In Air (% v/v)	Flammability Limits In Oxygen (% v/v)	Limits of Concentration Used in Anesthesia (% v/v)
Diethyl ether	34.6	2.6	1.9–48	2.0–82	3–20
Cyclopropane	−32.8	1.5	2.4–10.4	2.5–60	3–40
Trichloroethylene	87	4.5	None	10–65	2–7.5
Divinyl ether	28.4	2.2	1.7–2.7	0.8–45	2–12
Halothane	50.3	6.8	None	None	0.5–10
Halothane ether azeotrope	52.7	5.4	None	Lower limit 8	2–5
Ethyl chloride	12.5	2.3	3.8–15.4	4.0–67	2–6
Ethylene	−103	0.97	3.1–32	3.0–80	60–80
Nitrous oxide	−89	1.5	None	None	35–80
Methoxyflurane (Penthrane)	104.8	5.7	9.0–28	5.2–28	0.5–3.0
Fluoroxene (Fluomar)	42.7	4.4	Lower limit 4.2	Lower limit 4.0	1–5

[a]From Hill, D. W. (1976). *Physics Applied to Anaesthesia,* Butterworths, London, p. 411.

resistance of the floor shall be more than 25,000 ohms, as measured between a ground connection and an electrode placed at any point on the floor, and also as measured between two electrodes placed 3 ft apart at any point on the floor.

The extent of a hazardous area surrounding a patient is based largely on the fact that nearly all flammable anesthetics are heavier than air. For this reason the hazardous area extends from the floor to an altitude of 5 ft. The Association of Anesthesiologists of Great Britain and Ireland define the hazardous area as extending 25 cm around any part of the anesthetic circuit.

It must be remembered that the numerous rules, regulations, codes, and recommendations relative to anesthetic environments derived from the early days when explosive anesthetic gases were used routinely. At present fewer such anesthetics are used, and their use is diminishing with the passage of time. Whether these recommendations and codes will continue to have the importance they once had will be for the future to decide.

Although fires and explosions related to the use of flammable anesthetic gases are rare, they have occurred. For obvious reasons, there is relatively little information on this subject in the published literature. However, there are a few reports that describe the circumstances which contribute to this hazard. For a fire or explosion to occur, only three elements are required: (1) the presence of a combustible substance, (2) the availability of an oxidizing agent, and (3) a source of ignition. In some anesthetic procedures, it is necessary to use a flammable anesthetic which satisfies the first requirement. In all anesthetic procedures (and indeed in normal respiration) there is an oxidizing agent, oxygen. When these two elements are present in the proper proportion, all that is needed is the source of ignition which can be an electrostatic discharge or a spark from an electrically operated device used in the environment or the active electrode in electrosurgery. Walter (1966) stated that the energy required for an electrostatic discharge to ignite an explosive mixture of anesthetic gases is 0.1–1 mJ. An analysis of sources of the ignition in anesthetic explosions was presented in the United Kingdom by the Working Party on Anesthetic Explosions (1956). Table 10.2 lists the sources and their incidence during the period from 1947 to 1954 which identified 36 explosions. In the United States, Thomas (1961) stated that 60% of the anesthetic fires and explosions are due to ignition by static electricity.

TABLE 10.2. Causes of Explosion for Flammable Anesthetics[a]

	Number	Percentage	
Static spark	22	61.1 }	69.4
Static spark or open gas burner	1 }		
Static spark or electric heater	1 }	8.3 }	
Static spark or smouldering towel	1 }		
Diathermy[a]	5	14.0	
Spark in switch or cut-out	3	8.3	
Faulty valve in gas cylinder	1 }		
Foreign matter in valve	1 }	8.3	
Smoking (?)	1 }		

[a] From the Report of the Working Parts on Anesthetic Explosions (HMJO, 1956)

[b] Electrosurgical instrument in the United States.

Excellent descriptions of spark-ignited anesthetic gas fires and explosions were presented by Walter (1966). The remarkable characteristics of these accidents is their low incidence and their surprise occurrence. That they occurred is primarily due to a disregard for adhering to safety measures. Walter (1966) reported the explosion of an ether–oxygen nitrous-oxide mixture owing to a breech in the conducting pathway between the patient, anesthetist, and anesthesia machine. Interruption of this conducting pathway allowed the accumulation of an electrostatic potential that caused a spark that ignited the anesthetic-gas mixture. Walter (1966) described other ignitions of flammable anesthetic gas mixtures in which ignition was produced by a lighted cigarette, the switch on an examining lamp, contacts in a motor-driven floor scrubber, and starting contacts in a water cooler in an adjacent room, the door to which was open.

In an explosive anesthetic environment, the patient, the anesthetist, the medical staff, and the anesthetic machine are all grounded. Conductive tubing is used to the anesthetic machine. All of these and other precautions are taken to minimize the risk of an electrostatic discharge igniting combustible gases. However, if objects (or people) in the environment become ungrounded, or there is an interruption in the conducting path which is associated with the patient-anesthesia equipment, the stage is set for an explosion.

It is obvious that when anesthesia is produced with a flammable anesthetic gas and an electrosurgical instrument is used the conditions are right for a fire or explosion. For obvious reasons such accidents are unlikely to be reported; nonetheless, they must have occurred. The author has witnessed the use of electrosurgery in the thorax of a patient who was anesthetized with ether. Although the surgeon did not cut or coagulate lung tissue, he came perilously close at times. Recognition of the hazard is important because some flammable anesthetics are still used. When electrosurgery must be used in the vicinity of the respiratory system, flammable anesthetics should never be used.

BOWEL-GAS EXPLOSION HAZARD

Explosion of gas in the gastrointestinal tract, ignited by an electrosurgical cutting electrode, is by no means uncommon. Levy (1954) reviewed much of the previous literature to that time and presented important information on this phenomenon. For example, he pointed out that digestive processes, bacterial fermentation, diffusion of gas (presumably inhaled flammable gas) from the bloodstream, and swallowed gas are responsible for such accumulation. The composition of bowel gas is influenced by the amount of milk and legumes ingested. For these sources, hydrogen and methane are produced. On the average diet, the bowel content for hydrogen is about 21%; for methane it is about 7%; and the carbon dioxide content is between 9–69%. On a milk diet, gut hydrogen increases to about 44%, and on a legume diet, methane also increases to about 44%.

Hussey and Pois (1970) reviewed the literature on bowel-gas explosions from the time of Levy's report (1954) to 1970, and described a case of bowel-gas explosion which occurred when the large bowel was opened with an electrosurgical cutting electrode. The bowel was ripped by the explosion and required resection. Septicemia developed and the patient died. Prevention of bowel-gas explosion is possible and merely requires that attention be paid to the hazard. For example, opening the bowel can be achieved with a scalpel; thereafter the electrosurgical knife can be used. Some advocate purging the bowel with an inert gas. Obviously dietary management of a patient is important prior to bowel surgery.

POWER-LINE HAZARDS

There is a bewildering array of reports which describe electric shocks resulting from 60-Hz power-line current flowing through human subjects. Burns and death, owing to respiratory arrest or ventricular fibrillation, have resulted from accidental contact with the power line, usually in association with a piece of equipment connected to it. What is often missing in these reports is a clear analysis of why current flowed and the pathway through the subject. The following will provide the necessary information.

The starting point in understanding the reason for shocks from domestic power sources is a knowledge of the circuit behind the receptacle into which instruments are plugged. Figure 10.1 illustrates the basic plan for power distribution in buildings. Shown here is a sketch of the presently used three-contact outlet, into which a two-blade-and-rod plug is inserted to energize a device. The power source (E) is usually a nearby transformer, one side of which is grounded. The current-carrying conductor connected to this "neutral" or "cold" side of the power line is usually colorcoded white (WH). The other current-carrying conductor is described as "hot," and is usually colorcoded black (BK). These two conductors are connected to the rectangular contacts of the power outlet. The circular contact is connected to a grounded wire, which goes directly back to the point where the power system is grounded, usually at the point of entry of the power line to the building. The grounded conductor does not carry any of the current that is used to operate a device plugged into the power

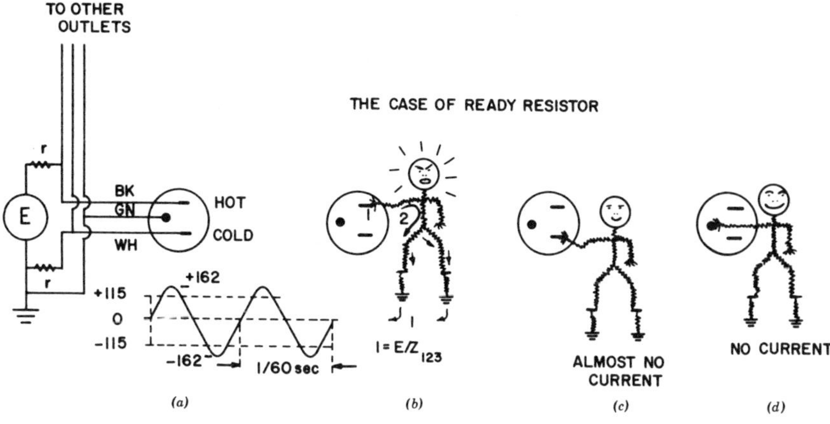

FIGURE 10.1. Shock hazard from domestic power outlet.

outlet. The important function of this green ground conductor will be described subsequently.

With a 115-V (rms), 60-Hz power distribution system, the voltage appearing between the two rectangular contacts of the outlet will rise to $115\sqrt{2} = 162$ V in the positive direction and fall to $115\sqrt{2} = 162$ V in the negative direction every one-sixtieth of a second as shown in Figure 10.1*a*. Now, if an inquisitive subject, Ready Resistor, takes hold of a bare metal conductor and places it in the hot side of the power outlet, current will flow through him to ground (*b*) because the other side of the power line is grounded. The amount of current that will flow depends directly on the voltage and inversely on his resistance to ground. Obviously, standing on a wet floor or in a bathtub while in contact with the hot side of the power line will reduce the resistance to ground, and result in a considerable current flow.

If Ready Resistor now places the metal conductor into the power outlet that is connected to the cold side of the power line (*c*), he may or may not receive a weak shock, depending on whether other current-drawing devices are connected to other outlets wired to the same circuit. Note in Figure 10.1*a* that the power conductors extending from the point of entry of the power system (where grounding occurs) are in reality resistors (*r*,*r*) having a low resistance. Now, if no other current-drawing devices are connected to the same circuit beyond the power outlet, there will be no current flow through either of these two resistors; consequently, there will be no voltage drop across them. Therefore, if Ready Resistor touches the cold side of the power line in this case, he will receive no shock (provided that the ground on which he stands is at the same potential as the power-line ground.) If, however, other current-drawing devices are connected to other outlets beyond the one which is connected to Ready Resistor, the current flow through the resistance of the conductors (r,r) will cause a voltage drop and the potential of the cold side of the outlet will not be at the same potential as the ground of the power system. Thus, Ready Resistor, who is at ground potential, will receive a weak shock by touching the cold side of the power outlet in this circumstance. It is to be noted that the voltage drop along power conductors is usually small, and in practice, the voltage of the cold side of the power line may only be from a few tens to a few hundreds of millivolts, above ground. Although this voltage may only be perceptible to the touch, it is more than enough to stimulate irritable tissue when directly applied.

If Ready Resistor places a bare metal conductor in contact with the circular terminal of the power outlet (Figure 10.1*d*), he will receive no shock because this conductor is connected directly back to the ground of the power system and current to operate devices is never drawn through this (green) conductor. Similarly, because all exposed metal parts of a power-line-operated device are connected to the circular ground terminal, there will be no potential difference between these surfaces and ground. It should be noted, however, that the small leakage current of appliances is carried by the green grounding conductor. However these currents are usually so small that the potential of the green grounding wire is very nearby at ground potential.

LEAKAGE CURRENT

The term "leakage current" refers to a flow of current which is not related to the principal mode of energizing a device. The following examples will illustrate various types of leakage current and also show why the term is difficult to define.

The source of most leakage currents is the electrical capacitance and/or conducting path between the power line and the metallic parts of a line-operated device. Perhaps the simplest example is offered by a motor or other appliance which is plugged into a power outlet as shown in Figure 10.2*a*. Because such devices are constituted by metallic conductors in a metal housing, there is a distributed capacitive coupling (Cd) between the conductors connected to the power line and the metal housing. Capacitors have the ability to pass alternating current by virtue of their reactance, which is equal to $1/2\pi fC$, where f is the frequency in Hz and C is the capacitance in farads. In Figure 10.2*b* the distributed capacitance has

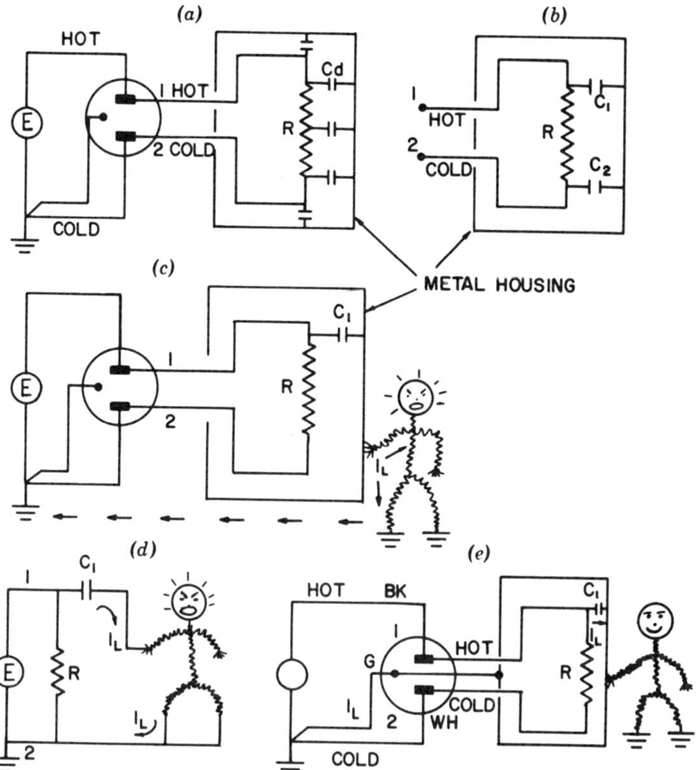

FIGURE 10.2. Leakage current due to capacitive coupling (*Cd*) in a power line operated appliance with its metal case ungrounded (*a*). The lumped equivalent circuit is shown in (*b*), and (*c*) illustrates the typical asymmetrical coupling where C_1 couples the case to the hot side of the power line. The equivalent circuit is shown in (*d*) which illustrates the current pathway. In (*e*), the condition for capacitive coupling from the case to the hot side of the power line is shown, with the case properly grounded.

been collected and represented as two capacitors (C_1, C_2) connected to the metal housing of the device. For illustrative purposes, assume that C_2 couples the "cold" side of the power line to the housing with a small capacitance. Assume that C_1 couples the "hot" side of the power line to the housing with a much larger capacitance. Consequently, the housing has the capability of sending current through any conducting path that joins it to ground. For example, if Ready Resistor touches this ungrounded or "floating" housing, a current will flow as shown in Figure 10.2*c*. If Ready Resistor has a resistance of 5000 ohms and C_2 has a capacitance of 1000 picofarads, the current flow through Ready Resistor (Figure 10.2*d*) is equal to the line voltage (E = 115 V rms) divided by the impedance of the circuit, $\sqrt{(5000)^2 + 1/2\pi \times 60 \times 10^{-9})^2}$. Performing this calculation provides a current of 43.4 μA rms. This leakage current could be barely perceived by the finger of Ready Resistor. However, if Ready Resistor improves his contact with ground very little more current will flow because it is determined by the reactance of the 1000-pF capacitance. On the other hand, if the metal housing is directly connected to an exposed nerve or muscle, it could stimulate it. Figure 10.2*d* illustrates the equivalent circuit.

It should be obvious that when a current flows through Ready Resistor to ground, the currents in the power conductors (1,2) will be unequal. With such a ground path, the current which flows in the hot side will exceed that flowing in the cold side of the power line. This fact is used in a variety of ground-fault detectors, which can be plugged into any power outlet and into which the appliance is plugged. Many of these ground-fault current indicators contain a circuit breaker that immediately arrests the flow of current to the appliance. Such devices are called GFCIs or Ground Fault Circuit Interrupters. At present, a variety of such devices is available commercially with a 5 mA rms differential current sensitivity; if the leakage current to ground exceeds 5 mA, current flow to the appliance is arrested within about 0.1 sec. If the leakage current is higher, current flow is interrupted in even less time.

The leakage current to ground can be prevented from flowing through Ready Resistor by connecting the metal housing directly to the circular (green-wired) connector of the power outlet, as shown in Figure 10.2*e*. The leakage current will then flow in the ground conductor and the exposed metal housing would be at ground potential.

Let us now suppose that the same appliance was plugged into the power outlet with a two-blade connector so that the conductor having the highest capacitance (C_1) to the case is connected to the cold terminal of the power line, as shown in Figure 10.3. In this case, the metal housing will be very close to ground potential and Ready Resistor would be unable to perceive any leakage current on touching the metal housing. Unfortunately, many appliances have only a two-conductor line cord, and in such a case, it can be seen that the power plug can be inserted with the ungrounded or hot side of the power line capacitively coupled to the metal housing. Moreover, there is no way of knowing which condition exists in a given situation. Many have had the experience of touching the metal case of an appliance and feeling a slight tingle, only to have the sensation disappear when the appliance plug is reversed.

The actual situation which gives rise to leakage current is slightly more complex than that just described. Figure 10.4 illustrates the worst-case condition in which there is both capacitive and conductive coupling from

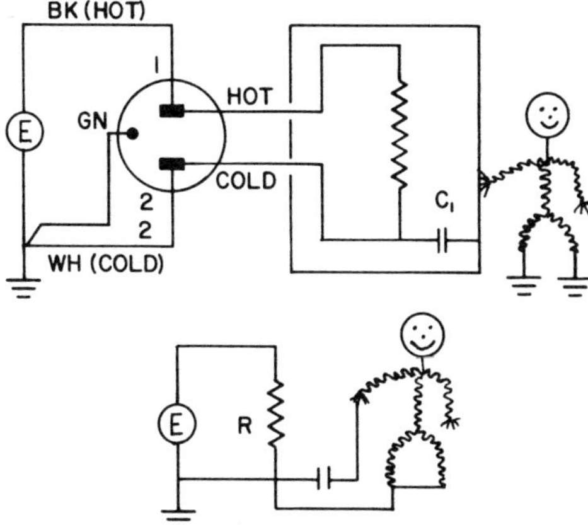

FIGURE 10.3. The safe situation when the asymmetrical capacitance C_1 couples the case of an appliance to the cold side of the power line.

the power line to the metal housing of the device. The capacitive coupling is represented by C_1 and C_2, as before; the conductive coupling is represented by resistors R_1 and R_2. The equivalent circuit that represents this situation is shown in Figure 10.4*b*. It can be seen that the metal housing (X) is connected to the midpoint of a voltage divider constituted by R_1C_1 and R_2C_2.

In practice, unless there is a fault which connects one side of the power line directly to the metal housing, the resistances of R_1 and R_2 are quite high. In many instances it is possible to measure the values of R_1 and R_2 by using a direct-current ohmmeter as shown in Figure 10.4*c*. With the appliance disconnected from the power line, the resistance between the metal housing (X) and one side of the power line connector is measured (R_{1X}); then the resistance is measured to the other side of the power line connector (R_{2X}). The two sides of the line connector are then joined together and the resistance is measured between this point and the metal housing (R_{12-X}). From these three measurements it is possible to measure the resistance of R_1, R_2, and R, the resistance of the device; the equations are presented in Figure 10.3*c*.

In a large majority of the cases, R_1 and R_2 are high for well-designed and constructed devices. However, the capacitance values for C_1 and C_2 in many devices are not negligible. To understand how these capacitances determine the potential of the metal housing, the following discussion is presented. Figure 10.5*a* illustrates the typical situation in which the leakage current is the result of capacitive coupling (C_1C_2) from the metal housing of a device and the conductors of the power line. In practical situations, the resistance (R) of a typical appliance is quite low. Referring

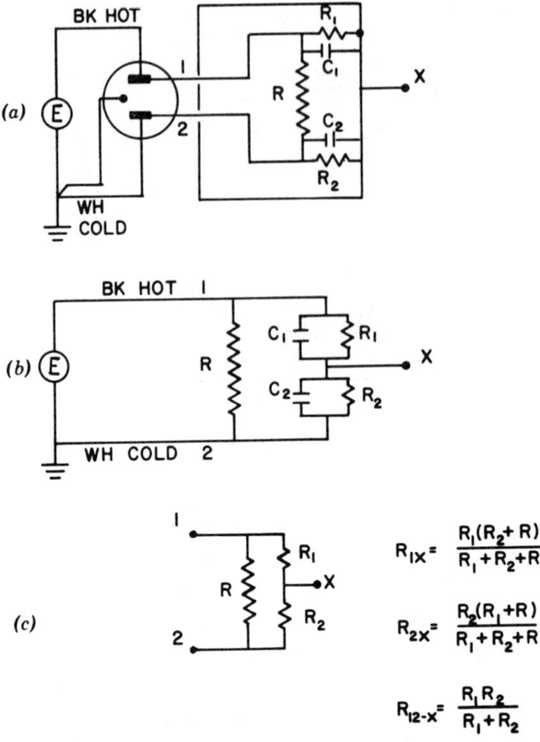

FIGURE 10.4. The measurement of leakage resistance and capacitance. (*a*) The coupling paths (R_1C_1 and R_2C_2) between the metal case and power line; (*b*) the equivalent circuit, and (*c*) the resistive pathways.

to Figure 10.5*b*, with the two terminals (1, 2) of the power connector joined together, measurement of the capacitance between this point (1,2) and the metal housing (X) provides a value for C_1 and C_2 in parallel. It is, however, necessary to make a different type of measurement to obtain data which will provide a value for the ratio of C_1 to C_2.

The test that can be carried out to determine the ratio of C_1 to C_2 is shown in Figure 10.5*c*. Note that it is necessary to connect the device to the power line with the metal housing not connected to ground. Using a battery-operated AC voltmeter with an input impedance of more than 10 megohms, the voltage between the metal housing (X) and sides 1 and 2 (E_1 and E_2, respectively) of the power line are measured. The ratio of E_1 to E_2 is equal to the ratio of C_2 to C_1 as shown in Figure 10.5*c*. Thus from the capacitance measurement described above, the value for $C_1 + C_2$ is obtained. From the voltage measurement just discussed, the ratio of C_2 to C_1

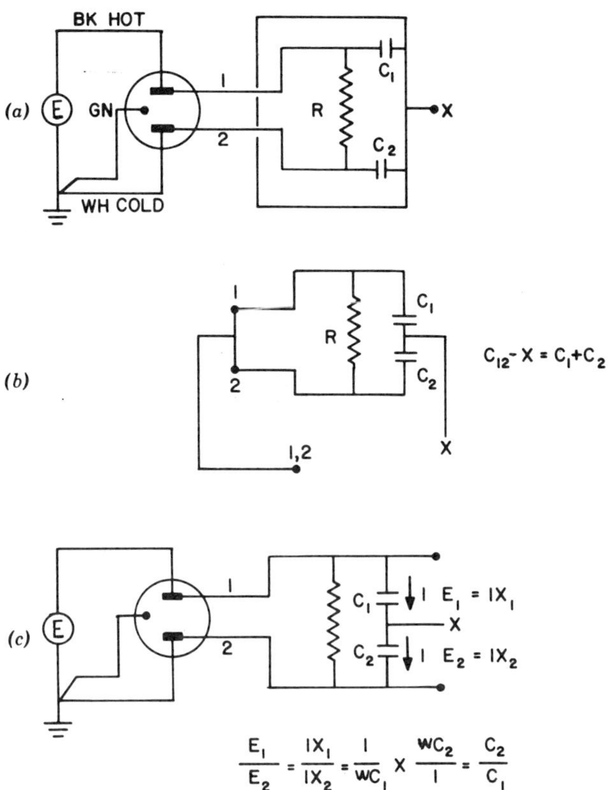

FIGURE 10.5. (*a*) The manner in which the case of an appliance is coupled to the hot and cold sides of the power line. (*b*) The method of measuring the sum of C and C_2. (*c*) The method of determining the ratio of C_2 to C_1. In all instances, point X represents the case which is ungrounded.

is obtained. Solving these two equations allows determination of C_1 and C_2.

GROUND-FAULT INTERRUPTER

A ground-fault interrupter (GFI) is a device that automatically arrests the flow of current to an appliance when the current in one of the power conductors exceeds that in the other. It should be obvious that when any appliance is plugged into the power line, the current is the same in all parts of the circuit, as shown in Figure 10.6*a*. If there is a conducting path to ground and current flows in it, the current in the two power conductors will differ by an amount equal to the ground-fault current. When a GFI is

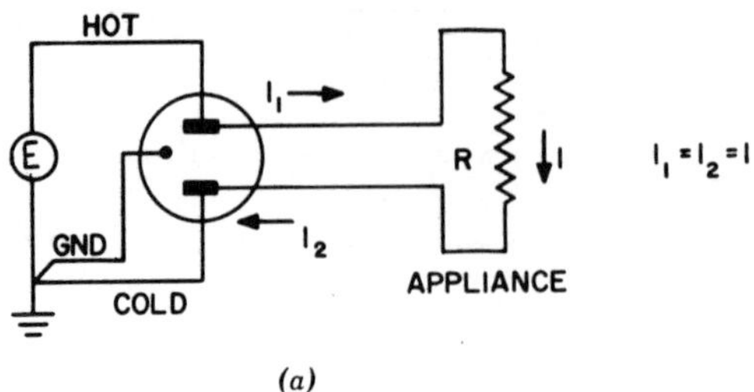

(a)

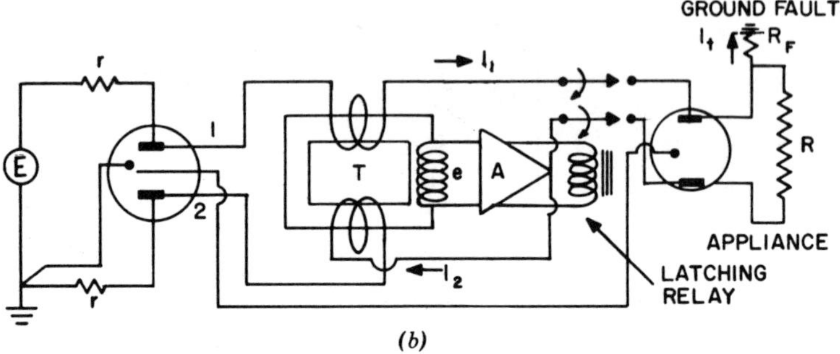

(b)

FIGURE 10.6. Ground-fault interrupted (GFI). (*a*) A nonfault condition in which $I_1 = I_2$. (*b*) Fault current (I_f) flows through the fault resistance (R_f); in this case, I_1 is greater than I_2. The transformer (*T*) is wound so that when I_1 is not equal to I_2, a voltage (*e*) is produced which is amplified (*A*) and energizes a latching relay which arrests current flow to the appliance.

interposed between the power outlet and the appliance, a ground-fault current can be detected and current flow arrested, as shown in Figure 10.6*b*. Suppose that a ground fault, represented by a resistance R_f in Figure 10.6*b*, occurs. In such a case the current in conductor 1, that is, I_1, will be larger than the current in conductor 2, that is, I_2, by an amount equal to the ground-fault current I_f. This inequality in current in conductors 1 and 2 is detected by a transformer (*T*) which has three windings, two for current and one for voltage (*e*). The connections are such that current flows in one direction in one current winding and in the opposite direction in the other. Thus, the magnetic field in the core of the transformer (*T*) is zero when the currents ($I_1 I_2$) are equal. In such a case there is no voltage (*e*) appearing across the voltage winding which is connected to an amplifier (*A*) and a latching relay with contacts in the normally closed condition as shown. Therefore, current flows to the appliance. However, when the ground fault occurs and I_1 becomes different from I_2, there is a net alternating magnetic field set up in the core of the transformer and a voltage appears across the voltage winding (*e*). This voltage, after amplification, activates the latching relay which arrests the current flow to

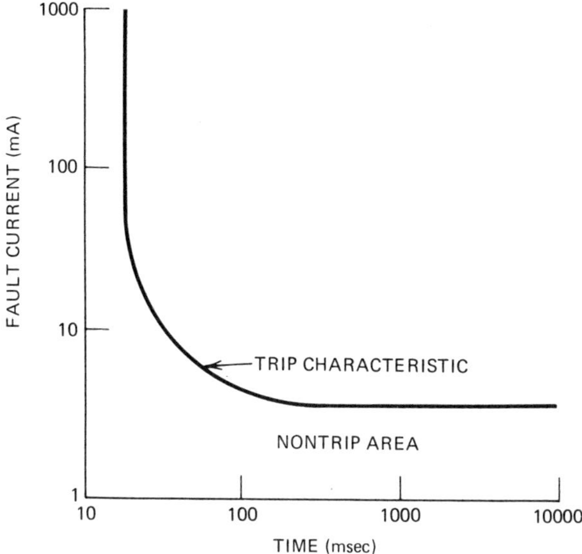

FIGURE 10.7. Performance characteristics of a typica ground-fault interrupter.

the appliance. The relay is designed so that its contacts stay in a locked-open position so that manual resetting is required to reenergize the appliance. If the ground fault has not been removed, the latching relay cannot be reset. Current can only be delivered to the appliance when $I_1 = I_2$, that is, when there is no excess flow of current in one of the two conductors to the appliance.

The rapidity with which a ground-fault interrupted operates depends on the magnitude of the fault current. Figure 10.7 illustrates the response (trip) time for a typical unit. The NFPA (76 BT-20641) recommends that the performance of a GFI for hospital use should have an interrupt time of 25 msec for a 2 mA leakage current.

ISOLATED POWER SYSTEM

An isolated power system is one in which neither side of the power line is connected to ground. An ideally isolated system would exhibit an infinite impedance from each side of the line to ground. Consequently, no current would flow in a conductor if it joins either side of the power line to ground. Obviously, owing to distributed capacitance, practical isolated power systems do not attain this goal.

Isolation in a power system is achieved by the use of a transformer in

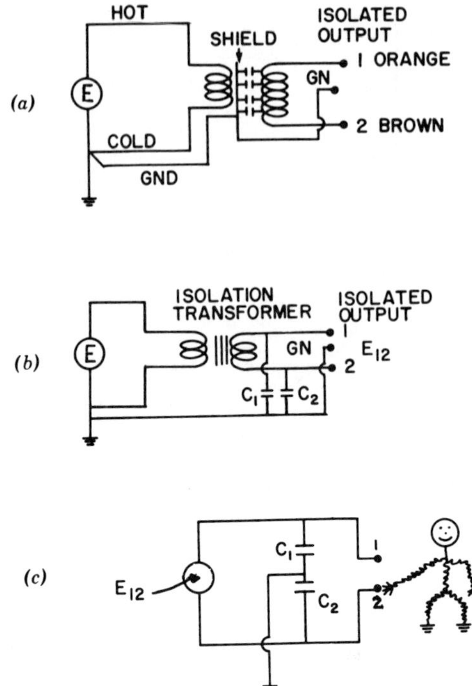

FIGURE 10.8. Isolated power system. (*a*) The use of a shielded isolating transformer; (*b*) the distributed capacitance (C_1, C_2) in an isolated power system; and (*c*) the equivalent circuit.

which the secondary (output) winding has a low capacitance to ground. Voltage is induced in the secondary by magnetic coupling which does not constitute a conductive path. Figure 10.8*a* illustrates such an isolated power system. Note that between the primary (input) and secondary (output) winding there is an electrostatic shield which is grounded; therefore, there is a distributed capacitance C_1, C_2 between the secondary winding and ground is shown in Figure 10.8*b*. In a well-designed and well-constructed isolation transformer, the capacitance is small and the insulation resistance is high. The equivalent circuit for such an isolation transformer is shown in Figure 10.8*c*, in which the distributed capacitance has been collected together and represented by C_1 and C_2.

The ungrounded, that is, isolated, power distribution system for hospital use became popular because of the many explosions of combustible gases that had been reported. The standards of performance for isolated power systems have been revised many times and the present recommendation appears in the National Electrical Code (Article 617) and in the NFPA report (Article 50) which relates to inhalation anesthetics. The

NFPA (76BM) has recommended that a different color code be used to identify the conductors in an isolated power system; orange and brown are used for the isolated output and green is used for ground.

The reduced shock hazard with an isolated power system will now be illustrated. In Figure 10.8*c*, if Ready Resistor touches either side of the isolated power line, the current that will flow through him will be small because the only connection from the power-line to ground is through C_1 or C_2 (depending on which conductor was touched). The 60-Hz reactance of these capacitors is high in a well-constructed isolation transformer. The NFPA (56A-22) recommends that the impedance (capacitive and resistive) from either conductor to ground should exceed 500,000 ohms (at 60 Hz) at the time of installation. Assuming that the impedance is capacitive, no greater than 0.005 μF exists from either conductor to ground.

The need for isolated power systems is a very controversial subject. There are very vocal supporters and opponents; the latter claim that by the use of good design practice in an instrument, isolated power systems are not required. An enlightened review of this topic is presented in Health Devices (1974).

GROUND-FAULT INDICATORS

In order to indicate the integrity of isolated power systems, a variety of ground-fault indicators has been created. All are designed to identify a loss of isolation of the system to ground, that is, C_1 or C_2 have become excessively large or a conducting path has developed between either (or both) conductors and ground. The basic principle underlying ground-fault indicators will now be described.

Perhaps the simplest and least expensive ground-fault indicator is shown in Figure 10.9. This device consists of two neon lamps (connected with series resistors (*r*) between each side of the isolated power line and ground. Obviously both lamps will glow when no ground fault exists. Grounding either side of the isolated power line will cause one of the neon lamps to extinguish. Simple and inexpensive as this type of ground-fault indicator is, it is very insensitive and quite a large ground fault can go undetected; it is also unable to identify a balanced or symmetrical fault to ground.

LINE ISOLATION MONITOR (LIM)

With the passage of time, ground-fault indicators became more and more sophisticated, and it was soon realized that certain types of ground-fault

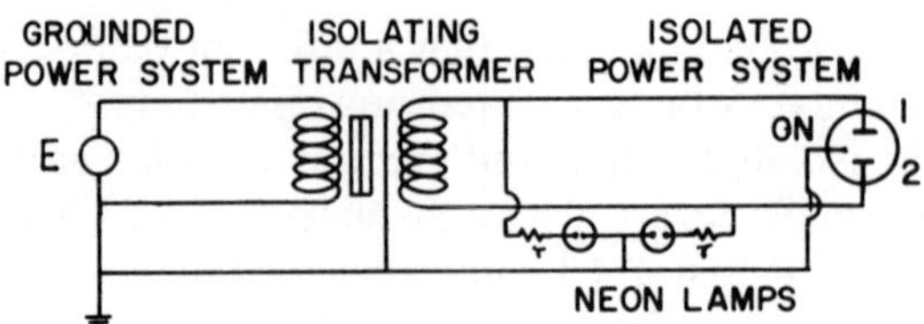

FIGURE 10.9. Neon-lamp, ground-fault indicator. With no fault, both neon lamps will glow. Grounding either side of the isolated power system will extinguish one neon lamp (τ = current limiting resistors, eg., 100K).

indicator were incapable of detecting a symmetrical ground fault, that is, one which placed an equal impedance from each side of the isolated power line to ground. For this reason it was recognized that there was need for a type of ground-fault indicator that would detect both symmetrical and asymmetrical faults to ground. Such devices were given the name, "line-isolation monitor" (LIM). Kusters (1958) developed one of the earliest LIMs and analyzed the performance of all the types of ground-fault detectors. Incidentally, he called his instrument a dynamic ground detector.

There is some confusion about the operation of LIMs, probably because there are so many different types. However, the function of each is to detect a ground fault from either or both sides of the isolated power line to ground. The manner by which they identify the fault is often not stated clearly. In the following, an attempt will be made to dispel this ambiguity.

Figure 10.10*a* illustrates the principle employed in an LIM. The switch S samples first side 1 and then side 2 of the isolated power line. Connected between the switch (S) and ground is an alternating-current-impedance indicator (I). If the power system is truly isolated, no current will flow through the impedance Z of the current indicator (I), because there is no return path. Now suppose (Figure 10.10*b*) that a low-impedance fault (Z_f) occurs between line 1 and ground. When the switch (S) is in position 1, virtually no current will flow through the indicator (I). However, when the switch in position 2, a current amounting to $E/(Z + Z_f)$ will be indicated flowing through the fault Z_f.

The example just presented illustrates that when a ground fault exists between one side of an isolated power line and ground, the other becomes live or hot. If Ready Resistor touches the unfaulted side (2) of the power line, a current will flow through him to ground as shown in Figure 10.10*c*. The current would be $E/(Z_f + R)$, where R is the resistance of Ready Resistor to ground.

It is the duty of a line-isolation monitor to indicate the hazard current that *would* flow if a subject having zero impedance touches the unfaulted

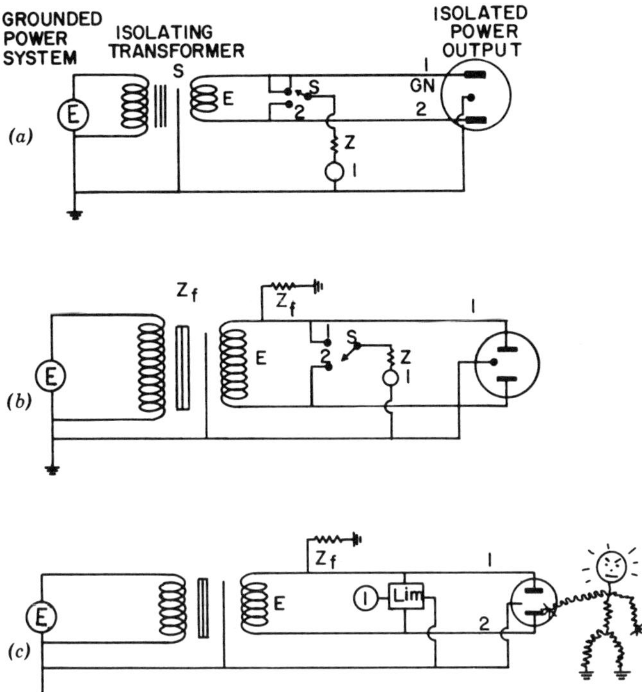

FIGURE 10.10. (*a*) Principle used in a line-isolation monitor; (*b*) a fault (Z_f) between power line 1 and ground, resulting in a current flow through the impedance (Z) of the indicator (I) and ground when switch S is in position 2. (*c*) If the unfaulted side (2) of the line is touched by a grounded subject, a current will flow and a shock will be received as shown.

conductor and completes a path to ground. The current that would flow in the example presented would be E/Z_f (because $R = 0$). Note that an LIM does not indicate a fault current, it predicts the fault current on the basis of E and measuring Z_f. In order to measure Z_f, the LIM must pass a small current by completing a circuit to ground from the unfaulted side of the power line to ground. LIMs typically have an internal impedance (Z) of several hundred thousand ohms. It should therefore be obvious that the addition of an LIM to an isolated power system reduces the degree of isolation slightly.

Many LIMs are equipped with both visible and audible alarms for excessive fault current, that is, when a fault impedance lower than a predetermined value develops. It is important to note that modern LIMs will detect both symmetrical and asymmetrical faults to ground in an isolated power system. The NFPA (56A, 3344) recommends that "an alarm is activated, when line-to-line ground impedances exits that would allow more than 2.0 milliamperes in a direct connection between either isolated conductor and ground.''

Certain important facts relative to isolated power systems and LIMs must be recognized. For example, an isolated power system is maximally isolated when no appliances are connected to it. From the foregoing, it should be recognized that all appliances have a capacitance to ground and the connection of additional such devices adds capacitance between the isolated power conductors and ground, thereby reducing the isolation. Moreover, addition of the LIM also reduces the isolation. Because a large number of LIMs contain mechanical or electronic switches to sample the impedance to ground of the two conductors, switching transients are often impressed on the isolated power line. In some LIMs, the switching is as low as 15/sec; in others it is as high as 60/sec. The frequency of the transient impressed on the isolated power line is that of the switching rate of the LIM. When bioelectric recorders (such as the EEG, ECG, EMG) are used on such systems and the patient ground is faulty, considerable interference can be encountered in the recording. Usually adequate patient grounding eliminates this type of interference. Kilpatrick (1973) presented a good description and evaluation of this problem. Perhaps the most important fact about isolated power systems and LIMs is that they are very controversial. Many believe that with adequate grounding and care in design and manufacturing of power-line-operated devices, isolated power systems and LIMs are not necessary. Others believe that the safety they provide make them essential in electrically susceptible patient areas.

EQUIPOTENTIAL GROUND

The term ''equipotential ground'' really means that all exposed metal surfaces accessible to a subject are at the same potential, which is ground. Achieving an equipotential ground means that all of the exposed metal surfaces are connected by heavy conductors to the same point that constitutes the patient ground. To do so requires the availability of a ground bus with multiple terminals to which all instruments can be connected. Detailed information can be found in the National Electrical Code 1971 (Article 517, para 51b), and in NFPA, 1971 (Article 56A). In general, the plan shown in Figure 10.11 typifies a method for equipotential grounding when used with an isolated power system. NFPA-56-A-25 requires that there be no more than 5 mV between all exposed metal surfaces accessible to a patient.

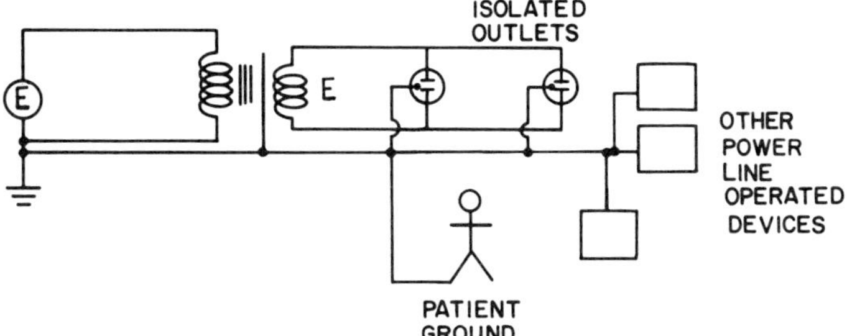

FIGURE 10.11. Equipotential ground.

LEAKAGE-CURRENT TESTING

From the foregoing, it is clear that there is the need to establish test procedures to quantify the 60-Hz leakage current that could flow through a subject connected to a power-line-operated device. Desirable as this goal is, there is no unanimity among the various standards-promulgating groups regarding the most representative electrical circuit that can be used to represent a worst-case condition for a patient in contact with ground. However, the differences between the standards groups is one of degree, rather than kind, and until the differences are resolved, it is useful to be aware that they exist.

Although many leakage-testing instruments can be purchased which measure power-line leakage current, as well as leakage current due to high-frequency generators (such as radio and television stations and electrosurgical instruments), it is useful to have a simple tester for 60-Hz leakage current testing. Such a device is illustrated in Figure 10.12 and is very useful for testing a variety of power-line operated devices.

The leakage tester shown in Figure 10.12 consists of a three-prong power-line plug that is connected via three switches to a three-prong receptacle to which the device to be tested is connected. The tester permits reversing the power line, opening the ground connection, and opening either side of the power line. The leakage current is caused to flow to ground from the device being tested through an impedance (Z), which simulates the subject's contact to ground. Associated with Z is the measuring device (preferably a battery-operated voltmeter with a high input impedance, that is, greater than 500,000 ohms).

The simplest equivalent for Z (Figure 10.12*a*) is a 500- or 1000-ohm resistor. The 500-ohm value was derived from the 60-Hz impedance between a catheter electrode in the heart and an electrode on the chest. The 1000-ohm value was recommended by the National Fire Protection Asso-

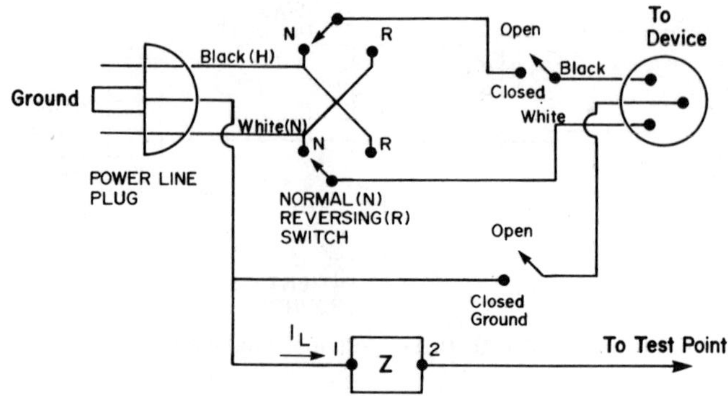

Z = EQUIVALENT SUBJECT

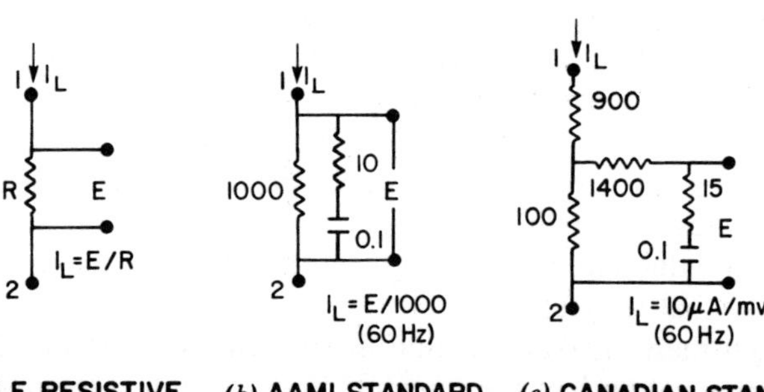

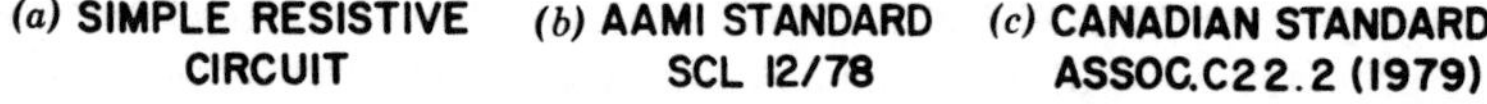

(*a*) SIMPLE RESISTIVE CIRCUIT (*b*) AAMI STANDARD SCL 12/78 (*c*) CANADIAN STANDARD ASSOC. C22.2 (1979)

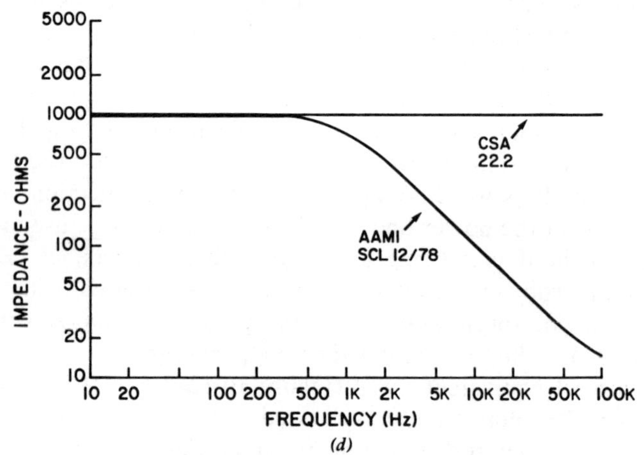

(*d*)

FIGURE 10.12

ciation (NFPA) (76BM-3042), which represented the impedance of a typical AC microammeter. With a simple resistor (R) used to simulate the subject, the leakage current is simply E, the voltage across the resistor, divided by the resistance (R) in ohms. As stated previously, a battery-operated AC voltmeter should be used to make this measurement.

The American Association for the Advancement of Medical Instrumentation (AAMI) developed a standard circuit for testing leakage current. Figure 10.12*b* illustrates the circuit which exhibits a decreasing impedance with increasing frequency, as shown in Figure 10.12*d*. At d.c., the impedance is 1000 ohms, the impedance is 10 ohms at infinite frequency. The impedance at 60 Hz is a fraction of a percent below 1000 ohms.

The leakage current is determined by measuring the voltage (E) across the circuit using a voltmeter with a high input impedance or an oscilloscope, with due precaution been taken to avoid ground loops. The leakage current $I = E/Z$, where E is the measured voltage and Z is the impedance at the frequency of measurement. Note that for the same leakage current, the measurement voltage (E) will decrease as the frequency of the leakage current increases.

Figure 10.12*c* illustrates the circuit recommended by the Canadian Standards Association (C 22.2, 1979). The impedance–frequency charac-

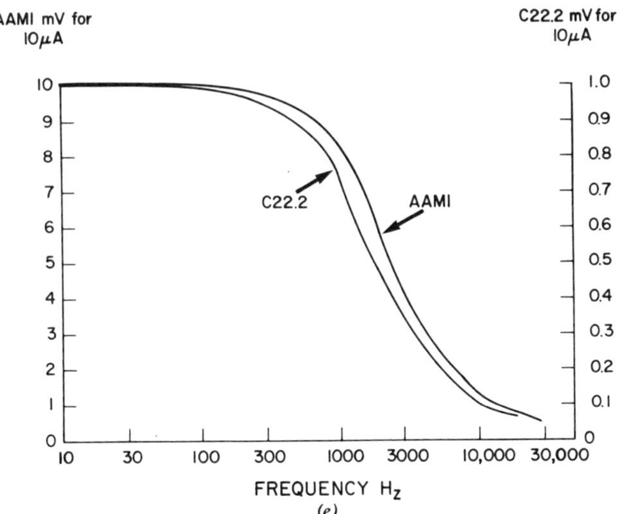

(*e*)

FIGURE 10.12. Leakage-testing circuit in which Z represents the equivalent circuit to ground. (*a*) A single resistor (500 or 1000 ohms), (*b*) the AAMI SCL/78 circuit, and (*c*) the C22.2 circuit. The impedance–frequency characteristics for (*b*) and (*c*) are shown in (*d*). (*e*) The measured voltage for 10 μA leakage current at different frequencies for the circuits shown in (*b*) and (*c*).

TABLE 10.3. Leakage Data

Test Conditions			Test-Site Leakage Current					
Reversing Switch	Ground Switch	Line Switch	To Chassis	1	2	3	4	5
Normal	Closed	Closed						
Normal	Open	Closed						
Normal	Closed	Open						
Normal	Open	Open						
Reversed	Closed	Closed						
Reversed	Open	Closed						
Reversed	Closed	Open						
Reversed	Open	Open						

teristics of this circuit is illustrated in Figure 10.12*d*. The impedance decreases only slightly with frequency, starting out at 1000 ohms at 0 Hz and decreasing to 993 ohms at infinite frequency. However, it is clear that the measured voltage (E) decreases with increasing frequency.

The leakage current for Figure 10.12*c* is indicated by measuring the voltage E. For frequencies below 100 Hz the scaling factor of 1 mV is equal to 10 μA of leakage current. Again, a battery operated AC voltmeter with an input impedance in excess of 150K ohms is recommended.

It is noteworthy that the American (AAMI) equivalent (Figure 10.12*b*) and the Canadian (C22.2) equivalent circuits (Figure 10.12*c*) are different in configuration and have different impedance–frequency characteristics (Figure 10.12*d*). It is important to recognize that it is the measured leakage current that is important. In Figure 10.12*e*, the voltage for 10 μA of leakage current is plotted versus frequency for both circuits. Although the two circuits are different, the frequency dependence for the measured leakage current is quite similar.

The leakage tester in Figure 10.12 permits performing eight leakage tests on a single test site (e.g., chassis, patient cable, etc.) in rapid succession by merely manipulating the switches in succession. Table 10.3 presents a document that can be used to log leakage currents.

The NFPA (76BM-30423) recommends that, in addition to testing leakage currents to ground, that leakage testing should be carried out between any pair of patient leads or combination of leads. In other words, the device should not send dangerous current through the subject. The current levels that can be tolerated and are dangerous are discussed in a following section in this chapter.

A useful DC leakage test for appliances has been proposed by NFPA

(76BM-30412). It states "Measure the DC resistance between both the current-carrying blades of the attachment plug of the line cord and the grounding prong of this plug with the power switch of the appliance in the 'on' position to demonstrate that a resistance greater than 1 megohm exists between these elements."

PHYSIOLOGICAL RESPONSES TO ELECTRIC CURRENT

Perception Threshold

It is of considerable importance to know the effects of various current levels applied to human and animal subjects. The lowest values (thresholds) for body-surface current for perception have been reported by many investigators. Although the various studies vary considerably, the data are similar in type. The threshold current for sensation depends somewhat on the electrode area in contact with the skin and distribution of sensory receptors on it. In addition, the duration of current application affects the perception threshold, particularly if its exposure time is shorter than a few seconds. Dalziel (1956) reported sensation thresholds for a thin copper wire on the middle finger and a polished copper plate as the indifferent electrode; his data are plotted in Figure 10.13. (crosses). A similar study was carried out by Geddes and Baker (1971), who measured the sensation threshold for 11-mm disk electrodes placed on the thorax and 0.25 in. aluminum-ribbon electrodes placed around the neck and abdomen; Figure 10.13 (dots) presents the threshold data obtained. Although these studies differ in their design, the data are surprisingly similar. The 60-Hz sensation threshold is between 0.2 and 1.1 mA for these electrodes. With increasing frequency the sensation threshold rises dramatically.

Cardiorespiratory Responses

Increasing the current above perception threshold produces effects attributable to the current pathway. With a head-to-foot passage of 60-Hz current, skeletal muscle contraction, respiratory arrest, vagal slowing of the heart, and ventricular fibrillation can occur. With the high levels of current, cardiopulmonary resuscitation and ventricular defibrillation are required to resuscitate a subject. The magnitude of current required to produce these effects depends on body weight, current pathway, and duration of current flow. For current applied between hands, or between a hand and a foot, the levels required for vagal slowing of the heart and for

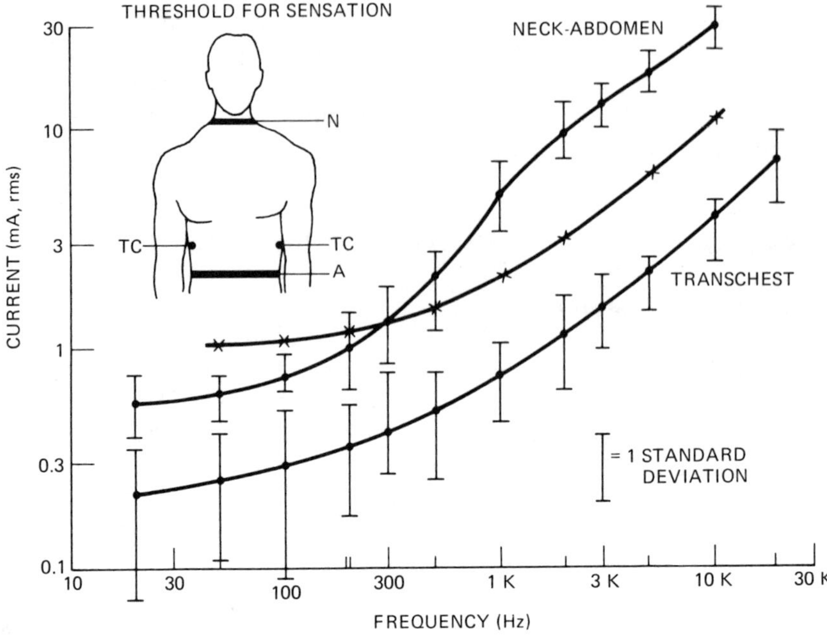

FIGURE 10.13. Threshold current for sensation. Dots represent data from Geddes and Baker (1971); crosses represent data from Dalziel (1956).

ventricular fibrillation can be deduced from animal studies by Geddes et al. (1971, 1973). Table 10.4 presents typical values for these responses.

Direct Myocardial Stimulation

The most dangerous situation for current flow through the body exists when catheters or electrodes are placed in the heart or vascular system, the former being the most hazardous. Considerable attention has been devoted to this situation by cardiologists, and there is some controversy over the amount of 60-Hz current required to produce ventricular fibrillation with electrodes in the heart chambers. The most sensitive situation occurs when a temporary pacemaking electrode is placed in the right ventricle and connected to an external pacemaker. In this case, a low-resistance conductor has direct access to the right ventricle. In the case of a fluid-filled catheter in a ventricle, there is a long and relatively high-resistance conductor between the heart and the outside. Monsees and McQuarrie (1971) reported that the resistance of a typical saline-filled catheter is in the megohm range. Hence, more voltage is required to pass the same current through the heart. For a catheter electrode, or a saline-

TABLE 10.4. Response to 60-Hz Current[a]

Current (mA,rms)	Direction of Current	Animal Weight (kg)	Physiological Response
50	Transchest	10–18	Slowing of the heart
50	Neck–Abdomen	10–18	Slowing of the heart
100	Head-to-Foot	10	Ventricular fibrillation
250	Head-to-Foot	70	Ventricular fibrillation
250	Forelimb	10	Ventricular fibrillation
630	Forelimb	70	Ventricular fibrillation

[a] Current flow for more than 1 sec. Data from *Principles of Applied Biomedical Instrumentation*, 2nd. ed. (1975), Wiley, New York.

filled catheter in direct contact with the ventricular myocardium, the threshold 60-Hz current for ventricular fibrillation has been reported by Weinberg et al. (1962) as 70 μA (40–140); by Whalen et al. (1964) as 258 μA; by Staewen et al. (1969) as 20–100 μA; by Starmer et al. (1971) 250 μA, and by Geddes and Baker (1971) as 60–450 μA. Figure 10.14 presents the current levels for 60-Hz and for other frequencies using dogs as subjects. These data are in agreement with the most recent values reported by Roy et al. (1977). Incidentally, the values required for precipitating ventricular fibrillation by directly applied (small) electrodes are not dependent of heart size above a critical lower heart weight (e.g., 50 g) in warm-blooded subjects. Very small mammalian hearts will spontaneously defibrillate; many cannot be fibrillated, although a short-lasting tachycardia can be produced in response to repetitive stimulation.

Two important facts must be borne in mind in the case of electrodes directly in the heart. The first is that if such an electrode or catheter is not in direct contact with the ventricular muscle, the current required to precipitate ventricular fibrillation is much higher, the increase being directly related to the distance from the device to the ventricular muscle. It is important to note that it is possible to precipitate ventricular fibrillation without the application of electric current to a catheter or electrode within the ventricle. This event can occur as the result of mechanical stimulation by the device as it flails within the ventricle while beating normally. In addition, the sudden injection of a fluid into the ventricles can cause an ectopic beat which can progress to ventricular fibrillation. When a catheter or catheter electrodes are being applied to the heart, it is very desirable to have an electrocardiograph running to identify any arrhythmias, and a defibrillator at the ready in case ventricular fibrillation occurs for any reason.

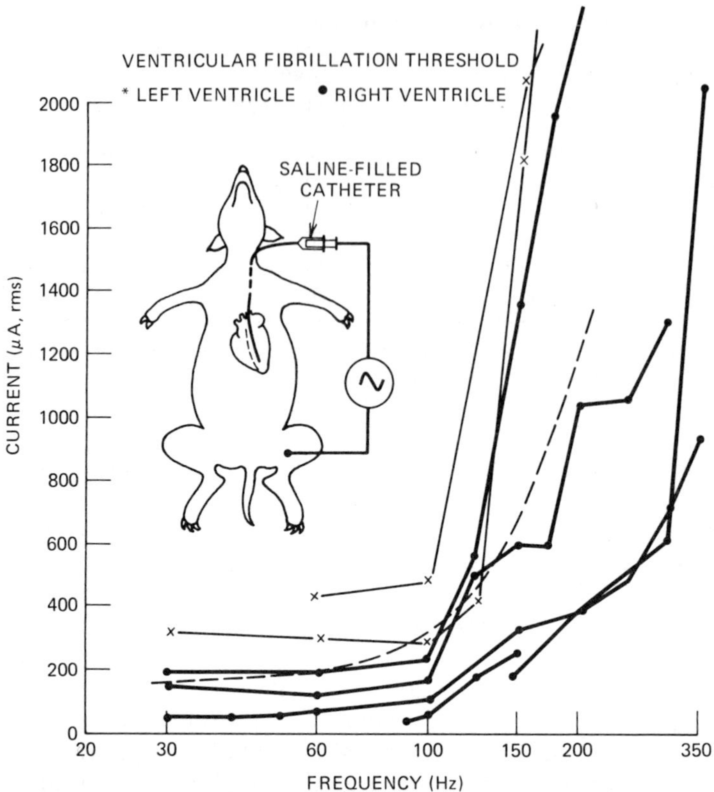

FIGURE 10.14. Threshold sine wave current (for 5 sec) required to produce ventricular fibrillation with a catheter electrode in the heart.

Indirect Myocardial Stimulation

With body-surface electrodes, the current intensity required to precipitate ventricular fibrillation depends on the frequency, duration of application, electrode location, and body size. Since 60-Hz current is the most hazardous, data will be provided to indicate the intensity required when the various factors are considered.

Figure 10.15 illustrates the threshold 60 Hz-current required for fibrillation as the duration of exposure is varied. Note that with this head-to-foot current pathway, the current required is higher as the duration of exposure is decreased. Also indicated on Figure 10.15 is the fact that for any duration of exposure, the current required for fibrillation increases as body weight is increased.

Figure 10.16 illustrates the level of 60-Hz current required to produce

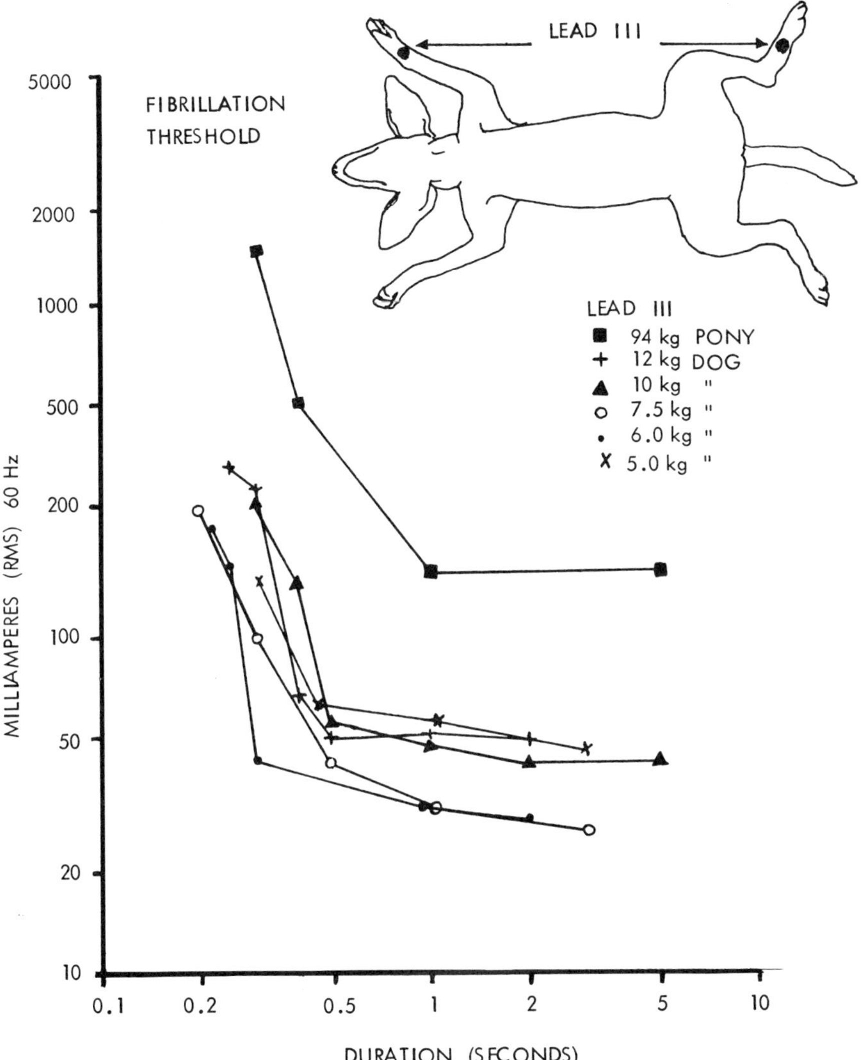

FIGURE 10.15. Threshold 60-Hz current required to produce ventricular fibrillation with different durations of current flow. [From Geddes et al. (1973).]

ventricular fibrillation with 5 sec of exposure in animals of increasing weight. The current required is least for the head–foot direction (leads II, III). Lead I identifies current application between the forelimbs. For any current path, the current required increases with body weight.

The body weight relationship for fibrillation is dependent on electrode location. In closed-chest cardiac pacing, where an active electrode is

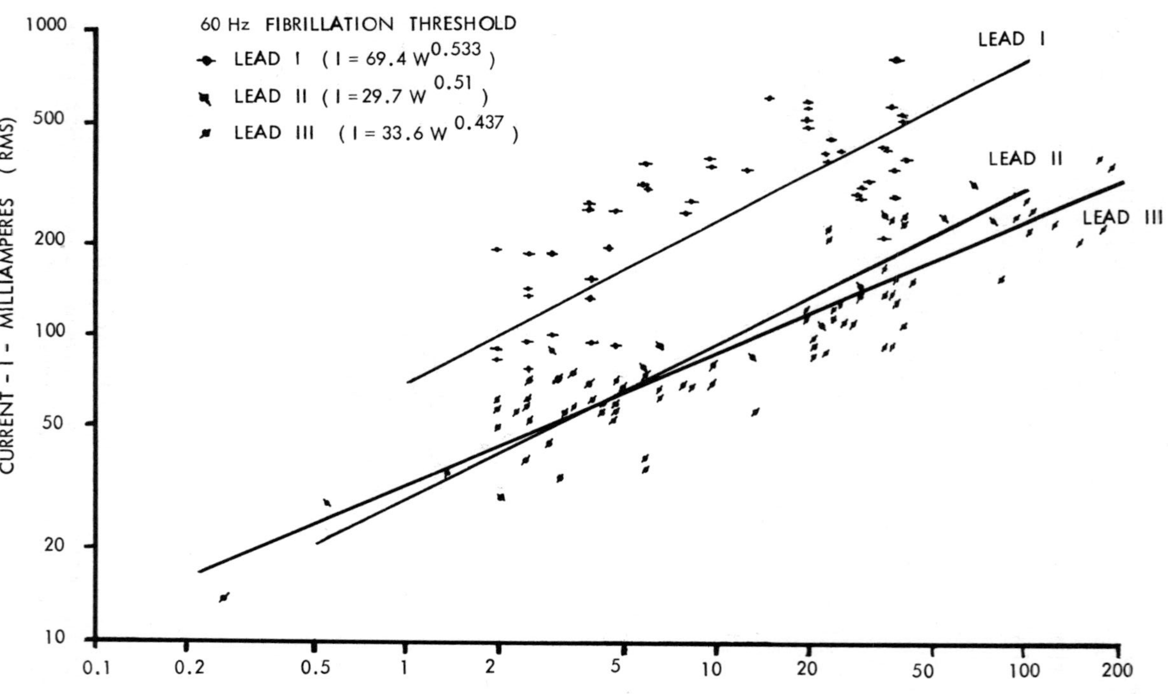

FIGURE 10.16. Threshold 60-Hz current required produce ventricular fibrillation in animals of increasing weight. Current application was 5 sec. [From Geddes et al. (1973).]

placed over the apex beat area, the threshold for pacing, (and fibrillation) is relatively independent of body weight, because the electrode has excellent access to the left ventricle.

Vulnerable-Period Stimulation

There is yet another important circumstance that can cause ventricular fibrillation; it is called vulnerable-period stimulation. The vulnerable period of the ventricular cycle is that period during the *T* wave of the electrocardiogram when a single strong stimulus will precipitate ventricular fibrillation. The stimulus must, however, be several times stronger than that required to produce an extrasystole; a discussion of this subject is in the chapter on cardiac pacing. The stimulus does not have to be delivered directly to the heart, although the least intensity of stimulus is required in this situation. Moreover, the stimulus can be electrical or mechanical. A discussion of the strength-duration and temporal characteristics for vulnerable-period stimulation was presented by Jones and Geddes (1977).

LEGAL ELECTROCUTION

Death by the passage of electric current through the body is designated electrocution. The method was first adopted by the State of New York in 1888. In 1890, the first criminal was electrocuted; details of this event have been reported by Bernstein (1973). In legal electrocution, the current flow is from head to foot. With the high level of voltage used, consciousness is apparently lost immediately and irreversible damage occurs within the central nervous system within seconds.

Both direct and alternating current have been used in legal electrocution. However, the majority of applications employ direct current. The technique consists of first applying about 2000 V to a head and leg electrode for from a few to about 10 sec. In a typical case, about 9 A of current flows. Then the voltage is reduced to about 500 and maintained at this value for about 30 sec. From this point on the programs of raising and lowering the voltage vary. However, in most cases the total period of current flow is about 2 min. To ensure that death has occurred, the law provides for a complete autopsy immediately after electrocution.

Postmortem examination of the bodies of electrocuted criminals reveals a variety of changes, most of which are attributable to an increase in temperature. The histological changes in brain tissue were reported by Hassin (1933) who examined the brains of five criminals electrocuted with

TABLE 10.5. Standards Organizations and Standards[a]

American Society for Quality Control
161 West Wisconsin Avenue
Milwaukee, Wisconsin 53203

American Hospital Association (AHA)
840 North Lake Shore Drive
Chicago, Illinois 60611

American National Standards Institute
1430 Broadway
New York, New York

Electronic Industries Association (EIA)
Health Care Electronics Section
2001 Eye Street, N.W.
Washington, D.C. 20006

United States Department of the Interior
Bureau of Mines
Washington, D.C.

United States Department of the Navy
Bureau of Ships (Navships)
Washington, D.C.

Code for the Use of Flammable Anaesthetics. Canadian Standard Z 32, 1963
Canadian Standard Association, 235 Montreal Road, Ottawa 7, Canada.
Normen-Verzeichnis und de- Vorschriften der Radiologie und Elektromedizin.
Verband Deutscher Elektrotechniker, 1958
Beuth-Vertreib GmbH, Berlin, W.12.
Safety Code for Electro-medical Apparatus, 1963
Department of Health and Social Security, Hospital Technical Memorandum No. 8. HMSO, London
Anti-static Precautions: Rubber, Plastics and Fabrics.
Department of Health and Social Security, Hospital Technical Memorandum No. 1, HMSO, London
Anti-static Precautions: Flooring in Anaesthetizing Areas.
Department of Health and Social Security, Hospital Technical Memorandum No. 2. HMSO, London
British Standards Institution, London
B.S. 2099: Part 1: 1960 Amendment p. 3786.
Castors for hospital equipment
B.S. 2050: 1961

TABLE 10.5 (*Continued*)

Specification for electrical resistance of conductive and anti-static products made from flexible polymeric material
B.S. 3353: 1961
Specifications for anaesthetic breathing bags made of anti-static rubber
B.S. 3398: 1961
Specification for anti-static rubber flooring
B.S. 2506: 1961
Anti-static rubber footwear
B.S. 3806: 1964
Breathing machines for medical use.

[a]Pacella, A. E. and Arnold, B. E. (1976). *The Guide to Biomedical Standards*, Quest Publishing, New York.

alternating current. Swelling, tearing, and liquefication of cells were found. In some instances the larger blood vessels were ruptured. The body temperature following electrocution was reported by Werner (1923) who measured a temperature of 120°F on the right leg, 145°F in the brain, and a slightly lower temperature in the lungs and abdomen. The blood was hemolyzed. Although the heart was not beating, it could be stimulated to contract. An indication that current may flow preferentially along blood vessels and nerve fibers was presented by Spitzka and Radash (1912), who reported tearing of vessel walls. They stated that "the maximum number of lesions are found in the most constricted part of the brain stem in the path of the current and are most numerous along the longitudinal fiber tracts and blood vessels."

There are many differences between legal electrocution and accidental electric shock. In the former, the current is directed in a head-to-foot direction and maintained at levels from 2 to about 9 A for up to about 2 min. In accidental electric shock, the duration of application is usually short and the current pathway rarely includes the head. Since tissue protein coagulates at about 120°F, it is clear from the temperature measurements that there occurs thermal death of the tissues due to the current flow in electrocution.

CONCLUSION

Perhaps the best way to conclude this chapter is to provide a list of agencies having an interest in personnel safety. Such a list appears in Table 10.5.

REFERENCES

American Association for the Advancement of Medical Instrumentation (AAMI) Safe Current Limits for Electromedical Apparatus SCL 12/78 (1978). AAMI, Arlington, Virginia.

Association of Anaesthelists of Great Britain and Ireland (1971). Explosion hazards. *Anaesthesia* **26,** 155–157.

Bernstein, T. (1973). A grand success. *IEEE Spectrum* **10,** 54–58.

Bruner, J. D. (1967). Hazards of electrical apparatus. *Anesthesiology* **28,** 390–425.

Dalziel, C. F. (1956). Effects of electric shock in man. *IRE Trans. Med. Electronics* **PGME 5,** 44–62.

Feldtman, R. W. and Derrick, J. R. (1973). The hazardous hospital environment. *Tex. Med.* **69,** 63–67.

Geddes, L. A., and Baker, L. E. (1971). Response to the passage of electric current through the body. *J. Assoc. Adv. Med. Instr.* **5,** 13–18.

Geddes, L. A., and Baker, L. E. (1975). *Principles of Applied Biomedical Instrumentation,* 2nd. ed., Wiley, New York.

Geddes, L. A., Cabler, P., Moore, A. G., Rosborough, J., and Tacker, W. A. (1973). Threshold 60-Hz current required for ventricular fibrillation. *IEEE Trans. Bio-Med. Eng.* **BME 20,** 465–468.

Hassin, G. B. (1933). Changes in the brain in legal electrocution. *Arch. Neurol. Psychiat.* **30,** 1046–1060.

Health Devices (1974). **3,** 238–267.

Hussey, T. L. and Pois, A. J. (1970). Bowel-gas explosion. *Amer. J. Surg.* **120,** 103–105.

Jones M., and Geddes L. A. (1977). Strength-duration curves for cardiac pacemaking and ventricular fibrillation. *Cardiovasc. Res. Ctr. Bull.* **15,** 101–112.

Kirkpatrick, D. G. (1973). Instrumentation CMRR and isolated power systems. *Health Care Engineering.* **1,** 16–22.

Kusters, N. L. (1958). The ground detector problem in hospital operating rooms. *Trans. Eng. Inst. Can.* (July) 3–10.

Laurence, J. S. and Bostress, E. K. (1959). Combustion characteristics of anesthetics. *Anesthesiology.* **20,** 192–197.

Levy, E. I. (1954). Explosions during lower bowel electrosurgery; method of prevention. *Amer. J. Surg.* **88,** 754.

Monsees, L. B. and McQuarric, D. G. (1971). Is an intravascular catheter a conductor? *Med. Elect. & Data.* (Nov-Dec) 26–27.

N.F.P.A. National Fire Protection Association, 470 Atlantic Avenue, Boston 07210
National Electrical Code (NFPA #70).
Essential Electrical Systems for Hospitals (NFPA #76).
Flammable Anesthetics Code (NFPA #56).
Inhalation Therapy, 1968 (NFPA #56B).
Nonflammable Medical Gas Systems, 1967 (NFPA #565).
Bulk Oxygen Systems at Consumer Sites, 1965 (NFPA #566).
Static Electricity, Recommended Practice on, 1966 (NFPA #77).

Parker, B. (1967). Electrical testing for safety of the operating room and intensive care unit. *Amer. Coll. Surgeons Bull.* **54,** 187–189.

Roy O. Z., Park G. C., and Scott J. R. (1977). Intracardiac catheter fibrillation thresholds as a function of the duration of 60 Hz current and electrode area. *IEEE Trans. Bio-Med Eng.* **24,** 430–435.

Staewen, W. S., Lubin, D., Mower, M. M., Tabaotznik, B. (1969). The significance of leakage currents in hospital electrical devices. *Mt. Sinai Hosp. J.* **15,** 3–10.

Stanley P. E. (1974). Safety in the electromedical equipment system. *Natl. Safety News* (Nov.) 71–75; (Dec.) 80–89.

Starmer, C. F., et al. (1971). Electrical hazards and cardiovascular function. *New Engl. J. Med.* **284,** 181–186.

Spitzka, E. A. and Radash, H. E. (1912). The brain lesions produced by electricity as observed after legal electrocution. *Amer. J. Med. Sci.* **144,** 341–347.

Thomas, G. J. (1961). Controllable hazards in the operating room. *Hosp. Progr.* **42,** 70.

van der Mosel, H. A. (1970). Electrical safety and our hospitals. *Med. Instr.* **4,** 2–5.

Walter, C. W. (1966). Anesthetic explosions: a continuing threat. *Anesthesiology* **25,** 505–514.

Walter, C. W. (1967). Explosion of an ether vaporizer. *Anesthesiology* **27,** 681–694.

Weinberg, D. I., Arley, J. L., Whalen, R. E., McIntosh, H. D. (1962). Electric shock hazards in cardiac catheterization. *Circ. Res.* **11,** 1004–1009.

Werner, A. H. (1923). Death by electricity. *Med. Journ. Med. Rec.* **118,** 498–500.

Whalen, R. E., Starmer, C. F., and McIntosh, H. D. (1964). Electrical hazards associated with cardiac pacemaking. *Ann. N.Y. Acad. Sci.* **11,** 922–931.

Index